PRAI
QUEST FOR LIFE

BY PETREA KING

. . . .

From her American colleagues:

"If there was only one book you could read to navigate your way through life-challenging illness, **Quest for Life** *would be the perfect choice. Petrea King has created an accurate, compassionate map that shows you both how to mobilize your inner resources for healing and also how to benefit most from modern medicine. More than a book that inspires hope and gives practical guidance, this is a course in how to live a loving, happy and fulfilled life."*
Joan Borysenko, Ph.D., author of *Minding the Body, Mending the Mind*

*"***Quest for Life** *is an outstanding, helpful book for those who are facing a life-threatening illness. I have personally observed Petrea King's work, and her work is both loving and beautiful."*
Gerald G. Jampolsky, M.D., author of *Love is Letting Go of Fear*,
director of the Institute for Attitudinal Healing

"Petrea King in **Quest for Life** *presents us with another transformative life experience following cancer. By learning from her wisdom and experience, we can all live a fuller life!"*
Dr. Bernie Siegel, author: *Love, Medicine and Miracles*;
Peace, Love and Healing; *How to Live Between Office Visits*

*"***Quest for Life** *is a bible of practical, down-to-earth advice for anyone who is sick and for those involved in their care....[It] does not encourage patients to abandon orthodox approaches such as drugs and surgery, but that they supplement them with proven or promising alternative methods — a 'both/and' rather than an 'either/or' approach."*
Larry Dossey, M.D., author of several books including *Meaning and Medicine*,
and co-chair, Panel of Mind/Body Interventions,
Office of Alternative Medicine, National Institutes of Health

"Petrea King radiates life—so does her wonderful book, **Quest for Life**. *Remarkably comprehensive in its scope,* **Quest for Life** *offers emotional comfort, wise practical information, and perhaps most importantly, spiritual sustenance. I am grateful that her work is now available in the United States."*
Dr. Paul C. Roud, author of
Making Miracles: An Exploration into the Dynamics of Self-Healing

"Petrea King works and writes from a rare level of insight. She understands that true healing is more than a question of physical life or death. In **Quest for Life** *she shares many practical tools for approaching serious illness as an opportunity for personal growth and increased understanding."*
J. Donald Walters (Kriyananda), author of several books including
Affirmations for Self-Healing

"**Quest for Life** *is obviously written through Petrea King's own experience and from her heart....* *The chapter about how to explain difficult situations to children would work well for any crisis not just those dealing with physical illness....She conveys very powerful healing methods for dealing with illness. Her story is inspirational and brings hope to those who suffer.*"

Barbara R. Findeisen, M.F.C.C.
President, Pocket Ranch Institute

"*Petrea King radiates love and wisdom and so does her heart-warming, sagacious book* **Quest for Life**. *She clearly shows how our thoughts, emotions and attitudes greatly affect our body's level of wellness and ability to heal itself. She also offers very practical guidance on how to unleash our personal power and inherent healing capacities. I will gladly recommend it in my work.*"

Susan Smith Jones, author of several books including
Choose to Live Each Day Fully

"**Quest for Life** *is a knowledgeable, practical, and accessible guide based on Petrea King's extensive clinical experience in combining traditional medical care with the best in lifestyle practices. Her case studies vividly illustrate her compassionate healing methods as well as her well-reasoned and wise approach to the patient/caregiver relationship.*"

Dr. Kenneth R. Pelletier, author of *Mind as Healer, Mind as Slayer*

"*This book presents many helpful suggestions in a balanced way that avoids -'doctor bashing.' It blends nicely with regular medical treatments and will be of benefit to physicians.*"

Dr. Peter Van Houten, Sierra Family Medical Center

"**Quest for Life** *is the best book of its kind I have ever read. I felt empowered by Petrea's message of 'Yes, you're on the right track. Here are a few more tools to continue your process.' In very human terms she supports the inner search to find your own place of healing.*"

Mary Jo Cleaveland, cancer patient and
director of Complementary Healing at the Children's Hospital of Denver

From her Australian associates:

"*It would be simplistic to say that if you told someone he or she was dying, that person would immediately learn how to live. But in the week I spent with Petrea King, I witnessed something very close to that maxim.*"

Good Weekend Magazine, Sydney

"*[Petrea's] support group is not about dying. It is about living. For these people, every moment is precious, to be savored and lived as vitally as possible. It is not the quantity of life that matters, but the quality.*"

Panorama Magazine, Melbourne

From her patients:

QUEST FOR LIFE

. . . .

A Handbook for People with Life-Threatening Illness

by Petrea King

Dedication

. . . .

In memory of my brother Brenden who taught me much in his search for peace and to all those who've enriched my life with their wisdom, courage, love, and faith. Many trials have you suffered and triumphs you've achieved, and I with you, both sorrowfully and joyfully. My deep gratitude to each of you.

DAWN PUBLICATIONS
14618 Tyler Foote Road
Nevada City, California 95959
United States of America

Published originally in Australia by
Random House Australia
First published 1988
Revised edition 1992
Printed in United States of America

ISBN 1-883220-05-X
designed by Sara Cryer
printed on recycled paper
10 9 8 7 6 5 4 3 2 1
First Edition

Contents

· · · · · · · · · ·

Foreword

. . . .

Although John Adams and Thomas Jefferson, the second and third presidents of the United States, were violent political enemies during life, they had something in common in death: Both men died on July 4, 1826, the fiftieth anniversary of the Declaration of Independence. According to his physician, Jefferson's last words were, "Is it the Fourth?"

A strange coincidence? Unlikely. Studies of hundreds of famous people in the United States reveal a "death dip" before their birthdays and a "death peak" in the four months following. "Death dips" have also been observed in Jewish men preceding Passover. Researchers suggest that this reflects the ability of people to "hang on" until a meaningful event has arrived, then "let go" after it has passed.

These observations are consistent with one of the tenets of *Quest for Life*—that our attitudes, emotions, and thoughts can make a major difference in health outcomes; that we can influence our fate to a considerable degree; that we ignore our own inner feelings at our own risk.

Evidence for this is impressive. Consider the "Black Monday" syndrome—the discovery that more heart attacks in the United States and other Western industrialized countries occur on Monday mornings around 9:00 A.M.—the beginning of the work week—than at any other time. Consider, too, that one of the best predictors of heart attacks in men under age fifty is the level in one's life of *job dissatisfaction*. The peak occurrence of death on a particular day of the week is one of the most amazing discoveries in the whole of biology—for, as far as we know, *no other species* manages to die more frequently on a particular day of the week.

This type of information could be multiplied *ad infinitum*. It is related to one of the great scientific insights of our day—that the body is more than a machine and that the "manifestations of our consciousness" can make the difference in life or death.

That doesn't mean that the body doesn't have machine-like qualities. Parts do wear out and break down; they can be tinkered with, repaired, and occasionally replaced. But human bodies can do things machines can't do. They can get well on their own; they can set their own healing processes in motion; they can experience spontaneous remissions of their illnesses and, occasionally, they can experience miraculous cures.

Quest for Life is an instruction manual for people who want to mobilize these healing capacities. It is a bible of practical, down-to-earth advice for people who are sick and for those involved in their care.

It should find a warm reception in the United States. Americans are ready for its message of hope and self-reliance, and for information about using alternative measures in getting well. This has been established beyond reasonable doubt. Dr. David Eisenberg and his colleagues at Harvard Medical School discovered in 1990 that one-third of the adult population of this country visited an alternative practitioner of some sort. This exceeded the number of visits to front-line doctors such as family physicians, internists, and pediatricians. The survey found also that Americans spent $14 billion for alternative care that year, most of which was not reimbursed by insurance companies. And, interestingly, 70 percent of those seeking alternative care chose not to tell their private physician they did so—probably because they felt the doctor might not understand, or because they felt they might be criticized.

Readers of *Quest for Life* will discover that Petrea King understands the urge of people to seek alternative healing methods because *she is a healer.* By "healer" I do not mean someone who "makes" another person well, but who demonstrates compassion, caring, and love for those she serves, and who helps the needy mobilize their own innate healing potential. She also has the talent of describing health care methods in clear, uncluttered ways. When valuable knowledge is dispensed with compassion and caring, the results can be magical.

Readers should realize, however, that "alternative" does not mean "substitute." *Quest for Life* does not encourage patients to abandon orthodox approaches such as drugs and surgery, but that they supplement them with proven or promising alternative methods—a "both/and" rather than an "either/or" approach. This complementary attitude is one of the qualities I admire most about this book.

In 1992 the United States Congress established the Office of Alternative Medicine within the National Institutes of Health, the most prestigious medical research organization in the world. The goal of the new Office is to scientifically evaluate alternative methods of healing. Many of the therapies discussed in *Quest for Life* are of great interest to the Office and will receive attention—imagery and visualization, nutritional approaches to cancer and other illness, acupuncture, massage and other body therapies, and many more. Until careful studies prove what works and what doesn't, patients would do well to follow the balanced approach recommended in *Quest for Life*.

Many of this book's central messages have recently been affirmed by a landmark publication—*Spontaneous Remission: An Annotated Bibliography*. This fifteen-year project describes over 3,500 cases of spontaneous remission in cancer and many other diseases. It is noteworthy that many of these cases involved individuals who engaged in many of the methods described by Petrea King. These findings should provide hope to anyone suffering from serious illness. It is evidence that the very worst diseases can, and often do, go completely away.

Persons looking for magic bullets or secret formulas will not find them in *Quest for Life*. The reason: there is no formula that could be applied to a specific disease that always results in a cure. As Gertrude Stein once said, "There is no answer. There never has been an answer. There never will be an answer. That's the answer." This is a way of stating that, in spite of the accumulated wisdom of healers through the centuries, and in spite of the achievements of modern medical science, there remains great mystery in health and illness. *Quest for Life* does not strive to eradicate these mysteries, it acknowledges and honors them. And unlike many New Age books on health, it does not try to provide slick, easy answers to those who are sick.

One of the most famous "quests for life" in Western literature is the Grail Quest. On one occasion King Arthur and his knights were sitting at the table, and Arthur would not let the feast begin until an adventure had occurred. Suddenly the Grail appeared, but it was draped and could not be fully seen. Gawain, Arthur's nephew, proposed that the knights embark on a quest to find the Grail and view it unobstructed. They agreed, but realized that it would be a disgrace to go in a group. Therefore they decided to journey alone, entering the forest at the place which to each of them seemed darkest—where there was no light, no path, and no guide. *Quest for Life* is like the Grail Quest in that it does not provide final answers or formulas. *Unlike* the Grail Quest, it contains an enormous amount of advice and information for anyone concerned with serious illness. That is why I am honored to endorse it.

Larry Dossey, MD.
1993

Dr. Dossey, co-chair of the Panel on Mind/Body Interventions, Office of Alternative Medicine, National Institutes of Health, is the author of several best-sellers, including *Space, Time & Medicine, Beyond Illness,* and *Recovering the Soul.*

Preface

. . . .

Quest for Life is written for those who face the many dilemmas presented by the diagnosis of a life-threatening or chronic illness. It's written for those who have a disease, for their loved ones, and for the health professionals who care for them.

Some of the sections within this book might seem irrelevant to you. For instance, if you don't have children, you might think chapter 10, What About the Children? is unnecessary reading. I encourage you to read the chapter anyway because there are many suggestions and ideas which overlap other areas. After all, we're all children to someone else. Likewise, read chapter 8, Burps, Burning, and the Dreaded Bloats (and Much More). Having read it, you'll know where to turn if, at some future time, you might need the information.

My hope and prayer, for you the reader, is that the thoughts within this book will instill a sense of a larger perspective and will provide many very practical steps which will give a sense of control in your life and, therefore, the experience of peace.

Introduction

. . . .

Since writing the first edition of *Quest for Life* in 1988, I've had
the opportunity and privilege of meeting many more people, in
person, by letter and telephone, who've shared their journeys of
self-discovery and healing. I work with the heroes of our times.
You might not see them often in our newspapers or on our television screens, though some have certainly been featured there.
Most of them are the unsung heroes—men, women, and children
who have the will and capacity to manifest all that the human
spirit can achieve. They've enriched my life with their stories of
love, courage, pain, hope, and humor. They are the true authors
of this book.

In the past nine years, I've counseled thousands of people on
a one-to-one basis and facilitated over two thousand support
groups for people with life-threatening diseases. One of the
things that constantly amazes me is how frequently we have a
group in which no one mentions their disease. Someone without
such an illness would probably find that extraordinary, believing
that surely the illness is the main problem.

The participants sometimes talk about the poor relationships
they have with their mothers and fathers; they talk about lack of
purpose, direction, or meaning; they talk about the extraordinary
beauty of the sunrise they witnessed that morning and how it
touched a central core within themselves; they talk about the
healing of their kinship with life or with God; they talk about
not asserting themselves in their relationships; they talk about
the unrealistic standards they've been trying to live up to all
their lives; they talk about the despair of being unable to control
and manipulate the world, and end by laughing at the arrogance
which led them to believe they ever could; they discuss their
struggles with faith and trust; they might acknowledge that all
their lives they've failed to give themselves any love and respect;
they talk of the guilt and shame they've held on to for so long;
they talk of forgiveness and its capacity to set them free from

pain; they talk about the peace and joy they have in every day lived, but mostly, they *do not* talk about cancer, AIDS, failed suicide, multiple sclerosis, scleroderma, HIV, anorexia, alcohol, or drug addiction, chronic pain, or whatever has brought them to one of our groups. It's not that they refuse to talk about the problem or disease; it's as if the disease or problem has brought sharply into focus the areas of their lives which aren't working well or are causing them pain.

A life-threatening diagnosis is often the first impetus we have for deeply contemplating the mysteries of our mortality. For some, it presents an opportunity to face, and then let go, their fears. When people are able to acknowledge that we all must die, they're more easily able to live fully, to celebrate every day above ground! Surely mindfulness of this fact is what gives us impetus and passion with which to live fully our lives.

People often ask me why I work with dying people. I can honestly reply that I don't know any *dying* people. I believe we're either alive or we're dead. While we're alive, we need to be given all the honor, respect, and encouragement due any living being, that's why I don't believe the word "terminal" should ever be used about people. Terminals are for buses, trains, and computers. Enough people have survived these "terminal" diseases for *all* people to be given the opportunity to be exceptions. This book is written for those who are living with a life-threatening disease, not dying with a terminal one.

It's not uncommon for people to say they're grateful for the experience of their illness. They often qualify that statement by saying they'd prefer the disease to go, but they wouldn't want to lose what they've gained by having it.

As one man expressed, "I've lived all my life trying to make my father proud of me. The experience of cancer has made me into a real, live, warm, loving human being and *I'm* proud of me!"

The diagnosis of a life-threatening illness can be a tremendous opportunity for personal growth and understanding. It certainly takes a conscious effort on the part of the individual to *see* it that way! If we feel we're the victims of a disease, it makes it very difficult to reestablish a sense of control over our lives.

We can't always change the outcome of a disease but we can change the way we experience that outcome.

It usually takes six to eight weeks for the initial shock of the diagnosis to wear off. Some people experience this time with a numbed awareness, some seemingly take it in their stride, some go into a blind panic, some become depressed and despairing, others become angry. Once this initial reaction has worn off, we can begin to look at what it means for us to be in this situation and what we're able to do to assist ourselves in our healing. For some, the positive result to an HIV test or biopsy will be a crisis, while for others it will only confirm what they had already suspected.

This book is brimful of ideas, suggestions, and techniques which will assist you in reestablishing a sense of control over your life. To be without hope, without choice or without influence over our lives, is the antithesis of being at peace. When we take an active part in our healing process, we have a sense of hope and control. It helps establish peace of mind as we create an environment for healing.

It is still commonly felt among doctors and society that treatment has been "successful" when a life has been "saved," and that medicine has "failed" when the patient dies. This criterion is a really inappropriate one. If we're to use the qualification of success or failure, then surely success must be people living with a good quality of life, with joy and fulfillment in every day lived, until they die with peace and dignity. Failure can only be living or dying in fear or in emotional isolation. If you decide, "I've been successful only if I overcome this disease," you're also affirming, "I've failed if I die."

If we make peace of mind our one goal, we're also creating the perfect environment for healing within our body.

To achieve peace of mind is a challenge at any time. To achieve it while living with a life-threatening illness is a victory indeed! Thousands *have* achieved this personal victory. Many who have done so are running late for their own funerals! Those who have achieved their life's potential and moved on have left a legacy of love within the hearts of those who cared deeply for them.

We don't value a life by its length. It is not how long we live but the spirit with which we live which is of importance.

We can choose to experience this illness as an adventure in exploring our inner nature; to find our abilities, talents, feelings, unfulfilled dreams, and aspirations. We can learn to appreciate life more fully by really enjoying every day lived, not worrying or being preoccupied with the future or the past but savoring each moment as it unfolds.

In these pages you'll meet many of those who've attained the victory of peace. You'll see that their stories are not unlike your story; their dreams, hopes, and fears not unlike your own. I've been privileged to journey with these heroes and I invite you to join with me in the celebration of their, and therefore our own, lives.

Chapter One

CREATING THE ENVIRONMENT FOR HEALING

· ·

In recent years, much has been written about the effect of stress on our bodies. More and more doctors are becoming interested in the theories about the connection between the mind and body. The branch of medicine which looks at this connection is called psychoneuroimmunology (surely one of medicine's most flamboyant attempts at communication!). Broken down into simple language this means the study of the physical effects of our thoughts and feelings upon our bodies.

Throughout the history of medicine, the recognition of the part the mind plays in a patient's recovery has always been acknowledged. In the twentieth century, particularly since the development of antibiotics, the sulfa drugs and refined surgical techniques, medicine has taken a more technologically based view of disease. In fact, medicine is now primarily learned by studying disease rather than exploring the ways in which health is gained and maintained. There was a time when every doctor knew that the basis of good health was contentment and peace of mind. When a person was subject to overwhelming stress— either through grief, depression, or continued discouragement— it was considered to be the breeding ground for disease.

Within the last fifty years or so, we've gained immense technological skills, many of which have their application in the field of medicine. The drugs which have given us the power to manipulate and control some diseases have tended to make it easy to overlook the relationship between the mind and body. Instead of concentrating on what ingredients create abundant health, we, as a society, have focused on how to alleviate disease. Patients often walk into the doctor's room wanting a piece of paper with a prescription written on it. Often they don't want to hear advice about their lifestyle. The common attitude of the patient is, "Let me do what I want, and you fix up the consequences." Whereas technological advances and new drugs can be subject to scientific means of appraisal, it's much more difficult to measure the effectiveness of a positive and enthusiastic attitude on the regression of a disease.

Traditional and Complementary Medicine

There wasn't a great deal of ideological difference between traditional medicine and "complementary" or "alternative" medicine in the early part of last century. It's since the advent of drugs and technological advances that we've moved away from consideration of the mind's potential to influence the health of an individual.

This difference is rather well demonstrated when we look at the life cycle of a bacteria. There are several essentials which must be available to the bacteria in order for it to reproduce. One of these necessities is a suitable host. It seems it's at this point that "traditional" and "alternative" therapies diverge. Traditional medicine concentrates on the elimination of the "enemy" (the bacteria). This elimination might take the form of surgery, drug therapy, and so on. The art is in finding what will eliminate the disease without eliminating the patient! Some wonderful drugs and techniques have been discovered in this way. Our skills in surgery are extraordinarily refined, as are many other areas of medicine.

Complementary or alternative medicine concentrates on increasing the health, fitness, and well-being of people so they're vibrantly healthy in mind, body, and spirit and would therefore also be unsuitable hosts for any bacteria or disease.

Health is not just the absence of clinical disease. Health is a dynamic state of being.

Self-Love Equals Self-Care

When we truly love and care for ourselves, we can expect every day to be challenging, satisfying, and full of vibrancy and health. Through our behavior we can gain a clear image of the extent to which we respect and love ourselves. Self-love could be a new or strange concept to some people, because it's a very misunderstood term. Over the years, anything with the word "self" in it has become suspect, as in "selfish" or "self-centered." To consider, and put self first, is regarded as unacceptable. You might find it easier to think of it as self-care rather than self-love.

By your actions you'll be able to see to what extent you love and respect yourself. If you don't eat healthily—what does that say about you. If you smoke? If you don't get adequate exercise? If you take on too many commitments? If you burn the candle at both ends—what does that say about you?

Many people give out very mixed messages. On the one hand patients with lung cancer might be doing many really positive things to improve their health by taking vitamins, exercising, improving diet, and so on. Yet they've only managed to cut back on smoking, when really it might make better sense to stop entirely.

There are also unseen and more subtle effects of this lack of self-love. The body is influenced by the thoughts and feelings of the mind. In some ways our mind is very much like a computer and it will only deliver in the way in which it has been programmed. It can only retrieve the information which has been fed into it. If the subconscious mind has only ever received messages of a negative, self-demeaning nature, then those are precisely the messages which will flow out to every cell within the body. This happens via our nervous and endocrine systems. It is unrealistic to expect the body to be healthy and run smoothly while the mind is full of depression, grief, anger, despair, or thoughts of unworthiness. If, silently in our minds, we have thoughts like, Life's a struggle, I can't cope, I just don't have what it takes to meet the standard, I'll never catch up with all this work, I'm so stupid, everyone else understands, then it's obvious every cell in the body is going to feel the stress of such thinking. It matters not to the body whether this thinking is in the conscious or sub-conscious mind. It will still have its influence.

Since writing the first edition of *Quest for Life* in 1988, much research has come out in support of the mind/body connection. It can now be readily demonstrated that thoughts and feelings have a measurable effect upon the body. People who have a chronic problem with low self-esteem, or who feel a failure, or who suppress anger, or who feel deeply discouraged and daunted by life, secrete into the bloodstream chemicals and hormones which suppress the immune system. These hormones and chemicals are often the ones which we secrete when we're under physical threat and are essential when we're required to make a physical effort.

The Fight or Flight Response

Back in the days when we lived in caves, we were frequently faced with physical threats to our lives. If a bear appeared in the mouth of our cave, our bodies had a distinct and essential physical response. Instinctively we pumped powerful hormones and chemicals into our bloodstream; these had a whole range of effects in our bodies. We immediately became very alert; our rate of breathing increased so we drew in more oxygen; our rate of expelling carbon dioxide escalated as our respiration quickened; the heart rate and blood pressure increased as did the blood flow to our arm and leg muscles. These responses enabled us either to fight the bear, if we considered our cave worth defending, or to run like mad—reassuring ourselves we were fortunate to have escaped so easily! If we chose to tangle with the bear, then our bodies were equipped as well as possible for that task. Likewise, if we decided our best chance lay in escape, then we also had the right internal environment to allow that to happen. In either case there was a great deal of physical activity.

This physical activity employs these hormones and chemicals, and eventually the body is returned to its usual physiological equilibrium. After the extraordinary stress of our encounter with the bear we could sit down and inspect our injuries and, if we'd been successful in fighting off the bear, reassure ourselves that there's no place like home. Or, if we chose to run, we could enjoy the respite from stress while cogitating over where to find another cave for the night.

The problem with this marvelous mechanism, known as the "fight or flight" response, is that it can become activated by stressful situations in which the answer is *not* intense physical activity.

Familiar situations that trigger this response are, for example, a motorist cutting us off in traffic; a law enforcement officer pulling us over for exceeding the speed limit; someone unfairly criticizing our child; the fact that *he* didn't take out the garbage for the hundredth time this year; that *she* nagged about the clothes on the floor in the bedroom yet again; and so on. I'm sure you have your own frustrating favorites. All these examples, and I'm sure your own, make us grit our teeth, tense our muscles or make our heart beat a little faster. If this is compounded with a poor self-image, depression, or feelings of failure or entrapment, then it's a very likely possibility our fight or flight response is permanently left "on." In fact, we can become so accustomed to the stimulating effects of these stress hormones that, should they ever decrease, we might deliberately go out of our way to reestablish what to us has become the "normal" equilibrium. Many of us only "feel alive" when our stress chemicals are flowing. In this way we educate our bodies to believe being stressed is "normal." It's rather like having a stimulating drug circulating in our bloodstream all the time. It wasn't until I was diagnosed with acute myeloid leukemia in September 1983 and given only a matter of weeks to live that I began investigating the patterns of behavior in my life. I realized I "thrived" in the midst of a crisis. If there wasn't one around, then sure enough I'd create one.

This tendency was evident in much of my behavior. One common example was my habit of procrastination. Many people thrive on being pushed to their limits and will create the situation in which they're pressured by time. We do this by leaving things to the last minute and then getting ourselves into a flap, trying to accomplish, in a short time, what we originally had lots of time to complete. One of the long-term effects of these chemicals and hormones circulating in our bloodstreams is the depression of our immune system's response.

The Immune System

The immune system is extremely complex in both its components and functions. Simply put, its function is to recognize what is "me" and what is "not me." One of the functions of the white blood cells is to recognize foreign cells, like bacteria and viruses, and to recognize imperfect cells. When it does find these cells—the "not me" cells—it sends out for the killer and scavenger cells who are then mobilized to dispatch the foreigners. I don't mean to oversimplify the complexity of the immune system. It's incredibly intricate and wonderful, quite awesome in fact.

This knowledge gives us tremendous cause for celebration. There's so much we can do to cooperate with our magnificent immune systems. We need to provide all the essentials, and then trust it's performing its task perfectly. This means controlling what we hold in our mind so the body receives positive, encouraging, and loving thoughts; that we affirm this thinking by giving our bodies the best and freshest foods and other substances for its health; that we exercise and rest the body adequately; that we choose appropriate treatments for disease; and that we lift and inspire ourselves frequently through the use of meditation and the many techniques within this book. In this way we create an ideal environment in which healing of body, mind, and spirit can take place. The characteristics of long-term survivors are:

- *A refusal to accept the fatality of the disease.*
- *A purpose for living.*

- *The ability to express feelings.*
- *A willingness to follow one's own inner guidance for healing.*

Self-Management of Stress

Through the regular practice of physical relaxation and meditation we allow the body to find its own chemical equilibrium. The hormones and chemicals created through stress subside and the body comes back to its "resting point" where it experiences an internal stability—often referred to as homeostasis. In the chapters on meditation and visualization techniques we'll explore more fully the means by which we can assist ourselves in the process of reestablishing this state.

The following questions from Shelley Kessler of Crossroads School of Mysteries, Santa Monica, California, are very useful in identifying or clarifying your thoughts and feelings about yourself. It's suggested that you answer these questions in your journal over a period of days or weeks. Answering the questions every six to twelve months is an excellent way to gauge your progress in appropriate self-management of stress.

1. *Who am I?*
2. *What are my needs, values, and goals?*
3. *Given the limitations of time, energy, and space, what are my priorities that reflect the above?*
4. *Can I accept my needs, limitations, and priorities?*
5. *How do I make decisions according to my priorities to minimize pressure in my life?*
6. *How do I read the signals of stress, overload, and misdirection in my life?*
7. *How can I cope with the inevitable and often unwanted change in my life in a way that promotes my growth and healing?*
8. *What are the techniques I use for relieving the tension and confusion that accompany the stress I do have?*

Attitudes to Life

There's a lovely story which comes from India about a man who was traveling from one town to another. As he entered a particular town, he stopped at the well to refresh himself. Sitting by the well was a very old man, and the traveler said to him, "What sort of people live in this town?"

The old man looked at him and asked, "What sort of people did you find in the last town you visited?"

The traveler replied, "Oh, they were a fine people; full of warmth, hospitality and kindness."

The old man nodded and said, "Yes, you'll find the people in this town very much like that also."

Shortly after, a second traveler passed by the well and, likewise, said to the man, "What kind of people live in this town?"

The old man replied in the same manner as before, asking what kind of people the traveler had found in the previous town.

The traveler replied, "Oh, they were a mean and inhospitable bunch of rogues. I didn't feel safe for a moment."

The old man nodded again and replied, "Yes, I'm afraid you'll find the people of this town much the same."

This story illustrates perfectly how our perception of things dictates exactly how we'll experience events in our lives. When we look at the world through the glasses of victim-consciousness, then rest assured our experience will be seen in the light of this perception. It's not always an easy habit to change especially when we've a disease which debilitates or frightens us. I well remember the panicky feelings which assailed me whenever I thought that there was some kind of monster running rampant in my body. Initially these thoughts were accompanied by a feeling of total powerlessness to change the situation.

Cause of Disease

At present, there's much written about people creating their own disease. This represents a terribly simplistic view of life. There's no point in blaming ourselves for creating our disease. There's great value in taking responsibility for our *response* to having the disease. There are so many factors involved in the formation of cancer, AIDS, or any other life-inhibiting disease—stress, genetic factors, viruses, smoking, environmental exposure to carcinogens and dietary considerations, to name some of the more obvious ones. The mind struggles to find reasons for having developed an illness and often resorts to some kind of philosophy in which life and its crises make sense.

I often refer to a Persian carpet in the center of our support group meeting area to explain my understanding of disease and its place in our lives. If I showed you a chocolate brown square centimeter of the carpet and asked you if you'd like a carpet in that color, you'd probably say, "No thanks!" If we could pull back further from the carpet and see that the brown is actually made beautiful because it has gold on either side, and then a warm russet color which enhances its shade, and that the emerald flash in the center of the carpet lends depth, character, and harmony to the whole, then you might say, "What a beautiful carpet and yes, I'd like to have it." Likewise in our lives. Sometimes we need to pull back from the momentary crisis in order to be able to appreciate the warp and weft of a lifetime. Only when we've a broader perspective can life become beautiful or meaningful. Often we're simply bewildered by the diagnosis and experience of illness and no explanation will seem satisfactory or appropriate. Sometimes I think that I'm just having one of *those* lives! My favorite bumper sticker is:

My karma just ran over your dogma.

To claim responsibility for having created the environment in which cancer or any other illness has formed could be much the same as claiming the responsibility for having created the color of your eyes. Does it really help to think you got yourself into this situation? To take responsibility for our *response* to a diagnosis gives us a sense of control and empowerment. How can I create an environment in which healing can take place?

It's not what happens to me, but how I respond to what happens!

Several years ago I was working as secretary/housekeeper to Swami Kriyananda, who lived about a thirty-minute drive from anywhere civilized. The very first morning he told me that an Indian saint was coming to visit and there'd probably be five or six people for afternoon tea. I happily went about finding the cups, saucers, teaspoons, and so on and made some cookies and banana bread. An hour later Swami returned and said there might be as many as ten for tea, but he didn't expect it to be more than fifteen. I happily found more cups and saucers and checked to see that there were sufficient cookies and banana bread. An hour later, he returned. "Perhaps," he said, "there might be as many as twenty, but I'm sure there won't be more than twenty-five." Swami continued throughout the morning in this manner and by lunch time, he *promised* there'd be no more than fifty people. I thought, "A promise is a promise, and from a Swami, it's better than a written guarantee!"

I was keenly aware throughout the morning of all the activity within my mind. Most of the time I was entirely content and was enjoying the preparations; sometimes I became panic-stricken as I thought, "What if we run out of milk or cookies?" and at other times was cross that Swami continued to invite more and more people ("Who does he think he is anyway?!"). It was impossible to remain cross with him because he was almost childlike in his enjoyment of the anticipated party.

The kitchen was slightly elevated over the main living area where the saint and the swami sat beaming at each other. After serving tea and cookies or banana bread to all *seventy-five* people present (a real loaves and fishes story, believe me!), I looked down upon the pair and realized, "This job isn't about being a housekeeper. It's about responding joyfully or willingly to what-ever situation presents itself." Just as that thought floated through my mind, Swami caught my eye and smiled sweetly.

Life's like that. Events, situations, accidents, diseases, catas-trophes present themselves in our lives and it's up to us how we respond to them. I could have blamed Swami for his lack of consideration but it wouldn't have changed the fact that seventy-five people came to tea. I had a choice in how I would respond. I didn't consciously invite leukemia into my life, yet I did have a choice as to how I would respond to my predicament.

A life-threatening disease has a hidden advantage. Although you can feel stuck between a rock and a hard place, often the old solutions either don't have any appeal any more, or they simply don't work. If we've always suppressed our feelings, have presented a facade of "I can cope," and try to continue this attitude when we're diagnosed, we could very well compound our problems. In fact, practicing old solutions could well have contributed to our poor state of health.

Inner Stresses

About five weeks after I was initially diagnosed, I really started to take stock of myself. Up until then I thought the diagnosis was incorrect and there was no way I could die—I just didn't feel as sick as that. Five weeks after diagnosis I began to adjust my thinking, as I experienced more weakness and inability to do the simplest things without complete exhaustion. At about this time I took to my room, not wanting to talk to anyone, and began to look deeply within. I was qualified as a naturopath, a yoga and meditation teacher, and had been a strict vegetarian and meditator for fifteen years. In fact, it was downright embarrassing to have cancer when I'd been teaching others about health!

One of my favorite Peanuts cartoons has Charlie Brown saying to Lucy, "I thought you'd achieved inner peace?"

Lucy replies, "I *have* inner peace but I haven't lost my outer obnoxiousness!"

Conversely, many of us project outer peace while we experience inner obnoxiousness. I appeared very "together," capable and peaceful on the outside, while turmoil festered and boiled within. Through my introspection at this time, I began to see that I had completely lacked self-acceptance. Life had always felt like a struggle and great efforts seemed necessary even to survive in the world. Ninety-five percent was five percent less than acceptable. This applied to every aspect of my life. As a child I was a gifted pianist and yet, when I had an exam looming in which I knew I'd get less than ninety percent, I became sick and was therefore unable to sit for it.

School, and being a teenager, were two insurmountable obstacles in my mind. I didn't feel I had the mental, emotional, or physical equipment to cope with them. This led to my leaving school just after I turned thirteen. I had many problems with my legs and, as I had several operations necessitating months in the hospital over the ensuing years, I never returned to school.

Clearly I didn't sit down consciously to figure out ways of making my body sick to achieve some underlying aim. Later in my life I didn't think, "Ah yes, a good dose of leukemia with a short prognosis is just what I need right now." Yet I firmly believe, at some more subtle level, that the particular disease and prognosis were precisely tailor-made for me. By that time in my life I was already adept at using my body to manifest illness as a coping mechanism. And, as with a lot of people, the six to eighteen months before diagnosis were particularly stressful, with the suicide of one of my brothers, a geographical move to another country, and the separation from my husband.

During this time of introspection, many long-held attitudes and beliefs gradually became clear and I felt as if I'd painted myself into a rather uncomfortable corner. Some of these beliefs and attitudes had developed as techniques for survival. Even though I had strong spiritual beliefs, I still basically felt life was a struggle. No matter how hard I tried I could never quite measure up to my own high expectations. I grew up believing we were meant to be "nice" all the time, at all costs. To feel anger, resentment, hatred (a word never mentioned in our home), let alone express those feelings, was the same as throwing mud pies at God. It was just unthinkable. I have been amazed since by just how many other people similarly view the world.

Because of my perceived need to keep all my feelings firmly under control and deeply suppressed, I lived more fruitfully in my head than my heart. If the most important thing was to be a likable person, then clearly the "bad" feelings would have to be kept locked up and only the "good" ones allowed to get an airing. Perhaps, if I only displayed the good ones long or often enough, I could fool everyone (maybe even myself?) that those were the only ones to which I was prone. Deep down, the conflict bubbled and fermented. Perhaps the last straw was the break-up of my marriage and the death of my brother.

To believe our bodies can be humming along healthily while our minds are full of hurtful and negative thoughts of failure defies common sense. How can we possibly have a well-functioning and enthusiastic immune system if our minds are full of fears, self-criticism, and harsh judgments?

A life-threatening disease has the possibility, if we're willing to allow it, of showing us how we have lived our lives up until now, and it gives us the opportunity to assess and decide if that is how we wish to continue. For myself, it was obvious that much of my thinking and attitudes were enough to make any immune system turn up its toes.

If there has been an underlying thread right throughout my life, it has been a great desire to understand. To understand the whole mystery of being human. How and why people get sick. Why we make the choices we do. How the intricacies of the entire universe come together to create perfect balance and harmony. Why humans have the extraordinary capacity to make choices—choices in thinking, in actions, in expression of feelings.

The Power of Choice

It's often said, "People don't change." I believe that statement is made only by people who don't welcome change in themselves. It's what sets humankind apart from animals. We have complete choice over the kinds of thoughts we wish to hold in our minds. What tremendous power!

In the shower, fairly early in my illness, I was devastated to see so much of my long, thick hair going down the drain. It really felt as if it was *me* going down the drain! My tears mingled with the water of the shower as I sank deeper into despair. One day, the thought occurred to me that I could experience the water flowing down over my body as a powerful torrent of healing light. It could flow right through my body, bringing energy and vitality to every cell. Just a simple change of perception. And yet, even though simple, one frame of mind was the antithesis of the other. One set of thoughts brought depression and a distinct feeling of powerlessness, while the other brought a sense of hope and positiveness.

We can't always change the outcome of a disease but we can change the way in which we experience that outcome.

When we make a firm commitment to life and to experiencing our connection with the flow of power and love in the universe, extraordinary and unexpected events begin to unfold. Greater peace, equanimity, and joy are experienced even in the midst of disease, and the experience of these states creates the perfect environment for physical healing to take place.

There came a time in my illness when I felt so lacking in energy that I wanted it all to end right then. Not in a few weeks, but right in that moment. I didn't want my children to see me going through what I perceived as the degrading, undignified scenarios which surround serious illness and death. Surely a phone call saying, "She's gone," would be preferable?

Obviously this thinking was going on at a time when I still felt completely powerless. During this time I prayed earnestly every night *not* to wake up in the morning. I was still panic-stricken because I didn't feel I had any control over my life. Perhaps I could have control over my death? Even this was denied me! Suicide was never an option for me—especially in view of my brother's recent death. So again I needed to look at my thoughts and see what could be changed. The beauty of being stuck between a rock and a hard place is that it forces us to find new ways of being. The old habits and patterns don't work and we seek new ones.

After a time I began a little ritual when I awoke each morning. I would visualize Christ sitting on the end of my bed. I thought to myself that Christ knows more about healing than anyone I'd ever heard about, so I concentrated all my attention on him. I would reflect on his life, his qualities. I guessed there were many times in his life when he thought, Do I really have to go the whole way? Couldn't I just slip away quietly, resume life as a carpenter or something? I reflected on his never-give-up attitude; his gentleness; his acceptance; his lightness and sweetness; his commitment to truth, his passion for life. Then I would visualize these qualities as light which radiated from his body. When I used every ounce of my concentration I could see that light extending out to fill the whole room. I could see it surrounding my body and I would begin to breathe in its radiance, each inward breath drawing more of those qualities inside my body, inside my mind.

No matter what state I'd awakened in—be it pain, discomfort, depression, or despair—within minutes I would begin to feel the peace, presence, and healing power of Christ, and it would always change my perception of how things were. In this way, I would survive each day. Throughout the day, and when assailed by fears in the night, I would wrap myself up in a cocoon of his light and presence, and feel comforted. It's a practice which I've continued. It's a way of handing over my perceptions to a greater power outside, or deep within, myself. It doesn't matter that perhaps I'm able to do this because I just have an overactive imagination. If it brings comfort and hope then I would rather experience those states than despair and powerlessness. This technique can become almost second nature after a while. Often I will visualize I am sitting inside the body of Christ while lecturing or talking with a patient. This has led to some unexpected experiences—unexpected both for myself and for the people to whom I'm talking. Intuition seems to increase manifoldly.

Recently I was invited to speak at an academic meeting of psychiatrists from two of our major teaching hospitals. The meeting was to be held from 8:30 A.M.-9:30 A.M. on a Friday morning. I knew which hospital the meeting was at and yet, written clearly in my diary, was the name of the other one which was about a twenty-minute drive further on.

I considered this meeting to be very important as it presented a rare opportunity for me to speak to senior professionals who are deeply entrenched in the orthodox medical system. This was the first time a non-academic had addressed their meeting. I'm usually very particular about punctuality and so I arrived fifteen minutes early at the wrong hospital in time to sit on the cliff tops overlooking the ocean. I finally arrived at the Department of Psychiatry just before 8:30 A.M. only to be told that I was at the wrong hospital. I asked them to telephone the other hospital and say I was on my way. As I sped (during peak-hour traffic) to the *right* destination I fluctuated between outbursts of, "I can't believe this is happening. Of all the meetings to be running late for! Damn, blast and bother!" (the last three words aren't an exact translation but they'll suffice), and, "Just practice what you preach, Petrea. Take some long, slow, deep breaths, feel the sunshine on the backs of your hands, relax your tummy. Damn! Blast! Bother! Breathing quietly in, quietly out, I can't believe this is happening! Gently in, gently out." And so it continued until my semi-flustered arrival at the right building twelve minutes after I'd left the first one.

There they were, all assembled, forty or fifty of them. I flew into a chair and while being introduced spent a moment visualizing that I was sitting deeply at peace inside the body of an angel. It works like magic for me. I never prepare lectures so I started to talk and finished on time fifty minutes later. There were a lot of wonderful questions asked, and several future connections and joint projects arose out of this particular lecture. One psychiatrist's comment really touched me. She said, "Of all the many impressive things you've shared this morning, the one thing I shall always remember was your ability to fly in here ten minutes late and be able to speak from a center of peace and calmness."

On another occasion a prisoner with AIDS taught me a great deal. One of the greatest lessons!

I'd been counseling several prisoners infected with HIV in

one of our main prisons for just over two years. One of the prisoners, Bruce, who up until then had shown no health problems, suddenly developed a lymphoma around the spinal cord, which ended his life within six weeks. (HIV attacks some of the T-cells in the immune system, resulting in a decrease in immune function.) This particular person had formerly had a high T-cell count, so it came as a great shock to the other prisoners that he should now be so very ill.

On this particular day, I went first to the prison to see "my boys" before going to the hospital to visit Bruce. I found them very angry and upset. They'd vandalized and set fire to Bruce's cell earlier in the morning and were now discussing his crimes, saying that he deserved to die painfully because he was a rotten "rock-spider" (child molester). I'd never particularly focused on the *reasons* for their imprisonment and, even though I knew Bruce was a child molester, my counseling had been more widely based than just on his crime. However, as they talked about Bruce's crimes I became more and more angry myself. I thought of my young son and what I might do to someone who interfered with him in the way Bruce had with a number of small boys.

When I arrived at the hospital to see Bruce, I wasn't in good shape to counsel *anyone!* He was very ill and I sat with him for a while, but all I could see was my own judgment of him as a child molester.

When I arrived home I was totally exhausted, something fairly rare for me. I went and sat quietly in my office and thought about my day and the reasons for my great weariness. Gradually I entered into a state of meditation and then it all became clear. I realized that "my boys" had been angry and upset, not because Bruce was a child molester but because he represented a fearful scenario to them since they had far fewer T-cells than he. What was to stop them from developing an HIV-related disease which might rapidly kill *them?* These men tend to express all their emotions through anger. Fear, sadness, grief, confusion, hopelessness, and so on are mostly expressed through anger, violence, or aggression. I'd become infected with

their fears which, for me, mostly centered around my son. In
their minds, they justified the severity of Bruce's illness on the
grounds of his crimes of the past. *They* weren't child molesters,
they were only bank robbers! *Their* thinking told them that only
really awful people would get such a severe illness. *They* had
plenty of time up their sleeves.

I realized that I was seeing Bruce wholly as a projection of
my fear and judgment. He wasn't being a child molester when I
saw him! He was sitting there feeling very frail and sick. I chose
to see something that didn't actually exist except within my own
perception. In a way, I kept him trapped as a child molester in
my interaction with him because that is whom I chose to see and
relate to.

Bruce lived another week and I again had the opportunity to
visit him. Before I entered his room I took some long deep
breaths and visualized I was standing inside the body of Jesus. I
would practice looking at Bruce with eyes of love rather than
eyes of judgment. We had a really wonderful meeting that was
full of warmth and acceptance. He spoke of his life, his own
childhood, his regrets, his shame. He said it was the first time
he'd been able to talk to anyone about his life. At one point, he
talked about his becoming a Christian and accepting forgiveness
for his crimes. My judgmental attitude leapt to the fore. How
dare he accept forgiveness! I was amazed to find a part of myself
which wanted him to suffer for all eternity! Again, I needed to
return to looking at him with eyes of love. We sat for some time
in companionable silence. When I took my leave of him we gave
each other a long, warm, and sincere hug. I truly felt I'd been in
the presence of a very special being and counted it a privilege to
have known him. He died very peacefully a few hours later. Perhaps the opportunity Bruce had to speak of his life, knowing that
there was no judgment, somehow completed his healing. I know
that when I'm able to leave judgment at the door strange and
unexpected things happen. I also know these techniques bring
comfort to both of us and, often, a new perception of life. It's
the essence of forgiveness to leave judgment aside and see the
person or situation afresh—letting go perceptions, expectations,

and simply allowing myself to be present without judgment.

When I was sick I knew if I continued my negative, self-critical, and fear-ridden thoughts, then surely I would die. If I practiced these other techniques, then regardless of the outcome of the disease, every day had the potential to be lived more peaceably. Even if I were to die, the peace and sense of hope these techniques gave were clearly going to make the experience of dying as emotionally comfortable as possible. I never claim to have cured myself. I'm grateful for every day which, for me, is a precious gift. My quality of life now is certainly much better than before I was diagnosed, because my level of self-acceptance, self-love, and self-respect is much greater. I'm in remission, and I expect to remain so for the next fifty or sixty years. The important thing is not *how* long we live but the *quality* of every day lived.

Question the quality in your life:

- *Did I have fun today?*
- *Did I feel challenged and fulfilled by my work?*
- *Were my interactions with other people genuine and satisfying?*
- *Did I experience love today?*
- *Am I fully alive?*
- *Is something missing from my life? If so, what?*

These are good questions to ask yourself on a regular basis. If you see from your answers that there's room for improvement, look into why you experience dissatisfaction and feel free to find more appropriate ways of living your life. This is the only life I'm currently aware of living and it's not a dress rehearsal. We're not warming up for the big event. This is it, this moment, here and now. I definitely want to give it my best shot. In this way, I expect the future will take care of itself.

To change the way we view the world seems a lot to ask, especially at a time when we're already under considerable stress. We need to find other ways of looking at life because the

ways we've been using up till now might not be helping us.
They could even have been causing the very problems we now
wish to overcome. We can be fearful of letting go habitual ways
of thinking or acting. Sometimes I felt it would be easier to give
up my life rather than to let go a cherished way of thinking. In a
way, I knew I could "do" a good death, but I didn't know how to
"do" a good life!

However, little by little, I began to let go and trust. It only
took a little willingness to do so. It even became fun as I explored new ways to "be." Meditation and visualization techniques formed the basis on which these changes began to take
place. I found I didn't have to be the same person any more. Life
became an adventure. Rather than thinking my way through this
process, I concentrated on "feeling" my way. I enjoyed *feeling* the
flow of warm light-filled air into my lungs, rather than *thinking* it
would be a healthy thing to do.

Instead of thinking what would be good and healing for me
each day, I started to feel what would be good for me. Gradually
my language changed to include far more feeling words than
thinking words. The mind is mostly preoccupied with the future,
or chewing over the past, whereas the body *always exists in the
present moment.* When we bring the attention of the mind to the
experience of the body, we're more easily able to enter the
realms of feeling.

In the next chapter we'll look at the many techniques which
can be employed to help create an environment for healing.

Chapter Two

TECHNIQUES FOR LIVING

. . . .

Kerry

My name is Kerry, and I'm a recovered cancer patient. I discovered a three-centimeter lump in my left breast on October 1, 1984. I was thirty-nine years old. Subsequent medical checking found a mass of tumors in the lymph glands under my arm, and several in my neck. Initial shock gave way to deep fear and despair. That "C" word had a powerful effect.

The first "good news" was that the disease hadn't spread to the bones, and the doctor told me they had many patients who'd lived for years with breast cancer. One woman, who did have bone metastases, was still alive after twenty years, and having regular checkups. My treatment was to be chemotherapy, radiotherapy, and more chemotherapy. He also suggested that I was the most important part of the treatment and suggested I attend relaxation sessions, eat wholesome food, have plenty of rest and fresh air. I immediately turned my predisposition to workaholism and obsession toward incorporating complementary therapies. Meditation, counseling, a local cancer support group, dietary changes, vitamins, spiritual healing, courses on cancer information, and assorted and sundry others, all helped me enormously. Even if now just writing the list makes me feel tired, I see, in retrospect, that all this activity really did keep me together emotionally. I also received more love and attention from family and friends than ever before. Though there were times I longed for someone to look after me, do the shopping or wash the "blankety-blank" juicer, I knew that taking the degree of responsibility that I did (and was physically capable of doing) was how it was meant to be.

Naturally there were moments of panic, depression, and sadness—especially when a new friend died. At the support group friendships deepened rapidly in the emotional intensity of sharing the really important things in life. We shared laughter, tears, pain, love, anger—as we expressed the full gamut of human emotions.

I kept a journal through this time, and in it I poured out my feelings, the happenings, my fears and hopes. It was invaluable to be able to look back and see how far I'd come.

After three months of chemotherapy and excellent results—the breast and neck lumps had shrunk away to nothing—only the underarm tumors didn't budge. They were then surgically removed. Radiotherapy followed to the tumor areas. Also my ovaries were irradiated because the cancer was hormonally responsive and this could assist in achieving a remission. No more chemotherapy was required, luckily. I loathed that treatment, but was aware of how well it worked.

"REMISSION" was the magic word!

Well, after all this frantic activity (over ten months) I settled down to—guess what? Incredible loneliness, feelings of isolation, depression, and panic attacks! Sorry folks, there was no walking off into the sunset smiling—or the equally mythic happy ever after. All the bargains I'd made with myself, like, "I'll never complain again," or "If I just get through this chemotherapy cycle nothing will ever be this bad again"—all gone!

I realized three underlying problems had been going on for many years before the cancer, and had sprung from a childhood characterized by fear and uncertainty with an alcoholic mother, and a severely depressive father. I masked the problems with alcohol for eighteen years before I found studying, and went from alcoholic to workaholic. Then ongoing stress of years of study, and a completed university degree, ended with a nervous breakdown, with severe mood swings, and the overpowering fear of "losing control." It was twenty months later that I found the cancer, and since that time I've worked with an excellent psychotherapist.

From my experiences with cancer and beyond, the following issues quickly spring to mind. Firstly, when I embraced, so enthusiastically, complementary therapies, and there are so many to choose from, I worried all the time, Was I doing enough? What about the things I wasn't doing? What about the ones I didn't even know about yet—was I going to worry about them too? Much later I finally understood that it was "fear" that kept me on my rigid diet for so long, even though I became allergic to half the foods I allowed myself to have. The "fear" of cancer returning if I stopped was so strong. Slowly, I've given myself permission to change, and again, hearing others deal with the problem has helped.

The reality is that my immune system is permanently depressed from the effects of the chemotherapy and radiotherapy; I've become environmentally hypersensitive, and have the herpes simplex virus.

So now I've finally stopped waiting for my white cell count to be normal—as if that were the magic sign. I do become easily tired, but I can see, hear, walk, talk, and feel. I do have anxiety problems with reading, writing, TV, concentration—and it's a life of limitations, but I've come a long way, and am still in remission!

I search for the meaning in my life, and feel the challenge is to look for the positives (they are always there). I'm endlessly fascinated by the great mystery of it all and have decided I don't have the answers, and that's O.K.

It's definitely one day at a time for me. Some days are a breeze, and on others I hold tight to the meaning of the beautiful serenity prayer: God grant me the serenity to accept the things I cannot change, courage to change the things I can, and the wisdom to know the difference.

Taking responsibility for our actions increases our feelings of self-respect and self-worth. When we're dealing with taking responsibility for our health and our treatments, it means we'll be informed to the best of our ability. Your doctor is clearly the most knowledgeable person to talk to you about your disease and its stages, and the medical treatments he or she can offer.

If we can accept that primarily we're spiritual beings who are embod-ied rather than bodies who happen to have spirits, then it can give us some meaning or framework in which to create our healing.

I believe the universe is entirely ordered and that nothing happens haphazardly. Leukemia was the best thing that ever came my way because I learned much more about myself, much more quickly than I ever could have without it. It is, of course, only because I'm sitting here *above ground* that I'm able to say such a thing. However, this experience of illness has been re-stated many times by others who've viewed their disease and healing process in the same way.

When we've a life-inhibiting disease, it's essential that we take responsibility for the establishment of peace of mind: to have peaceful and harmonious thoughts; to acknowledge and release past hurts, angers, resentments, and feelings of unworthi-ness; to ensure the body receives all it requires for abundant health and healing. When we can cultivate an overall feeling of life being a game, or fun, and learn not to take it all so seri-ously, it makes the heart lighter.

Once, when I was sick, I was given a rose. I dissolved into tears, thinking that this was probably the last rose I'd ever see. Then I realized that this was simply a beautiful rose. Right here, right now. Me and the rose. It became a perfect moment rather than a fearful projection into the future.

When we've taken 100 percent responsibility for how we conduct our lives, how we think, how we feel, then we learn to trust. Trust healing *is* taking place, trust everything is unfolding as it should, trust that if healing occurs in mind and spirit but doesn't include the body, then that will be O.K. too. To achieve this state of mind takes considerable effort, as we so much want healing to be done on our terms. If we view our illness or death as a monster lurking in the corner, and we desperately seek ways to "buy him off," we're generally not successful—especially in achieving peace of mind. When we learn to trust that whatever happens to us is for our highest good, it can give us the courage to look at disease, death, or negativity and make really fundamental changes to the way in which we perceive life. Once I'd looked at death and all the parts of me that were so scared to live, I was better able to deal with those aspects of myself.

To affirm life in every way—through relationships, through thoughts, through the healthy expression of feelings, through diet, through exercise, through laughter, through facing challenges—is to create the perfect environment for healing. For the rest, we trust.

If all our efforts are going into staying in a body at all costs, then we may be destined for disappointment. If our efforts go into healing ourselves of all that prevents us from truly living in each moment, then the rewards are certain and abundant.

Love, peace, faith, hope, and acceptance are attainable, and in the presence of these qualities all things are possible. My work is not to keep people alive, but to help them to live.

Self-Esteem

Many people have a real problem with self-esteem. In Western society it's often more common to put people down than build them up. We do this with our children, too, unless we're watchful. If our self-esteem is low, its effect will be felt in every part of our lives. Many of us excel in one area of our lives, and we work quite hard to convey the image of being equally successful in all aspects.

Where does this crushing need to be perfect come from?

Is it a childhood in which our best efforts were never quite good enough; where parents berated us instead of encouraging us? Perhaps as we came to adolescence we had demeaning nicknames thrust upon us—Fatso, Poofter, Squirt, Pudding, Pin-head, Bus-face—or whatever. We longed to be like the popular, good-looking members of our class or school, not realizing they, too, probably had their hang-ups and uncertainties. Perhaps our low self-esteem came from a father who, though a good provider and therefore in the eyes of the world a good father, was always at meetings, out to dinner, and never at home when we longed to talk to him about what was happening in our lives. What could this tell us? That other things were more interesting, more worthy of his attention than being with us? Perhaps it wasn't long before we got the message—"I'm not important, I'm not interesting, I'm not worth much."

A broken relationship, where a lover has rejected us, could translate into "I'll never have a successful relationship," "Men don't like me," or "I'm not attractive to men" (or their equivalent counterparts). Sure enough, the subconscious programmer gets to work and this is what we begin to project.

I remember when I was about eleven or twelve overhearing two teachers talking about me. One was trying to describe me to the other, who didn't know me by name. She said, "Oh, you know the one. That mousy-haired, sickly looking girl." It was like a dagger through my heart! The fact is, maybe they weren't talking about *me* at all! Maybe it was my sensitivity "out there" looking for confirmation that I wasn't up to scratch. But I certainly "owned" what was said. Sadly, our projected images of ourselves are so powerful that they can be extraordinarily difficult to change, even if we want to. These images inhibit our reaching out to others, developing our skills, building relationships, embarking on careers.

Our personalities can become corroded and we might never realize our full potential. We go on giving out negative estimations of ourselves and people take us at our own face value—the value we've been at pains to project even if deep down we know we're "not really like that." This further builds our "victim-consciousness" because we also begin to think, "Why can't they see what I'm *really* like? I must be the way people *think* I am." This self-perpetuating circle brings more and more pain. It often leads to a breakdown in our health. However, often out of breakdowns come breakthroughs.

Many people have said they're grateful for their illness because with it have come insights into themselves, previously unsuspected, and they come to realize with joy that "I'm not so bad after all." At one stage, it occurred to me that thinking I was somehow worse than everyone else was just the flipside of thinking I was better than everyone else: You think you're unworthy;

well, I'm much more unworthy than you!

So what can we do about this sick kind of thinking?

Firstly, we need to acknowledge that we *have* this kind of thinking and that it's no longer appropriate for us to continue in this way.

Secondly, we become willing to see things in another way. A simple willingness to let go the perceptions and judgments we hold about ourselves. This little poem gives a lighthearted understanding of the art of becoming more fully one's self.

On Being Yourself

You must learn that you cannot be loved by all people.

You can be the finest apple in the world—ripe, juicy, wet, succulent—and offer yourself to all.

But you must remember that there will be people who do not like apples.

You must understand that if you are the world's finest apple, and someone you love does not like apples,

You have the choice of becoming a banana.

But you must be warned that if you choose to become a banana, you will be a second-rate banana.

But you can always be the finest apple.

You must also realize that if you choose to be a second-rate banana, there will be people who do not like bananas.

Furthermore, you can spend your life trying to become the best banana—which is impossible if you are an apple—

Or you can seek again to be the finest apple.

So how do we begin to relinquish who we are not and become more fully ourselves? A good place to start is in our choice of words. We'd all benefit by leaving out the following words:

- *Can't*   (*Usually means won't*)
- *But*   (*Looking for an excuse*)
- *If only*   (*Wanting it to be different from how it is*)
- *Should*   (*Who says?*)
- *Ought*   (*Who says?*)
- *Impossible*   (*Start thinking possible*)
- *Try*   (*Just do it!*)

When we look back through history at the great people who continue to inspire and uplift us, they weren't the kind of people who would have used any of those words. Imagine if Beethoven had said, "If only I wasn't deaf, I'd keep writing music!" Or if the Wright brothers had decided after their first unsuccessful attempt that it was impossible for humans to fly....

We each know people in our own lives who've inspired us to go beyond our usual limitations. Listen to their vocabulary. You'll find it's full of positive statements. They're usually positive people who have the capacity to create what they want in their lives.

For those with a religious background, incorrect interpretation of the word "humility" can be the start of low self-esteem. Humility is not self-belittling and yet it's sometimes interpreted that way. Often this attitude is carried by people long after they leave their church. We've been told "to love others, as ourselves." This certainly implies we must honor, respect, and love ourselves if we hope to be able to do likewise with others.

We can renew ourselves by consciously taking opportunities to do things we enjoy—going to a play, a concert, a film, for a walk. Take time out to watch the waves on a beach, a sunset, sunshine on new leaves—surround yourself with uplifting things.

Check also to hear when you're putting yourself down, and stop, even if it's in mid-sentence. Change it to a positive.

Learn to accept and give a compliment. Be open to the love others extend to you and return it in full measure. Take every opportunity to listen to, and help others—even if the help seems minimal. The right motive makes the degree of help irrelevant. It's the desire to help that often heals.

Our self-esteem is helped as soon as we start looking outward instead of inward. When we're less self-absorbed by our faults and practice giving love to others by being genuinely interested in their welfare, life begins to take on a richness and depth not previously felt. After a time, we don't need to practice this consciously, because it becomes second nature to us.

At my very lowest emotional ebb, I was in a monastery outside Assisi in Italy. I felt totally useless, extraneous to the world's activities. My children were managing all right without me and there didn't seem to be anything that grabbed my attention and made me feel worthwhile. Frankly I was groveling in a morass of self-pity. It was terribly painful and there seemed no light at the end of the tunnel.

One day I was eating grapes outside the "cave" where I used to meditate. The day was clear, cool, and sunny. The surroundings, though very beautiful, didn't seem to jolt me out of my depressed state. Before long, a beautiful blue and black butterfly landed on my knee. Without much thought, I squeezed him a drop of grape juice which he lapped up enthusiastically. Within two minutes, another butterfly of the same coloring landed upon my other knee. Likewise, I squeezed him some juice which he seemed to enjoy. The butterflies and I sat in companionable silence eating grapes.

It might sound very strange to you, but suddenly I thought, I *am* useful. I'm a good landing place for butterflies.

Perhaps only those who've scraped the bottom of their own world and survived will recognize the impact that such a realization can make. It was yet another turning point.

This wasn't the first or only low point in my life. I've had times when just beginning the day seemed an insurmountable task. The depression was paralyzing, making all endeavor virtually impossible. On another occasion, to rescue myself from the pit of despair, I created a timetable for my day. It was a very tight schedule broken up into blocks of ten to fifteen minutes. It looked something like this:

7:00 A.M.——7:20 A.M.	*get up/have shower*
7:20 A.M.——7:30 A.M.	*make bed/tidy bedroom*
7:30 A.M.——7:45 A.M.	*have breakfast*
7:45 A.M.——8:00 A.M.	*clean up kitchen*
8:00 A.M.——8:30 A.M.	*tidy house*
8:30 A.M.——9:00 A.M.	*vacuum*

...and so on

I include this simply because I know I'm not alone in experiencing despair. When a sense of hopelessness begins to descend it can be difficult to shake off its influence. For those who experience such dark moments, take heart, you're not alone. It's a lonely road to walk because reaching out to others is made almost impossible by our own paralyzing pain.

It is possible to change our experience of depression:

- *First, we need to acknowledge we're in a pothole.*
- *Second, we need to want to change our perception.*

We can implement small changes to our daily program, things like:

- *Getting out of bed by a certain time*
- *Showering every day*
- *Tidying up one small thing each day (for instance, the top of the dresser, a drawer, corner, bookshelf, or cupboard)*
- *Putting fresh sheets on the bed, a clean towel in the bathroom*
- *Eating at the table with a tablecloth and cutlery*
- *Dusting one room*
- *Placing flowers throughout the house*
- *Playing music that's new to you*
- *Washing the dishes, drying them, putting them away*

These simple things are the beginnings of affirming that we're worthy of love and respect. Don't let yourself become overwhelmed by what needs to be done. Just accomplish one new thing each day and acknowledge you've achieved something. Don't focus on what's not right, focus on and approve of your efforts to change. Endeavor to see the glass as half-full rather than half-empty. As soon as you feel you can reach out to someone, make a phone call to a help-line, a support group, or a counselor. I know it's scary, and I also know it's possible to pass through the darkest hours and emerge into a brighter way of perceiving life. It takes courage and you have what it takes. You'll notice it becomes easier when you find good company in which to make your recovery. Good company includes books, music, and nature, as well as people.

Positive imaging can bring our desired goals very close indeed and give us confidence to go on believing. There's information on this aspect of the technique of visualization in chapter 6, In My Mind's Eye (see pages 140-146). Be prepared to give up your unrealistic expectations of yourself or others' expectations of you. This is *your* life. This is it, *this* moment, *right* here, *right* now.

What you're living now is the real thing, so feel challenged to take the risks which come with changing your way of thinking. Understand that you don't have to be saintly. You're perfect and acceptable just the way you are. Give yourself permission to make mistakes. Celebrate your mistakes as a valuable means of learning something. A so-called mistake then takes on a new meaning. If you've acknowledged there's a better way of doing something, then you've gained new and valuable knowledge. Self-flagellation is out! Self-congratulation is in!

Love your imperfections as much as the things for which you allow yourself credit, because they're all part of the same you. Stop judging yourself. One cannot release thoughts of negativity through rejection, only through love. So be nice to yourself and stop scaring yourself. We spend so much time and money on scaring ourselves half-silly. We do this by watching scary movies, reading depressing articles about our disease, and so on.

Create a safe, warm, and loving world around you, not one where you perceive attack lurking around every corner. Many people perceive their cancer cells, multiple sclerosis, HIV, or whatever, as "out to get them." Change your perception. Cancer cells are weak, unintelligent wimps! They've forgotten how to behave appropriately.

Often we're assailed by emotion in what seem to be the most inappropriate places. For instance, while pushing a shopping cart around the supermarket, your eye is caught by something which triggers a memory and suddenly you're overwhelmed by powerful emotions. We struggle to maintain control, suppressing our feelings once more. I have a fantasy that all those half-filled shopping carts you see in supermarkets have been abandoned by shoppers who fled in tears!

Some people feel there *is* no safe place in which they can freely express their emotions. It's important to recognize that we *have* feelings; then to give ourselves *permission* to have those feelings; then to find a place in which we can experience the feelings. I often need to retreat into the silence of solitude in order to allow these feelings to be recognized, "felt," and thus released. This is often in meditation or prayer, or it might be in the form of a walk along the beach, a visit to an empty church, time out in the country or on a park bench.

This simple formula works well in all situations. Mostly the problem arises when we *resist* the feelings we have. *Then* we have to suppress them in order to continue functioning "normally." Once we can give ourselves permission not to cope, to feel fearful, to feel angry, to feel overwhelmed, or whatever else might be applicable, then we can move through those feelings which will enable us to feel peace once more.

Try using the following formula:

1. *Acknowledging the feeling,*
2. *Giving yourself permission to have the feeling, and then*
3. *Simply experiencing the feeling.*

For instance, the steps might go something like this:

1. *"This is how it feels to be Petrea feeling fearful."*
2. *"It's O.K. for me to feel this way."*
3. *"This is how fear feels."*

Paradoxically, acknowledging that I'm afraid, then giving myself permission to feel afraid, is the first step toward being released from fear! Likewise, to acknowledge that I'm feeling overwhelmed, and that it's not surprising that I'm feeling overwhelmed, is the first step toward feeling back in control.

The fastest way out of feelings is through them.

Many people are afraid to express how they feel to someone else because they fear ridicule or abuse of the trust they've extended. It's important to be respectful of our feelings and to choose wisely those with whom we seek to share our vulnerability.

When we realize our life has been one of self-criticism, doubt or despair, and that there *is* a better way, it's as if a light has been switched on and we take our first steps out of emotional darkness into our true self. Then we can be comfortable but not complacent with our imperfections.

To find the light within ourselves is a wondrous experience, and yet we cannot find the light until we've acknowledged the darkness. When we acknowledge the light in others, our own begins to shine more brilliantly. Trust in your own ability to find peace, joy, and self-love. There's no room in our lives for ancient history. Forgive the past, release its influence, and move on. Ultimately we take responsibility for ourselves by dealing with what's causing us pain, ridding ourselves of guilt or any other negative emotion, and proceeding with greater self-acceptance. With self-acceptance comes acceptance of others, and of the events in our lives.

Sometimes the mind goes on a rampage of panic and despair. It's good at such times to have techniques up your sleeve to deal with these situations.

Try an exercise for a moment:

Close your eyes and concentrate all your attention on the big toe of your right foot: not thinking about it, but actually feeling your big toe. You may need to wriggle it a little to locate it more fully in your awareness. Notice its temperature, the texture of your sock or the pressure of your shoe, or the touch of the air. Bring all of your awareness to your big toe, right now.

You probably found, when you did that simple little exercise, that your mind became still and receptive to sounds around you, to atmospheric temperature, and to the soft touch of the air against your skin; an overall awareness of your immediate surroundings. This experience is not dependent on your thinking process, but on your feeling ones. It has a remarkable capacity to clear the mind of any thought, even thoughts of panic and despair. This very simple technique, of focusing our attention on the sensations in our bodies, can give us the opportunity to let go unwanted or undesired thoughts and can help move our reality to more neutral ground.

Everything in our culture is geared to overload us with information. To stop, to listen, and to feel is a totally new experience for some people, and is the beginning of meditation. It can become quite intoxicating in its effect, and can lay foundations for a new way of experiencing life. This way includes a freshness and spontaneity so often lacking in our lives. It connects us with each unfolding moment—each one new, never to be repeated; each one precious and full of potential. The heart understands these words easily. The mind questions, tries to distort, attempts to complicate. The heart is still by comparison. Learn to trust stillness and the knowledge which arises out of it. Allow yourself the luxury of peace. Learn to value it as your most precious asset. With this attitude it's surprising how many worries take care of themselves and dissolve back into quietude. When panic or anxieties assail you, put them on hold and spend some time with the techniques of relaxation and letting go. If they're important concerns or panics, rest assured they'll be there for your attention later. Don't fight them off. They're like wayward lost children who are tired and irritable and they clamor for your attention right now. Like overtired children, they need reassurance and putting to bed. Having done that, practice being at peace, practice trusting that everything *is* all right, that everything is unfolding in its own perfect time. In the beginning, it could seem an insurmountable task. Fear makes its presence known. Reassure the fear; put it to bed. And practice feeling peace once again.

Many people find it helpful to develop a little ritual around these fears or panics. Perhaps you could visualize putting them into the basket beneath a hot-air balloon and then, loosening the ropes, letting them soar up and away. Or, as suggested above, putting them to bed and simply turning off the lights. Or seeing those fears surrounded by light, melting away into light. Or placing your problems in a small boat at the edge of a river and giving it a push until the current bears it away downstream. One man, Graham, who tried this image, said that by the time he had put his mortgage repayments, car, and relatives into the boat, it sank to the bottom of the river! Find something which seems appropriate for you, perhaps some method which jumps out from your own lifestyle.

If you have any affinity with Christ (or some other teacher), you might wish to use the technique mentioned before: visualize you're sitting inside the body of that teacher, letting his or her love and light protect and heal you of your fears. Further techniques for visualization are given in chapter 6 (see page 140-146).

Anger

Many of us are afraid of our own anger. I didn't think I had any anger! I thought I was a peaceful person who didn't get upset about things. What I realized was that I was a peace at any price person and that I was sitting on a volcano of anger and resentment. I don't think I even knew what anger was and I would substitute other expressions like, "I feel irritable or moody." Much of my depression was a shield for anger. I realized that in my childhood I'd never seen healthy anger cleanly expressed. If my mother was angry, she spoke more quietly with a certain threatening tone in her voice. I found it very scary.

My daughter, Kate, has taught me a great deal about the healthy expression of anger. At the age of sixteen, she's got it mastered! My inexpert way of dealing with anger would be to walk down the hallway hurling angry accusations at her over my shoulder. Kate will have none of that. She'd say, "Don't walk away from me! We're having an argument. Now come and look me in the eye and say that!"

Kate's school was organizing an excursion to the Middle East. (When I was a girl, *our* school excursion was to the local dam to visit the filtration system!) Egypt is a favorite part of Kate's world and she was looking forward to it enormously. They were going to travel with an archaeologist and historian up the Nile by boat, later visiting Israel to climb Mt. Sinai at dawn, as well as touring all the fascinating places where so much history was made. Then came the crisis in Kuwait and we knew her excursion might have to be canceled.

About this time, Kate had been doing a lot of work on an extracurricular project for her school. This involved her spending many hours at the computer in very exacting work. She'd spent the whole of one weekend at it and most nights until quite late, making sure there were no errors.

One afternoon she returned home to find the letter that finally canceled her trip to the Middle East. She didn't say much at the time because she had to continue her work on the computer.

Later that evening, we were both working in my office, she at my desk and I at the computer. Suddenly she thumped the desk and said loudly, "I'm feeling really p...d off!"

Before she could continue, I immediately leaped in. "Kate, I won't have that language in..."

She rushed on with, "You be quiet and listen. I feel angry that everyone expects me to be able to get this program done for school and not make any mistakes, as well as doing all my homework and other projects, and I come home and Egypt's been canceled and I've been sitting on tears ever since, so now I'm going to have a good cry!"

And she did. I sat in awe and wonder. I apologized for interrupting her at the beginning of her outpouring.

She replied. "I didn't need you to get involved. I just needed you to listen! I feel fine now."

How often do we leap in and react to another person's anger when it isn't necessary at all? If I'd blazed on with my insistence that her language wouldn't be tolerated, we'd probably have ended up having a major argument where hurtful things could have been said, with doors slammed and the unresolved anger left to fester. At a later time, we talked about her language and my preferences with regard to choice of words! Then she could hear what I was saying, but to insist upon it in the middle of her outburst was inappropriate.

On another occasion, I had come home after a long and sad day. Several people in my AIDS group in the city were sick, had died, or were in the hospital. I was feeling sad and powerless. Instead of saying *that* to Kate when I got home, I attacked her with, "Why are you watching television? Have you done your homework? How many times have I told you not to have afternoon tea in front of the television?"

Kate looked completely dismayed and hit back with angry words. I realized what I was doing and I had to make a conscious decision to say to her, "Kate, I'm sorry. I'm not angry with you at all. My boys are sick and dying and that's why I'm upset and I shouldn't have dumped it on you." She's so forgiving, she simply said, "Why didn't you say so?" and then came and gave me a hug.

It's so hard when one is in the midst of wrongly targeted anger to stop and apologize. I'm having so much fun just getting it out that I don't seem to care who gets bruised! If I feel bruised, then why shouldn't I make someone else feel bad? I can't believe my own immaturity. We can certainly learn from our children. I don't give myself a hard time over it, though. I figure that I'm learning how to be a healthy human being who can express her emotions and that it takes time to grow up. I never saw anger expressed healthily as a child, so where would I have learned how to do it?

One of the participants in our group, Jennifer, was talking about the way her mother expressed anger: she'd never explain what was wrong and would say, "If you don't know *I'm* not going to tell you!" She'd then stalk off in silence, which she'd sometimes maintain for months. This group participant has had to learn both how to acknowledge and express anger in a healthy way.

Some people are easily able to transcend their anger through the techniques of meditation and forgiveness, while others need to find other outlets to really get their emotions moving. There's nothing negative about experiencing anger. It's a natural emotion. What *is* negative is to keep the anger inside where it can only fester and cause resentment. Anger changes the chemical balance in the body and is certainly detrimental when not discharged. These chemicals are the same ones which trigger our fight or flight response. To find an appropriate way for your anger to flow out is important. It can be difficult sometimes within our suburban environments to freely express anger without causing neighbors concern, or at least raised eyebrows. It's inappropriate to express our anger through physical violence, but there are many excellent ways of getting it out without causing offense to other members of society.

Expressing Anger

The following are a few suggestions for physically expressing anger in ways which won't cause damage to yourself or someone else.

You might find, because this is an unaccustomed way for you to behave, that initially you feel self-conscious, or a bit foolish. The mind will probably jump in and say things like, "I'm not really *that* angry about the way my ex-partner belittled me and undermined my relationship with my children; it was so long ago now; what's the point in being angry?" even though at the time you felt outraged by those actions and were frustrated by your feelings of powerlessness. Persevere until you really get in touch with the outrage within. This exercise only works when you really have conviction in what you're doing. If you're beating a pillow with your fists, then you must believe the pillow *is* your ex-partner. It's often very hard for people to get into this type of exercise without supervision and assistance. Hitting the heck out of your ex-partner isn't what we're really doing (though I'm sure, for some, that would be tempting!). It's simply a means by which we can let out the anger, and often it's the image of the person which can stimulate the rage. It helps to voice the feelings at the same time as doing the action. You might want to say, "They're *my* children too and I won't have you interfering with our relationship. I hate you for jeopardizing *my* relationship with *my* children! I hate you for putting me down to them!" or whatever. By doing this, we're ridding ourselves of the anger and helplessness we still feel about those actions. In using these techniques, the potency of those emotions can be accessed and freely expressed.

There are many such events in our lives when we feel infuriated, and yet we may never have expressed the feelings long held in. What about an ex-spouse who's making things very difficult financially; in-laws who are forever interfering with our family; a boss who constantly derides or puts us down; a parent who abused us (sexually, emotionally, physically, or psychologically) when we were young? These situations are often a potent source of outrage and feelings of helplessness, and it can be quite confusing to feel murderous rage toward someone for whom you once felt (or feel) love or respect. Many people then feel guilty, ashamed, and frightened by the intensity of these feelings. To express the anger in a safe environment is essential to its healthy resolution.

One young mother expressed her anger toward a father who had sexually abused her as a child by beating the blankets and carpets on the clothesline with a broom! The important thing is really to put your heart into what you're doing.

When all the emotion of anger is spent, there are usually

tears of sadness mixed with relief; a feeling of release and contentment; a sense of having passed through the storm rather than having just skirted its edges; a sense of completion.

It's not until we've access to the subconscious mind that many of our negative, fearful or long-held attitudes become apparent. The subconscious mind is what really dictates how we'll react to a situation. Our subconscious mind is that part of our awareness which remembers every past experience and has made personal laws or rules which filter all future actions and thoughts.

A common statement made by people who have difficulty in expressing their anger is, "What's the point of being angry. It isn't going to change things anyhow!" People who can express their anger in a healthy manner are able to recognize that even though their anger might not change anything, it's important that it be *acknowledged* and *expressed*. Those who have difficulty in expressing anger tend not even to acknowledge it.

Many people feel really uncomfortable with the idea of expressing anger in a loud or aggressive way. These people might benefit by persevering until they lose that fear, or they might prefer to find some other activity which will assist them in acknowledging and expressing their anger. You can write a letter to your ex-partner (whether alive or dead), expressing exactly how you felt when you were belittled constantly, behind your back, to your children. Expressing your anger through the written word can be very useful. You might wish to send the letter (if appropriate) or you can burn it. Likewise, you could "paint" your anger or "dance" it or "sing" it or "scream" it.

Many years ago I stayed with some friends in the mountains of Wales. Every afternoon as the gentle sun sank toward the Irish Sea, my hostess would wander up the mountain behind the house. About half an hour after she'd left, an eerie scream would filter down through the mists as she divested herself of the day's tensions. At first it was a little unnerving for me, being the house guest and wondering if in some way I had contributed to her distressed state. She'd return to the house looking refreshed and revitalized, ready for another day's trauma in the Welsh hills.

Some people find that sporting activity gives them a physical outlet for their emotional energy.

Matthew, a champion swimmer before he lost his leg to osteosarcoma, found that swimming now gave him the environment in which he could get in touch with, and express, his anger and frustration. Before he entered the pool, he'd remember his moments of frustration and then "swim out" his aggression.

The most important thing is for us to learn to recognize when we *are* angry; to acknowledge and find expression for it appropriately.

Guilt

The most destructive, useless, and stagnant energy of all is guilt. It paralyses our actions and achieves nothing. It brings only oppression and fear: fear of punishment. To feel guilt presupposes we believe we've committed actions not acceptable to the mores of our society, church, or family. If we believe we've erred, it reinforces our sense of unworthiness, that we're somehow not acceptable as we are. If we've done something for which we feel shame or are genuinely sorry, then let there be remorse. Honest remorse comes from the heart, not from the mind. Once we've felt, acknowledged and apologized for what we did, if that is appropriate, we can learn from it and go on enlightened.

Until my illness I felt a terrible guilt because I believed people were meant to be perfect and I knew I wasn't. I tried so hard to maintain an image to the world which said, "I know who I am; I know where I'm going; I'm a capable, efficient, intelligent person and everything's just fine." However, I felt like a fraud and a hypocrite, knowing none of these things were true. It was far from a happy way to live. On the outside I tried to maintain the image of coping with everything, while on the inside there was the constant voice of self-criticism: "You spoke for too long; not long enough; too loudly; too softly; you probably confused people; you're making a mess of everything; you're just not good enough!"

It has taken a lot of determination not only to become aware of this negative, self-defeating tendency, but also to control it! For some of us accomplishing self-acceptance is a lifelong task. When I was first asked to write a book, my immediate reaction was, "I can't do that! I left school at thirteen. I've only ever written a school composition! Everyone will see I'm uneducated!" Believing we're somehow worse than everyone else is exactly the same as believing we're somehow superior. "So you think your heart is full of imperfections—huh, mine's the blackest on the block!"

These days I can go to bed with the attitude, "Oh well, I made some assumptions today. I'm sorry, especially if I confused anyone. I might have spoken too loudly, too softly, for too long, or not long enough." Of course, we're going to keep doing some or all of these things. Being aware and more accepting of myself helps me to be able to say, "I know my heart's in the right place, and I'll be out there tomorrow doing my best." And instead of self-criticism, I go to sleep with a peaceful heart. I feel more responsible for my life and my actions, and yet I don't feel the weight of the world resting on my shoulders, or that the bogey man (or God) is out to get me. Self-acceptance makes self-forgiveness unnecessary. It's O.K. to be human. It's O.K. to make mistakes. In fact, if we didn't acknowledge mistakes, we'd just go on making them. When we take total responsibility for our actions we're free to leave the darkness of guilt and to move into the light. Guilt is negative and keeps us bound while taking responsibility is mature and liberating. For some of us, the advent of a life-inhibiting disease is the impetus to free ourselves from guilt and fear.

I realized that I had needed my guilt in order to stop me from living. Once I'd made a commitment to life, to living fully, the armies of guilt were on my doorstep. But I had to be willing to let go my guilt. I had to be willing to accept myself and my actions as they were. In accepting them, they no longer kept me prisoner. This is healing. To heal ourselves of our past judgments, criticisms, and self-hatred, we need to be willing to be made new and whole *now*. Healing is the relinquishing of guilt and fear. Health is the experience of peace and acceptance.

Guilt and fear, who were twins, had been my constant companions. To be willing to let them go and replace them with forgiveness and love was the healing of my life. Regardless of disease, these two represented all that was truly sick. I don't have to live a long life in order to be healed. Each moment presents the possibility of healing. It would be more of a tragedy to live to ninety-nine with guilt and fear as my companions than to die at a younger age with peace and acceptance in my heart.

Blame

It can be easy to blame others for the predicament in which we find ourselves. This exemplifies victim-consciousness and needs to be eradicated from our being if healing is to take place. It's easy to feel victimized and, at one time or another, we've all felt so demeaned. Blaming others is the antithesis of taking responsibility. Thoughts which we hold in our minds will dictate the reality we experience, and it becomes our choice as to what we wish to hold there.

People can use blame for many different reasons, but each and every one will come back to not wanting to own their responsibility. Society reinforces this attitude in many ways. We blame the weather. We blame circumstances. We blame other people. We blame society or the government. We go out of our way to avoid taking responsibility. When we accept responsibility it means we can decide to make changes in our lives. If we continue to blame outside circumstances, what we're really saying is, If only *you* or *it* would change, I'd be happier.

Change is often resisted because it's new and unfamiliar. I recently read these words:

Change is often desirable, frequently necessary, and always inevitable.

We adhere to old routines even if they make us sick. If it were not so, we'd all be eating nutritionally perfect food in just the right amounts, exercising regularly, thinking peaceful and harmonious thoughts, and stepping out into the world with boundless confidence and enthusiasm to meet all the challenges which come our way. A lifestyle of personal responsibility opens the way to greater health, peace, and vitality.

Many people who've developed cancer or AIDS blame someone or some situation for their disease. They're often angry with themselves also for having allowed the person or situations to have such an effect upon them.

A friend of mine taught me a lot about not blaming himself, the weather or any other circumstance. He was traveling to the skiing fields in his fairly new car. The roads were icy as he wound his way up into the mountains. He was traveling behind a tourist bus of skiers, also on their way to the snow-fields, when his tires began to slip upon the ice and he slid right into the back of the bus. His car wasn't able to be driven but the bus was virtually undamaged. Some of the tourists from the bus helped him to push his car off the road. He then climbed onto the bus with his ski gear and continued on the journey to the snow-fields. The tourists remarked that the incident hadn't seemed to have bothered him at all. His reply surprised them. "In five years time I'll look back on this incident and smile. Why waste time now by being upset?"

Bargaining

Many people approach the various healing modalities with the underlying attitude of, "If I'm good enough, if I meditate deeply enough and long enough, if I never miss a juice, if I take all these vitamins and herbs, if I exercise, if I pass the test by doing all these things, then maybe my reward will be that I get well." This bargaining attitude stems from fear. The same old fear of "Maybe I won't be good enough," the fear of a standard which I have to meet and yet fear I lack what it takes to measure up. It's not an easy thing to trust all is well when physically we're unwell. When we're willing to change, to embrace what is new and unexplored, life can become an adventure. To continue with the old criterion of "Do I have what it takes?" is to perpetuate a pattern all too familiar to some of us. Remember, a lot of us are high achievers and we could well fall into the trap of finding a diet or other program so rigorous that it could almost make failure a certainty. Don't misunderstand me. I'm not saying diet, even rigorous diets, are not beneficial. What I *am* saying is that the attitude *behind* the diet is of paramount importance; the attitude *behind* the practice of meditation is of paramount importance.

For example, you can drink carrot juice because you're afraid you might die if you don't, or you can drink it because you love life and you can *feel* it doing you good. The carrot juice is the same. It's the attitude that is different. Much is written on the attitude behind, and the application of, a healthy diet in chapter 7, Recipe for Life (see pages 152-180).

Many people come to me looking for the rosy path to healing. They want to be told all the things which they must *do* in order to heal themselves of their disease. Many do not want to hear about the thorns; the anguish, fears, angers, resentments, guilts and shames, the unresolved relationships which need to be addressed in order to truly heal their *lives*.

In healing our lives, all we ever wished to accomplish becomes real to us. We live, "healed" of our anguish, or we die, healed of our anguish. I've known many who died "healed" and this accomplishment is every bit as miraculous and wondrous as those who healed and continued to stay in their bodies. Sometimes I think we celebrate too much those of us who didn't die on time. We need to celebrate *life* and to honor all those who gave life their best shot. This is what is truly wonderful about the human spirit: to have the odds stacked against us and give it our darndest anyway!

We don't value a life by its length. It's not how long we live which is of importance. It's the spirit with which we live that will continue to nourish the hearts of those who knew us.

Healing Relationships

We often believe, mistakenly, that a painful relationship from the past is best forgotten. Yet more often than not it isn't forgotten: the painful memories are just buried deep inside ourselves. We could say we don't wish to be reminded of the pain it caused us. But the fact is it's *still* causing us pain and we're therefore *still* in a relationship with that person or situation. The person perhaps is no longer physically present in our lives, yet their influence is still there. Quite likely, at the time of being hurt, we made some "laws" about how we would henceforth live our lives, "laws" like:

- *Never trust men or Never trust women.*
- *Don't let anyone in too close or I'll be hurt.*
- *I'd better get my needs met first, otherwise I'll miss out.*
- *Never trust a stranger.*
- *All women want to change men.*
- *All men just want sex.*
- *Mediocrity is safe.*
- *If I'm not too ambitious then I can't fail.*
- *Life's hard.*
- *I'll never get it right.*

Take a look at which ones you've created for yourself. When there's someone in our life who's hurt us—even though that person might now be dead—we remain in a relationship with them. It's as if there were a rope stretched between that person and ourselves; we're still holding on hard to our end of the rope. When we let go of our end, it sets free a lot of energy previously trapped by the negativity of that relationship. We might need to let go that rope a hundred times before we're successful in totally forgiving, but we can then learn from the experience and move on. Many people have no desire to forgive those who've hurt them in the past. They almost savor their hurts as opportunities to feel righteous indignation. To let go of the resentment or bitterness also means to let go of the righteous indignation.

One man, Jeremy, had a long and difficult relationship with his mother. He used to become extremely agitated over her neglect of him. They battled constantly when he chose to see her. His mother represented all he hated in the world.

When he was diagnosed with cancer, he continued for some time in his lamentations about her. Finally he accepted that his life span could be seriously curtailed, and that his anger exhausted and depressed him. He decided that if he were to die within a few months, as his doctor said he would, he didn't want to maintain his rage against his mother because it was destroying the quality of his life. This was the impetus for his healing his relationship with her, and since then he's learned to keep his sense of humor and perspective when in her presence. He learned to accept that she couldn't give love to him in the way he'd always demanded, and that he needed to accept her and the love she gave on her terms. Physically he has gone into remission.

By forgiving the past, we can cultivate compassion for others, the compassion which we'd like to have extended to ourselves. We all make mistakes. Recognize them as opportunities to learn something new. They're there for our education, not to carry around with us for an eternity. Acknowledge the resentment, forgive the person or situation, accept it, and move on. In this way, you will continue to grow. Long-held resentments and bitterness cause stagnation and disease.

Forgiveness

To forgive is to let go the past, to respond wholeheartedly to the present without the pain or clutter of what went before. Sometimes forgiveness is easy and sometimes exceedingly difficult!

I was at a conference on burnout among AIDS workers in San Francisco in 1988. One of the participants gave this as her definition of forgiveness:

Forgiveness is giving up all hope for a better past.

To forgive is to let go of the past.

John had a long and bitter relationship with his father, Eric. The relationship had gone sour over business dealings many years before. Eric had never forgiven John and, at one time, wrote an angry, bitter letter to him, disowning him as his son. Even though John knew that Eric was receiving help from a psychiatrist for some emotional problems, he was deeply hurt and shocked by the poison expressed in that letter. He couldn't easily put it out of his mind and he resolved never to be alone with his father again. Because he was fearful of the effect his father had on him, he moved interstate to avoid any confrontation.

Sometime after John was diagnosed with AIDS, he became aware of how much pain and unresolved grief was bound up in his relationship with his father. He was afraid to forgive his father because he felt it might make him vulnerable to emotional injury once more. He was angry with his father for having made his life so miserable, and at himself for being susceptible to his criticism. Since his illness there had been no word from his father.

Christmas was drawing close and John was reflecting on the number of Christmases he might have left. In his words: "I suddenly felt weary of the pain and grief I'd been carrying so long. I didn't want to take the sadness of this relationship to my grave. For the first time I felt a kind of pity and compassion for my father and realized how much I desired his love and acceptance. Perhaps that was all he required from me. I decided then and there to release the past, to accept it as it was, and to extend to my father what I so much wanted from him. For Christmas I had delivered to him a large basket of fruit with a simple note that conveyed my love to him. The release I felt and the weight it lifted from my shoulders was enormous. My Christmas was complete when he telephoned saying it was the finest present he could ever wish to receive."

John experienced a tremendous sense of peace and serenity from letting go the past. He'd completed his relationship with his father and had given both of them the possibility of a more amicable future. To forgive someone is very different from condoning the behavior.

We sacrifice the possibility of peace today while ever we carry the trauma of the past into each present moment. Allow yourself the opportunity to let go the pain of unforgivingness. It's *you* who suffers while you hold on to the pain.

Technique for Forgiveness

Many people have found the following technique valuable:

Sit quietly and take some long, slow, deep breaths, breathing in peace and relaxation, breathing out all tension and anxiety. Let your breathing return to its own natural rhythm. Allow the image of someone you love to come into your mind's eye. Feel the love and warmth you experience when visualizing that person and allow it to flow out from yourself to the person. Enjoy the experience, noting how easily the love flows to that person. Then let the image of the person fade gently away.

Now allow the image of a person to whom you feel quite indifferent come before your eyes. Perhaps it is someone like the girl in the local paper shop, the gas station attendant, or someone with whom you aren't closely associated. Visualize the person strongly, and again allow your love and compassion to flow out to that person. It might be quite a strange experience for you, but persevere. Just allow warmth and kindliness to flow out from your heart to that person. Then in your own time, allow the image to fade and replace it with the image of the person who has hurt you in the past. Again, see the face clearly before you. Notice what is happening in your body, and let the tension soften. Visualize that person, and allow whatever love and forgiveness you are able to muster to flow out from your heart to that person. If you find it difficult, that is all right. Allow whatever understanding and compassion you have for that person to flow out from yourself. You've been angered or hurt for so long, just let those feelings soften and melt into light and ease. Let go the pain of unforgivingness. Your natural state is love. Even though it might be very difficult for you to feel any truth in the following words, say them anyway:

"I forgive you for all the things I thought you did, in word or thought or action. Please forgive me also."

If it's easier to start with people or situations which are less threatening for you, then do so. The important thing is to keep practicing. The day will dawn when you'll feel only light and love flowing out to that person, providing that's what you desire. You can see, by your resistance to forgiving a person, how much energy is bound up in that relationship. This energy, when it's set free through forgiveness, is truly amazing. Now liberated, it can be used for your greater healing. We have to be ready and willing in order to be able to forgive. Be gentle and don't push yourself. Forgive yourself for being human! Open your heart to your own closed-heartedness!

Forgiving the person is *not* the same as condoning the behavior or action. The behavior might be totally unacceptable, but that doesn't make the person unacceptable. Perhaps it's easier to understand if we think about a young child who's learning about appropriate behavior. A child might do something which is very cruel and it's right that we should express our anger at that behavior. To disapprove of the behavior while maintaining love for the child is quite possible. We seem to forget this as people grow older, believing that they should know how to behave. If we believe *they* should know how to behave, we're affirming that *we* should know also! This kind of thinking may well lay the foundations for further personal guilt and judgment.

To forgive ourselves is perhaps the greatest challenge of all. It's extraordinary to me to see how incredibly harsh and unforgiving I used to be when I made a mistake. If anybody else did the same thing I wouldn't hesitate to tell them that it was O.K. to make mistakes. Just pick yourself up, apologize if necessary, learn from the experience, and move on. Is that what I would tell *myself* when I made a mistake? No way. Self-flagellation was my automatic reaction! I'm gradually learning to extend the same compassion to myself as I do to others.

If I constantly drag the past into the present, then I'm always living out my past. And in so doing I ensure my future is a replica of my past. To forgive myself means to let the past be buried. In this way I can learn from experiences and then approach each moment as being fresh and new. To constantly judge myself for my "wicked past" is to sacrifice the present and future to the fears of yesterday.

Dreams and Their Interpretation

Our subconscious mind is what supplies our dreams with their images. In our dreams many unresolved problems are played out, so it can be very beneficial to work with someone who's familiar with interpreting dreams. If you choose to do this, it's necessary to describe in detail the substance of the dream. Even if you're working only on your own with your dreams, the process of writing them down can be very helpful.

Many people say they have no recollection of their dreams. We can train ourselves to remember them. If you go to bed with pen and paper close by and a firm commitment to remember your dreams, you'll find they begin to become clearer. You might find it easier to scribble things down in the dark rather than to put on the lights and then try to remember. Bernie Siegel, an American cancer surgeon, has written much in his book, *Love, Peace and Healing* (see Recommended Reading), about the role dreams can play in diagnosis and treatment of disease. Many people have received major clues to their lives through their dreams and their interpretation.

Keeping a Journal

Keeping a journal can be a wonderful way of getting in touch with your deeper thoughts and feelings. This would be not so much a journal of events and happenings in your life, but a record of how each day unfolded for you at a "feeling" level. It's also a valuable way of uncovering feelings about things rather than thoughts about things. Reactions to conversations, people, and situations can be noted. The journal is invaluable as a tool for discovery about yourself. Even long after you're well, you'll continue to learn much about yourself from its pages. To share your journal with a trusted loved one, friend, or therapist can also be beneficial, and can provide a base for further discussion. It's important to find a means of expression for the thoughts and feelings usually kept within. Once they're expressed in words, dance, drawings, and so on, the issues begin to be resolved.

Drawings

Much has been written in recent years about the value of drawings as a means to access the subconscious mind. I've used drawings extensively with adults and children with life-threatening diseases and they've provided valuable shortcuts to understanding the innermost feelings of the person. What we acknowledge and express through our conscious mind can be completely different from what we truly feel in our innermost being. It's impossible not to give away what's happening in the subconscious when we draw. This applies even if we wish to cover up what's there. One of the values of drawings is that something is put out there for us to discuss. Unless we gain access to those hidden feelings which empower our actions, choices, and decisions, we continue along in our habitual way.

I often ask people to draw pictures of themselves, their disease, their immune system, their treatment, their family and any other drawing of their choice. Sometimes I ask them to draw themselves and their family when they were children of five, or to draw any other relationship which may be fruitful for exploration. Many people complain that they can't draw. This in no way inhibits the process. It can even enhance it, because what we *do* put down on paper will not be contrived. The only "rules" for drawings used in this way are:

- *White paper*
- *Crayons or colored pencils—no felt tips*
- *A wide range of colors to choose from*
- *No stick figures*

Sometimes we'll have a drawing morning in one of our

support groups when each of us works on another person's draw-ings. These mornings are enormously insightful and enjoyable. Many realizations have been made and unexpected messages conveyed by the drawings. Often people will show clearly what's stopping them from healing themselves. This creates an opportu-nity for choice and decision.

One doesn't need to be a trained therapist in order to bring insight to a drawing. Having an interested person to ask ques-tions about the drawing will bring out much that is there. The very act of drawing is creative and valuable in itself. It gives the person the opportunity to bring to light something from within, which is therapeutic in itself. To have feelings and thoughts churning around in our mind isn't helpful. Drawing provides a way for these thoughts and feelings to be expressed, aired, un-derstood, and released.

Colors

Colors are a valuable indicator of how people perceive their situation. This applies not only to colors used in their drawings, but also the colors in which they dress, or which they use to decorate their homes. To change deliberately the colors around us to uplifting and cheerful ones can have a marked effect on how we feel. If you're someone who habitually wears subdued or somber colors, try wearing some harmonious but brighter colors, just for a change.

Marion had always worn black. She looked elegant and so-phisticated but her entire wardrobe was composed of just this single color. She was a very striking and beautiful woman who could wear black with grace and style. She had twenty-three pairs of black shoes. For casual wear, she had black boots and black runners. She relied on gold and silver to highlight and contrast the black, but would wear absolutely no color.

Her job was a senior one in the corporate world and in-volved a lot of business meetings and travel. She believed she enjoyed it. She worked incredibly long hours, had few friends, had never married, and lived in a high-rise apartment which was decorated in black and silver.

Marion developed cancer of the breast at the age of thirty-
eight. She took a week's vacation from her job, had a
mastectomy, and returned to work. After her surgery, she used
to drive to the hospital to have her radiotherapy on her way to
work. Friday afternoons, she entered the hospital, had chemotherapy on Saturday, felt sick on Sunday, and was back at work
late Monday morning.

When I saw her the first time, very early in the morning, she
constantly consulted her watch so that she would be out on time for
her first meeting of the day. No one in her life knew she had cancer:
not her mother, not her employer, not her secretary, no one.

It took time for Marion to "make time" to have cancer. It
took even longer for her to begin to question her lifestyle, her
philosophy, her goals. In time, she *had* to slow down as her
treatments and schedule began to take their toll. She had lived
her life by "centrifugal force." If she kept everything spinning
fast enough she wouldn't notice that she wasn't happy.

One Saturday while waiting for her chemotherapy to begin,
she sat out on the hospital balcony in the early springtime sunshine. The balcony was drab, the hospital uninspiring as far as
beauty was concerned. On the balcony stood a cracked terra-
cotta pot with a withered and miserable geranium which
struggled for life. It grew in a place where attention to its needs
was half-hearted and haphazard. Its leaves were withered, some
of its roots exposed, the soil in which it grew lacked vitality and
nourishment. It seemed to cry out for care with little expectation
of receiving it. She reflected on how similar their lives were.

During that day and the next the thought of the plant struggling for life often came to her mind. It even entered her dreams
as she dozed.

On Sunday, when she was ready to be discharged, she turned
back to the nurse and, feeling a bit silly, asked if she could take
home the plant on the balcony. The staff gladly acquiesced.

Even though she still felt unwell, Marion stopped off on the
way home at a local nursery to buy a new ceramic (black!) pot,
fresh soil, and fertilizer. She repotted, watered, and fertilized

the plant as soon as she arrived home.

Strange as it might seem, this was the turning point for Marion. She began to take care of another withered being and in so doing gave permission to do the same for herself. The plant thrived in her care. She too began to blossom. As Marion changed, she softened, she smiled more. It was difficult for her to let go the lifestyle with which she was so familiar: the rush, the "buzz" of business, the aloofness and detachment. Gradually she began to make space in her life for other things. Books, music, and crafts came into her life. At first it was a book about geraniums. She was fascinated by what color bloom *her* geranium might produce. She telephoned me like an excited child the day it burst into red flowers.

As she changed, so did her home. She bought other plants to keep her geranium company. Her life began to include more color, more textures, more depth and feeling. She even went to the pound and chose a stray cat. It wasn't a beautiful cat but it was warm and affectionate. It had half an ear missing and was a mixture of colors and heritage. She named her Patches. She wasn't allowed to keep a cat in her apartment but she took it home anyway.

In her years of working, Marion had accumulated several houses among her assets. One of them was a cottage by the sea which she'd rarely visited. This cottage became her hobby. She redecorated it during weekends once her chemotherapy had ceased. She painted it white with blue trim and put geranium flower boxes at the sills. The garden became her creative outlet and she began to experience a sense of serenity and connection to life. In time, her values and priorities changed as she found a peace and serenity within herself. She also experienced a sense of community among those in the seaside village near her cottage. Within a year, this house became her home.

Music

Like color, music can lift the spirit and brighten our day. Choose music *you* find enjoyable. If music represents a fairly new adventure for you, then take note of what you enjoy on the radio and perhaps purchase copies for your personal collection. Don't be shy about going into a whole new area of music.

If your only musical world has been popular music up until now, consider investigating your likes and dislikes in classical music. Likewise for those steeped in classics, investigate jazz or popular music. As with all things, there's no one right way or, in this case, no right music. You enjoy what you enjoy. Be liberal in your investigations. You could surprise yourself by what you *do* enjoy. Just as there's no right music, so there's no right way of listening to it. I've enjoyed popular music with a very strong beat through headphones as I worked out on a rebounder (a mini trampoline), and I've experienced classical music while in a deep state of meditation. During my recovery I spent some time living in a very large geodesic dome in the foothills of the Sierra Nevada mountains in California. A large part of the dome had been replaced by glass and the outlook was straight out over mountains with not a house, light, or road in sight. In the evenings it was possible to lie on the floor of the sitting room and stare straight up into the heavens with the myriad stars twinkling in the clear night sky. I would put on a selection of music, turn out the lights, stretch out on the floor, allow myself to melt into the carpet, give myself over to the music's influence, and surrender totally. In this way I didn't experience the music through my intellect. It felt as if my body also became an instrument, and the music was played through me. Just letting the notes play through me, rather than making sense of them with my mind, was a powerful experience. It felt rather as though my consciousness had become a vast ocean in which these vibrations rose and fell, ebbed and flowed like waves. So allow the limits of your musical enjoyment to stretch. Be open to new forms of music and new ways of listening.

Pets

Some people have deeper relationships with their pets than they do with people! Most of us have had times when it's easier to communicate with the cat or dog than it is with our teenagers (or partner). One of the loveliest things about the companionship of cats or dogs is that they accept us just the way we are. Even when we're so confused and bewildered that we don't know what to think, ol' Fido or Puss will be there to nuzzle, cuddle, or sit on us to reassure us of their love. Pets can be great company when we're feeling out of sorts and they can help us to relax and calm ourselves. It's difficult to stay frazzled for long if you sit down and stroke the cat.

One of my cats was a psychotherapist in disguise. If I had a very agitated or angry client with me, she would often scratch at the door to be let *in*! Most cats don't like being around angry people, but she was the exception. What's more, she would jump onto the client's lap and settle herself there. The client would often begin stroking her unconsciously and, sure enough, within a few minutes, between the cat and the client they sorted out the problem. I saw it so many times that I stopped being surprised. For others, birds are of particular importance. Apart from making wonderful pets, they are a source of joy and peace in the garden.

One woman, June, who was having chemotherapy for her cancer, said she always felt better the moment she got to her weekend home. In the garden she would feed the brightly colored parrots and other birds. She said it made her feel whole and at peace and connected with all life.

If animals, pets, or nature are important to you, then remember to have contact with them. So often we let slip by the little things that bring us so much contentment. Life is really made up of many moments. It's often the simple things which enrich our lives and make those moments magic.

There's every reason to have your pets around you when you're unwell. The animals will probably love it as you'll be *their* captive, providing pats, strokes, and conversation whenever *they* desire. Cats and dogs particularly seem to know when you're feeling unwell and will often deliberately "gentle" themselves to your level of activity.

They can also be a wonderful distraction when you're in pain. A warm furry friend can soothe and comfort without words or side effects!

Communication

Communication is the lifeblood of any relationship. Much of what's discussed in this chapter is about communication. Sometimes that communication is with ourselves—for instance, when we recognize and acknowledge our own needs and feelings. Sometimes it's in acknowledging our feelings and needs to those we love. The intricacies of communication between family members is often very complex. As much is conveyed through body language, lack of affirmative action, intonation, emphasis as with anything which is actually put into words.

Communication within most families reflects how each of the individuals interact in the world, outside of the family situation. I always enjoy visiting people in their own homes in order to learn how they interact with each other. Sometimes what is said flippantly can indicate a great knowledge of the personality beneath the exterior. One teenage friend of mine, Beth, conveyed much information about her father and her relationship with him, when she good-humoredly said, "I wanted to get out of there before what was written on his face came out of his mouth."

For some, communication flows effortlessly. For others, it's a difficult and painful process. Those for whom communication is difficult have often come from families where emotions weren't aired or were inappropriately expressed. If this is your background, be gentle and compassionate with yourself. Don't put yourself down because you feel unskilled in the use of words. Practice with a loved one. You might need to exert yourself if talking about your feelings is unfamiliar to you. Turn it into an adventure by taking small risks; then celebrate your accomplishment!

It's very common for people to want to keep a stiff upper lip when they're first diagnosed with a life-inhibiting disease. These people often feel that so long as they're keeping their feelings under control they'll be able to cope. Sometimes shared tears are more healing than all the medicine in the world. They give us the opportunity to experience a deeper and more profound intimacy, in which we can communicate our distress and fears. To communicate at such a level is the first step towards healing. I believe that "health" is the experience of peace, and that "healing" is the relinquishing of fear. There are many eighty-year-olds who experience every day with fear and trepidation and who grasp at life with each breath. Yet I've known young children who've achieved all that we honor and consider heroic in the human spirit and who, having truly lived, were able to pass lightly from life into the mystery of death.

Communication, of course, isn't always verbal. Words are constructions of the mind. More often, it's the subtle inflection, emphasis, posture, or gesture which touches or repels us. On occasions, silence conveys more than volumes of clever speech. When we're faced with the pain of another and feel helpless to effect any change, another language becomes appropriate. The language of touch, a meeting of the eyes, a smile or hug can speak more eloquently than words. In such circumstances, if you listen to the language of your heart, it will guide your actions and words, so that they convey love, understanding, and compassion.

The gentle touch of a loving hand conveys much to those who are too weary or ill to speak. Hands of love can convey all we've ever learned of compassion, trust, peace, and acceptance. Let your hands become a channel that conveys your wisdom, serenity, and faith. Your touch can be far more eloquent than mere words.

Communication with Doctors

Some doctors are great communicators, some aren't so fantastic, and others are abysmal. Remember, they're human just like us and come from families where communication may have been excellent, haphazard, or nonexistent. Skills in communication aren't formally taught in their medical course and oncologists/ immunologists often have a very sad and difficult job to perform. We *can* improve our communication with our doctor if we're willing to do so.

I encourage all people to write a short note to their doctor. Express your appreciation for your doctor and what he or she does for you. Acknowledge the difficulties and pain he or she must experience in his or her work and be appreciative of his or her encouragement and support of you and your efforts. Thank your doctor for answering your questions and helping you to understand the treatments.

I can hear many of you saying that *your* doctor doesn't do *any* of those things. If you write to your doctor and encourage him or her to be the doctor you'd like him or her to be, you could well find he or she will be more amenable to questions on your next visit. Imagine the impact it would have if thousands of people wrote to their doctors to acknowledge their difficulties and to encourage them in their efforts! We all grow through encouragement more readily than through criticism. If your doctor continues to be unsupportive, then consider seeking another. After all, your doctor is in *your* employ. You're not only *his* or *her* patient, he or she is *your* doctor. Your doctor is being well paid for a service, so make sure you receive what you're paying for. If you feel you've been treated very poorly or insensitively, again, write a letter expressing your concern (or anger). Unfortunately it often falls to the patients to educate their doctors in the art of supportive communication. One of my jobs now involves occasionally lecturing medical students on communication with and support for patients with life-threatening illnesses.

A participant in one of our groups, Jeanette, has a very supportive oncologist. When, after ten years, she was found to have secondary spread from a melanoma she became very depressed and felt her self-esteem plummet (a common reaction after a diagnosis of a secondary cancer). After several weeks of tears and depression, her oncologist actually *telephoned* her and said she was practicing dying and that she must start practicing living instead. He gave her the telephone number of a doctor who worked with nutritional medicine and vitamins and the number of the Quest for Life Center. She wholeheartedly adopted the dietary and vi-

tamin program and, after one session of counseling, became a
keen member of our weekly support group. Sometimes we need a
kick start and who better to receive it from than our doctor.
She's now living every day with confidence and enthusiasm and
is supporting others in their endeavors to live with their life-
threatening illnesses. Because of her oncologist's support she
feels she has the best doctor in the world to help her to *live*.

When I was a teenager, I had considerable reconstructive surgery to my legs. It required cutting through the bones above and
below my knees and rotating the legs in an attempt to straighten
them, then plating and pinning the bones in place. Over the
years I've had continuing problems with them, ranging from arthritis to torn cartilages and so on. The joint in my right knee is
close to being worn out and in the coming years I'll probably
need a knee replacement.

Recently I consulted an orthopedic surgeon to see how I
might extend the period between now and when such a replacement might be necessary. His registrar took down my long and
complicated history of surgery, examined the X-rays and my
legs, and declared I was certainly a candidate for a knee replacement, now or in the next few years. He then asked if there was
anything else he should know about my medical history. I told
him I had leukemia in 1983. He put down his pen, raised his
eyes to the heavens and said, "Well, that changes everything!"
He went on to ask what the prognosis was. I told him the doctor
had said I'd only live three months from diagnosis, but that now
I was in remission I expected to stay that way for another fifty
or sixty years. His reply startled me. He said I'd have to have a
bone marrow biopsy before they could consider a knee replacement! Somewhat bewildered, I said, "I beg your pardon?"

He repeated what he'd said, adding that there was no point
in giving me a new knee if I was only to get a couple of years
wear out of it!

I'm a poor communicator in such circumstances of shock and
dismay and was astonished at his lack of tact. When he repeated
to the orthopedic specialist as well as two or three trainees my
knee history, he concluded by saying, "She's certainly a candi-

date for a knee replacement; however, she does *have* leukemia, so
we'll need a bone marrow biopsy to establish a prognosis before
we decide the viability of surgery." I was half-naked and lying
down on an examination table during all this. (Why is it that we
seem to be trapped in the most vulnerable positions at times like
these?) However, my basic communication skills had surfaced to
some extent and I was able to interrupt and say, "Excuse me, I've
had two bone marrow biopsies. They're painful and uncomfortable and the prognosis has been wrong both times, and I'm not
having another one. If I need a new knee, then I'll jolly well [not
a literal translation] *have* a new knee!"

They were all slightly stunned. Frankly, so was I! The specialist looked at me, and I looked at him (so did his trainees),
and then a sparkle came into his eye as he perceived that I was a
human being in need of his help, rather than a leukemic with a
bung knee. He then readily agreed to surgery.

If I'd been the kind of person to be thrown by the comments
of doctors, I could easily have been deeply upset by the
registrar's comments.

On another occasion a year or so ago, I was just surfacing
through the mists of anesthesia after an arthroscopic procedure
to this same knee when the surgeon said, "I'm sorry, the prognosis is very poor!" *He* wasn't to know that I was immediately cata-
pulted back into another doctor's office where he was talking
about my life expectancy rather than just a knee.

Many people find they feel intimidated by the surroundings
of their doctor's office and that they forget everything he or she
said the minute they walk out the door.

If at all possible, take a friend with you when seeing your
doctor so you're better able to comprehend and absorb what *has*
been said. Feel free to ask questions. If you feel your questions
aren't being answered to your satisfaction, then you can say
something like, "Excuse me, Doctor, would you mind repeating
what you just said in a simpler way? It's really important for me
to understand my position so I have clear choices and can then
make good decisions." Many people write out their questions be-
forehand and then work steadily through their list. You could

say, "I'm not much good at remembering all the things you tell me, so do you mind if I write down the answers to these questions?" Many people find that to record their consultation with their doctor on a cassette player is tremendously helpful. This gives you a record of the explanations and can serve as an invaluable reference to jog your memory when you're at home. Most doctors will be more than happy to cooperate. We need to be mindful that specialist doctors are in very heavy demand and often have a waiting room full of people to see. However, it's important you create a rapport with your doctor so you feel you have every confidence and trust in his or her ability to help you.

If you'd like a second opinion about your physical health or the treatment suggested for you, it can easily be arranged. Ask your doctor or his secretary for all your reports, results, X-rays and so on, and make an appointment with the doctor of your choice. You might need a referral from your general practitioner, and you might need to be quite definite in your request. Occasionally a doctor will be unhappy about your request, but this is your life and you're entitled to the care you choose for yourself.

A Word to the Medical Profession

It's a difficult job to balance diagnostic and treatment skills with continuous compassionate care of patients. Evaluating and dealing with people's needs on physical, psychological, emotional, and spiritual levels is asking a great deal from anyone. However, many patients will expect *all* those needs to be met by you.

The following list of requests from patients has been compiled in order to let you know their needs.

Please:

- *Look me in the eye. Make eye contact with me and my family (if present).*

- *Talk to me honestly and directly, remembering that I have limited medical knowledge but a great desire to understand. After all, this is my life we're discussing.*

- *Speak slowly, making sure I understand what you're saying. A diagram*

often speaks more clearly to me than words, and I can take it home to
share with my family.

- Give me options rather than dictating to me what must happen. You
  might not be aware of factors other than my health.

- Encourage me in my efforts to help myself. Tell me that whatever positive
  steps I take will make a difference.

- Answer my questions even though they might seem silly, repetitive, or
  inconsequential to you.

- Offer me hope and encouragement even when things seem bleak. Affirm
  any small improvement and assure me of your continued support in
  maintaining my quality of life.

- Be patient with me. I've never been in this situation before. I could be
  feeling bewildered, angry, frustrated, or frightened.

- Understand that I don't expect you to have all the answers. Maybe I'm
  medically unfixable but I'd still like your support in living as well as
  possible. After all, I might be expecting a miracle—they do happen; so
  don't destroy my faith.

- Choose your words carefully. I have on my supersensitive ears and am
  listening intently to your intonation, inflection, and emphasis.

- Remember, I have a life outside of my illness. I'm also a mother, son,
  breadwinner, lover, etc. Treat me as a person with a problem rather than
  a leukemic, AIDS, or cancer victim.

- Don't tell me how long you think I've got to live. Remember, I believe I
  can make a difference.

Chapter Three

SHOULD I OR SHOULDN'T I?

Bob

I had always taken my health for granted until 1986 when I suddenly developed acute sciatica. I went from being a very active person who did lots of physical activity to a virtual cripple barely able to get out of bed. I had not needed to see a doctor for more than ten years.

My wife, Deidre, wanted me to visit our local physician but I was reluctant as I thought it would probably improve within a few days. However, my back and leg became more and more painful and it reached the stage where I could no longer do more than get to the bathroom and return to bed. A couple of small lumps had appeared in my groin and finally Deidre insisted that a doctor visit us at home.

Initially, the doctor diagnosed sciatica and gave me some painkillers. The painkillers certainly helped, but only for a short while, and the pain would return once more. I had an x-ray which proved normal and then an ultrasound which showed a 'mass' low down in the pelvis. By this time a couple of weeks had passed and I was enormously worn down by pain and increasing fear about whatever was wrong with my body.

After a biopsy of the lymph nodes in my groin and a CT scan, I was finally told by the surgeon I had been referred to that there was little that could be done except to 'make me comfortable.' He told me that I had very advanced melanoma which had already spread to my lungs. It was an unpigmented melanoma so there wasn't a change in a mole on the surface of my skin. The surgeon said it could have started anywhere inside my body. He quoted statistics about longevity, offered me chemotherapy if I felt I wanted it, and made arrangements to see me again in three months. He removed the glands in my groin and told me to enjoy the rest of my life.

Deidre and I cried on and off for days. Friends inundated us with books, tapes, and stories about people who hadn't died when the doctors said they would. We felt enormously bruised and battered by the diagnosis and the blunt approach of the surgeon. I vowed I would never return to him.

Petrea's name was mentioned by many of the people who wanted to help us as someone who could give us a positive direction in which to proceed. Our visit to her home gave us the first glimmer of hope. She didn't talk about curing melanoma, but she gave us a belief in ourselves and in our ability to handle the situation we were in, in a positive manner. We came away from that first appointment with a sense of being better equipped to deal with the many decisions which seemed to surround us.

Petrea had suggested we see a particular oncologist who spends time with his patients and encourages questions and discussion. Petrea also said he had a strong belief that patients could make a difference to the outcome of the disease by their positive attitude and the practice of meditation. Even though he wasn't a specialist in melanoma we decided to make an appointment.

'Dr. David' was a marvelous man who listened patiently to our story and answered the many questions we had. He actively encouraged us to continue with the advice Petrea had given us and told us he believed meditation and attitude played an important part both in the quality and quantity of a person's life.

Gradually, the nightmare of melanoma became an adventure in healing. We found how important it is to research as much as possible before making any decision. I found that I need to honor my own power to choose and I learned to respect the wisdom within myself. Deidre and I became closer than ever and our efforts have brought many gifts not only to ourselves but to our friends and loved-ones. Our priorities have changed and we have a much more relaxed life style.

Now, seven years after my diagnosis, I feel really good about my life and have learned so much about myself. I have had to have several lymph nodes removed from my neck but, so far, I haven't needed any chemotherapy. The tumors in my lungs have gone and my quality of life is good. I know that I might die as a result of melanoma but I cannot see that happening for a long time.

After much thought and discussion with Deidre, I did return to the surgeon I had first seen as he's an expert in his field. However, I employ him for his expertise and not for any psychological or emotional support. He's reluctant to give any hope and thinks I should be grateful for the time I've had so far. I still visit 'Dr. David' and Petrea after each visit to the surgeon as I find they always 'pick us up' and give us hope for the future. Deidre and I feel we have a good healing team: our meditation, the support groups, the diet, supplements and juices, our faith, and the people who love and encourage us in our efforts to be fully alive.

When you have a life-threatening illness, so many decisions need to be made right from the beginning. Some decisions leap out at you and you know then and there that you don't need to make a choice. But there are many other decisions which aren't so clearly delineated and they can be much more difficult to deal with.

The Decision-Making Process

The choices about your illness begin from the moment you know something's wrong in your body. Many women have felt a lump in their breast and decided "to keep an eye on it" instead of taking themselves to their doctor to have it investigated. Likewise, some men have known they felt "out of sorts" or have found a swelling which they've chosen to ignore and have been reluctant to go to their doctor. The problem with this approach is that it niggles away in the back of the mind and undermines our ability to live life fully *now*. If the lump, swelling, or feeling out of sorts is due to something other than an illness, then there might be some other appropriate treatment which can be undertaken so we can get on with our lives. If the diagnosis is cancer, infection with HIV, AIDS, or some other serious illness, then we're confronted with a whole range of new choices.

As was mentioned in the introduction, it usually takes six to eight weeks for the initial shock of the diagnosis to wear off. Some people experience this time with a numbed awareness, some seemingly take it in stride, some go into a blind panic, some become depressed and despairing, others become angry. The problem is that you probably have to confront choices and make decisions during this time when you don't feel your usual self. Well-meaning friends and relatives can sometimes increase our confusion. Suddenly our home is transformed into a library of books and tapes on healing our particular disease. Everyone seems to know someone whom we *must* talk to or see. Your positive-minded friends probably know someone who had your disease and recovered while your negative friends (if you haven't already got rid of them) and/or your relatives (who are sometimes more difficult to get rid of) knew someone with your disease who didn't recover. The more we read, the more bewildered we can become. Our greatest enemy is confusion. It undermines all our good intentions and makes us feel powerless. But sooner or later, you come to the realization that *you're* the one with the disease and *you're* the best person to decide what's right for you. No one else has your *particular* disease; no one knows just how it feels to be you, right now.

You might need to make decisions about who is the right doctor for you. Do you require a second opinion? Remember, it's your right to have a second (or third, fourth, or fifth) opinion if that's your wish. It's your body; it's your choice. Different hospitals sometimes have different approaches to the same disease and one approach could suit you and your lifestyle better than another.

Is the doctor you've chosen likely to be a person in whom you have confidence, and with whom you feel comfortable? One of the major factors in the process of healing is the relationship with our physician. We need a good working relationship with

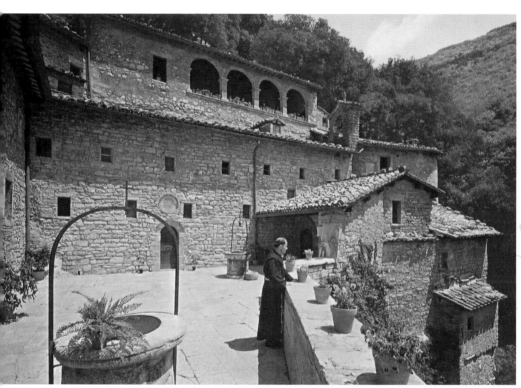

he Hermitage outside of Assisi. It was in this monastery that I sought spiritual guidance rough long hours of meditation.

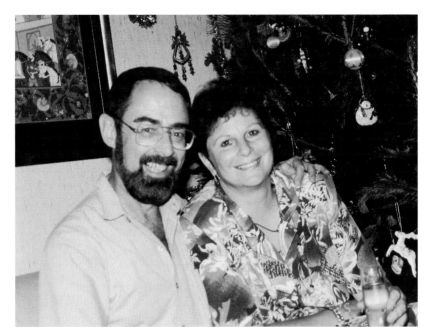

Peter and myself at our orphans, waifs and strays party held in my home each Christmas.

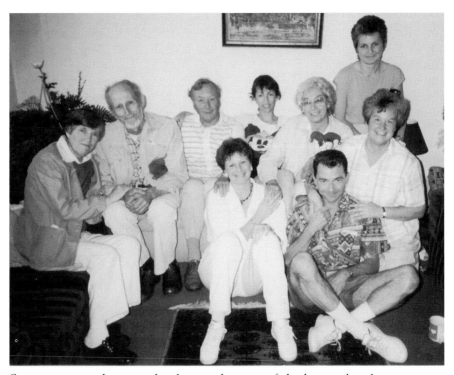

Support group photograph taken so that one of the hospitalized participants could keep us 'next to him.'

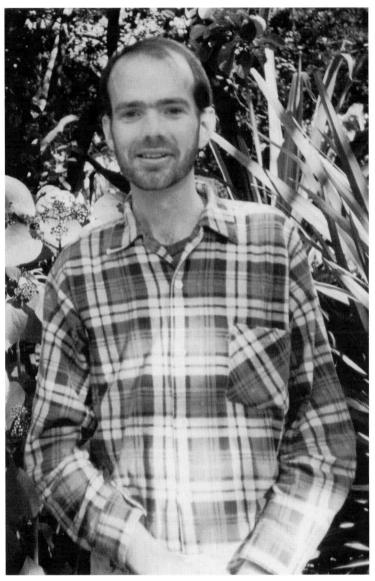

George mentioned on page 338.

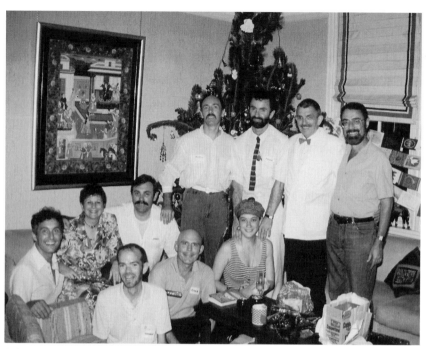

The orphans, waifs and strays Christmas party at my home.

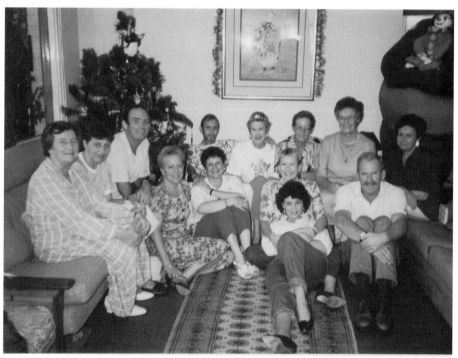

Friends for life. Our Monday support group.

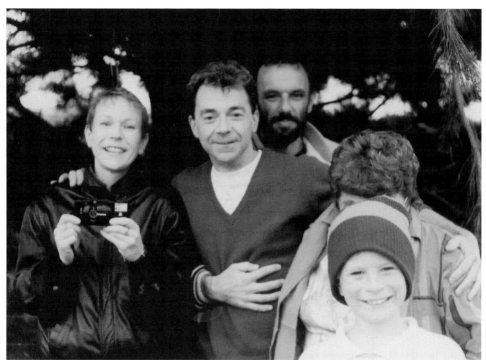

Members of our winter workshop for people with life-threatening illnesses.

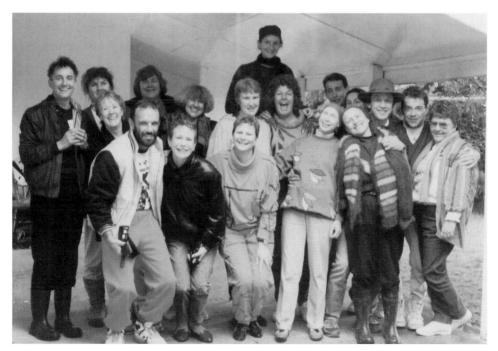

Participants at a residential workshop in the country.

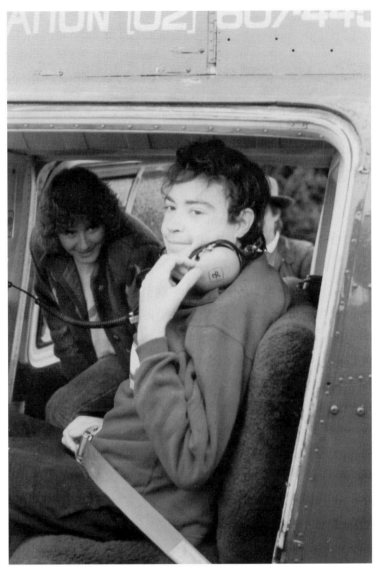

Craig, arriving by helicopter for a residential workshop in the country. (pages 82-84)

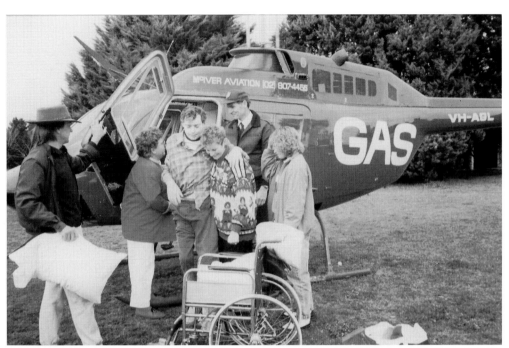

Craig being lifted very gently into a wheelchair.

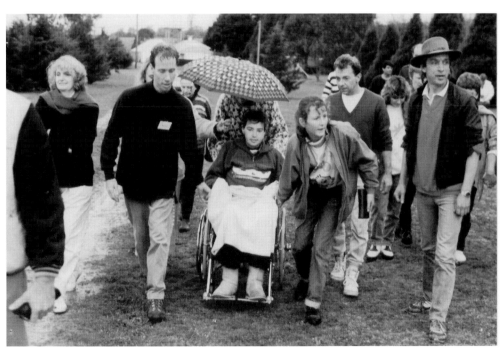

Craig's wheelchair being carried to the seminar room by other participants.

Lois and Roger sharing a hug after a support group.

our doctor in which we feel free to communicate and ask questions. We, as patients, aren't looking for statistics. We're looking for positive healing through the establishment of hope and a loving supportive environment combined with expert medical treatment. Unexpected healings take place frequently. These are called spontaneous remissions by the medical profession. If we call a disease terminal we eliminate the possibility of the exceptional. There's no harm in changing your doctor if you don't feel comfortable with the one you have.

One morning I saw three clients who all happened to be the patients of one particular professor of oncology. To the first one he'd said, "Oh, you're just another whining cancer patient!" To the second one, "When are you going to give up hope—there isn't any!" To the third, "We can't have patients making decisions about their own lives!" This man has a high reputation as an oncologist, but I would add it is a high and mighty one as well! We need doctors, immunologists, and oncologists who believe each person is an individual with a life beyond his or her disease. Choose a doctor who will help you to live up to your full potential with your own brand of courage and spirit. More and more doctors are understanding the need for this, so make it your priority to find one. If it's not possible for you to find a doctor who meets these requirements, then decide you'll employ him or her for his or her expertise and seek your emotional support elsewhere.

You might wish to explore other therapies which will complement your medical treatment. Where do you begin? Which diet will you adopt? Which meditation technique? So many questions. Often there's an underlying feeling of urgency which compounds our bewilderment.

If peace of mind is your one goal, then your choices and decisions will be in accordance with that.

The formula set out in this chapter will help you in making your decisions while keeping that goal of peace in mind.

Peace is not a passive, don't care, sickly sweet kind of attitude. It is a dynamic state of being. It is FULL of possibilities and free of the encumbrance of fear.

By using the formula for decision making, we can take back full responsibility for the treatments and therapies which *we* decide to utilize. We employ the expertise of our oncologist, immunologist, naturopath, meditation teacher, nutritionist, or whatever, rather than blindly following advice. In this way, we can orchestrate our healing team.

New choices will present themselves along the way. New books, new therapies, new ideas from other patients. Learn to listen with your heart as well as use your discernment, so you can ascertain which things will be of benefit to you.

When we take responsibility for our lives and our health, we emerge from the quagmire of confusion into the crystal-clear light of certainty.

Once you have made the necessary decisions, act as if the benefits are already on their way to you, trusting implicitly. Believe you *have* the very best doctor in the world; the diet you've chosen is the perfect one for you and for your state of health; your meditation techniques have been designed specifically for you, and all the support, encouragement, and benefits are already being experienced.

Many people, acting out of fear, have traveled all over the world, forever seeking some new therapy or clinic which might benefit them. In the beginning it's a good idea to spend time assembling information on the therapies and therapists with whom you feel comfortable and in whom you trust. Once you've done so, it's essential to give your chosen therapies your concerted attention, trusting that healing is taking place right now.

To be constantly changing doctors' therapies or therapists suggests that the right choices weren't made in the first place, or the person making the choices doesn't trust his or her own ability to discern wisely what's best for him or herself.

Peace of mind is our greatest healer. It must become our primary goal.

Feeling clear and comfortable about the decisions we've made is essential to peace of mind. Some decisions which you'll need to make could also have drawbacks attached to them—for instance, chemotherapy or any other toxic drug treatments, radiotherapy, and surgery.

Even some diagnostic tests have drawbacks attached. If you've decided, after going through the decision-making formula, that the benefits outweigh the drawbacks, then make a firm commitment to concentrate on the benefits and minimize any of the side effects. Sometimes even drawbacks can be turned into positives.

One of my clients, Peter, suffered for several months with very persistent diarrhea. He wrote to me, saying: "One day I retreated yet again to the bathroom. When I found the toilet seat still warm from my last occupation, I decided to do something about it! I chose a "safe" time—when I didn't think I'd need to go to the toilet for at least an hour—to go shopping for the most exotic orchids in bloom I could find. Now my bathroom is filled with exquisite color and beauty and I can sit and gaze at the intricacies of their patterns for hours!"

If you've decided on chemotherapy as your best avenue of treatment, then visualize it pouring perfect healing light into your body, filling it with vitality; the light so strong and pure that any old or diseased cells wither away to be replaced by vibrant, energetic, and healthy ones.

The same applies to whatever additional therapies you choose. For instance, if you decide to include vegetable juice in your diet, then drink it with enthusiasm and the belief that it's providing all the essentials for perfect health. I believe your attitude will make a difference as to how you benefit from the therapies you've decided to employ. On the one hand you could be meditating because you believe it's beneficial in assisting you to achieve peace and you can *feel* it doing you good; or you could be sitting there reluctantly, hating every minute but persevering nonetheless because someone said it was good for you.

Are you meditating because you love life, or because you don't want to die? The technique is the same, but I'm convinced your attitude will make a difference to the benefits your body receives.

The Decision-Making Formula

This formula has many applications. It can be used in almost every situation. Tailor the formula to *your* particular requirements, but keep in mind the principles set out here.

1. *Make a date with yourself for the decision to be made. Allow a suitable length of time to gather and assimilate your information.*

2. *Gather as much information as possible about the subject on which you need to make a decision. Talk to others who've had experience, read books, find out what facilities are available in your community to provide the necessary information.*

3. *Let this information gradually distill within you. Use some of the time after your meditation to tune in to what is truly helpful to you. Remember, within you there's the absolute knowledge of how to bring about your healing. You only need to find the right combination to establish the perfect environment for that healing to take place.*

4. *Make your decision on the date previously decided upon and make an absolute commitment to the course of action you've chosen.*

5. *Trust completely in the decision you've chosen, believing it to be a perfect one for yourself at this time.*

6. *Believe that healing is taking place right now.*

7. *Set a period of time wherein you wholeheartedly implement your decision.*

8. *At the end of this period of time, evaluate your progress and make any adjustments or additions which appear necessary.*

9. *Maintain your program while listening to the voice within. This allows flexibility in your decisions.*

10. *Repeat steps 7 and 8 regularly.*

For some people the decision-making process is quite new and unfamiliar—and these are *major* decisions that have to be made. So, for those people who have difficulty in this area, be gentle with yourselves and concentrate particularly on trusting you've made the right choice.

With this formula, flexibility, and listening to the "still small voice within," we can find our way through the most awesome and bewildering circumstances and go on with renewed vigor and belief in our chosen path.

Chapter Four

FRIENDS FOR LIFE

. . . .

Zelma

I am Zelma, fifty-six years old, in the "afternoon" of life. Three years ago I underwent surgery to remove the portion of my pancreas which contained a tumor. When giving me the report of this operation, I was very aware of my doctor's body language, and knew, before he spoke, that his news wouldn't be good. The tumor was malignant and small secondaries were visible on my liver.

Because of my family history I had occasionally considered the possibility of cancer for myself, but it came as a shock when I heard the news. The fact that it took me by surprise gave me a jolt—I realized that I didn't really know myself as well as I thought.

I vividly recall my initial response to the doctor on that warm, humid February morning as we sat on the verandah of the hospital: "How will I ever tell Mom?" (she and I were the only remaining members of our family), and his reply, "Well, I think you need to give some time to yourself first." I smile now when I remember my flurry of confused thoughts about what to do first—clean up and organize my belongings so that others wouldn't be left with the task? How would I tell others? What would be their reaction? On that morning everything seemed unreal, and yet I found some comfort in the blue sky outside and the normal activities of people in the hospital and outside on the street.

But the bewilderment, perplexity, and helplessness of those first weeks gradually yielded to a calmness within as I resolved to face up to the cancer and not allow it to create fear or discouragement. I'd seek ways of making it a positive, rather than a negative influence in whatever span of life remained to me. In times of prayer, and talking with those who weren't threatened by the open expression of my feelings, I realized that my anxieties and periods of depression were because I'd lost control of my life. I was being asked to surrender my tight grip on life, to let go of what I'd considered to be important and necessary.

Several events occurred one year after my diagnosis. I emerged from another bout in the hospital physically weak and in a state of psychological exhaustion. During the recuperation period my mother died—the deepest grief I've ever experienced. Then I attended my first support group.

This combination of illness/fatigue and Mom's sudden death, together with the opportunity of sharing my thoughts and feeling in the safe, accepting atmosphere of the support group, has steadily altered my way of dealing with life. These events happened two years ago, and now I can only breathe a profound and peaceful THANKS for all that those twenty-four months have given me.

The support group was, and is, a most influential factor in helping me to live more fully, to achieve greater peace of mind, to grow in self-knowledge and awareness that I have something to contribute to others. My former goal of working tirelessly and faithfully, while inwardly struggling to overcome my insecurity and feelings of inadequacy, completely collapsed with the onset of illness. Serious illness was something I'd never experienced in my fifty-three years of living. Through sharing these experiences with others in the groups, and discovering similarities in their stories, I'm learning to accept myself for what I am, not for my acquired skills. I'm particularly grateful for guidance in learning meditation and relaxation techniques, and dealing with anger, guilt, resentment. Three years ago I'd never have thought it possible to enjoy freedom and peace of mind to the extent I do now.

I'm learning to be content with what I have, to live in the now, without anxiety for the future, to recognize and then dismiss negative thoughts, to live through periods of turbulence, anxiety, fear, prejudice, which still rear their heads but don't have their former power to dominate my life. The secret I had to learn was to ask for help,

*acknowledge my incapacity to deal with aspects of life, and trust that
my plea would be heard. So simple, and yet so hard to do because of
my independence and self-sufficiency.*

*These reflections on my experience give me confidence that I'll con-
tinue my inner journey and become the person I was meant to be—in
other words, to name myself. The following quote from Mary
d'Apices's book* Noon to Nightfall *is a fair summary of my journey
thus far:*

*"Perhaps the answer to all our questioning about the mystery of
human pain can be found in the discovery of the Little Prince: 'What
makes the desert beautiful is that somewhere it hides a well....' And
de St. Exupery writes: 'And as I walked on so, I found the well, at
daybreak.' "*

As I said in the introduction, "In the past nine years, I've counseled thousands of people on a one-to-one basis and facilitated
over two thousand support groups for people with life-threatening diseases. One of the things that constantly amazes me is
how frequently we have a group in which no one mentions their
disease. Someone without such an illness would probably find
that extraordinary, believing that surely the illness is the main
problem.

"The participants sometimes talk about the poor relationships
they have with their mothers and fathers; they talk about lack of
purpose, direction, or meaning; they talk about the extraordinary
beauty of the sunrise they witnessed that morning and how it
touched a central core within themselves; they talk about the
healing of their kinship with life or with God; they talk about
not asserting themselves in their relationships; they talk about
the unrealistic standards they've been trying to live up to all
their lives; they talk about the despair of being unable to control
and manipulate the world, and end by laughing at the arrogance
which led them to believe they ever could; they discuss their
struggles with faith and trust; they might acknowledge that all
their lives they've failed to give themselves any love and respect;
they talk of the guilt and shame they've held on to for so long;

they talk of forgiveness and its capacity to set them free from
pain; they talk about the peace and joy they have in every day
lived, but mostly, they *do not* talk about cancer, AIDS, failed suicide, multiple sclerosis, scleroderma, HIV, anorexia, alcohol, or
drug addiction, chronic pain, or whatever has brought them to
one of our groups. It's not that they refuse to talk about the
problem or disease; it's as if the disease or problem has brought
sharply into focus the areas of their lives which aren't working
well or are causing them pain."

There's nothing quite so reassuring and comforting as to be
among people who understand and can empathize with our
situation.

A support group, effectively facilitated, creates a safe, warm,
and supportive environment in which any issues can be discussed
with complete openness and frankness. Often there are problems
or concerns which we feel unable to share with our family or
partner, perhaps because it will be too upsetting for them or
perhaps because they can't or don't know how to respond in any
really helpful way. Even though we live so closely with family,
it's often said by participants in the group that those nearest to
them physically don't really know or understand what they're
going through. Such groups give us the opportunity to explore
and verbalize our innermost feelings and, often, the courage to
express them to our loved ones.

Sometimes people have an unsympathetic home environment
where the family thinks that because one has a good doctor
there's no need for any additional support. Sometimes this happens in homes where the wife, who's always been the one who
has to "cope" in the family, is the one who's sick.

One woman, Jean, said that when she was diagnosed with
breast cancer, her husband retreated into himself and wasn't able
to give her any emotional support. She said *he* looked so miserable she realized she would have to give *him* a hug. She added
wistfully, "How nice it would have been if he'd been able to give
me a hug." She wasn't being critical of him, but she was certainly
expressing the sentiments of many copers.

The family's attitude can sometimes be, "If she looks all right

then she must *be* all right." This can also be the case when we
have a long or protracted illness during which we often don't
look particularly sick. At times when we appear well, everyone
breathes a sigh of relief, believing that everything can return to
normal again. "Isn't it great! You're better now." It's often at *this*
time that the full impact of what's happening to us hits home.
Everyone goes back to work, back to familiar routines, and we're
left feeling everything is *not* all right at all!

Frances expressed this very well in one of her groups. She'd
had fairly extensive surgery for bowel cancer which had spread
into her lymphatic glands and liver. She has three young children and a very busy husband who is the managing director of a
large company. She recovered well after her surgery and re-
sumed her responsibilities gradually as wife and mother. Her
husband would spare no expense in indulging her. He bought
her a new and expensive car with a car phone (just what *he'd*
have liked if he'd been in her position!). Initially, he did his best
to make sure her duties were light, but as time progressed and
she *seemed* well, she ended up doing more and more of the
heavier duties like carrying the shopping, and the baby up the
stairs, and so on. Frances was very keen to feel and act as normally as possible because she, too, wanted to believe that all was
well.

It's often difficult to find the balance between "Am I a sick
person?" or "Am I a well person?" Often we don't want people
asking us, "How are you *really*?" Yet there are times when it
would be so nice for someone to inquire how we truly are. It's
very difficult for the support person to know which frame of
mind we're in, and how we'd like them to respond.

By talking it through with the group, Frances was able to
acknowledge that her husband loved her dearly and that perhaps
she needed to give him some kind of guidance as to how she
was really feeling. She realized that in giving her the car he was
saying how valuable and important she was to him, and that *he*
had every confidence she'd be around for a long time.

She was able to go home and reopen discussions about what
was and wasn't appropriate for her to be tackling physically.

This led into deeper and more emotional issues. Her husband expressed gratitude that she'd brought the whole subject up. He'd been loath to do it, because she always seemed so capable and he was afraid he might upset her by raising issues he thought she wanted to forget.

Many times the dilemmas we create for ourselves stem from a simple lack of communication. Sometimes raising the issues which cause us pain or stress is a challenge; we all tend to want things to be fine. We don't want to face painful issues. They *can* sit on the back burner—until we feel the heat is so strong that we're beginning to get singed! Often when we take this attitude, we find we're sitting on a hotbed of emotion. Inflamed discussions are rarely anticipated with joy. If we can acknowledge and deal with the small brush fires, we could well avoid the towering inferno.

Frances was encouraged to talk through her disgruntled feelings and resentment in the group and thus was able to sort out the issues in a calm, nonjudgmental environment. Had she not been able to do so the situation could well have escalated into a towering inferno, where hurtful things might have been said quite unnecessarily.

Communication is the lifeline of all relationships but never more so than when we're thrust into a situation which feels like a *nightmare. We* need to have our fears heard and acknowledged. We're then able more easily to live comfortably with them, or let them go entirely.

By continuing to participate in your support group, you make a statement to your family and friends about who you are and what your needs are. In this way they can gain some understanding and respect for your situation. Many a partner has said they're really happy their loved one has the group with whom to talk over fears and anxieties. They're extremely supportive and encouraging of the person's participation in our group. Of course partners, support people, and friends are also welcome to attend most support groups and, indeed, are encouraged to come and share their own perspectives and experiences. It can be very valuable for the support person to meet other people who are in

the same situation. Support people need support, too. Chapter
13, The Tender Trap, is entirely devoted to caring for caregivers
(see pages 349-363). Nevertheless very often the person attends
the group without their partner because it's not uncommon for
partners to feel quite frightened of being confronted with a
group of people who have life-threatening illnesses. There's no
point in applying pressure to them and the most you can really
say is, "It's really important to me that you come to one of these
groups."

You must respect the fact that people have different ways of
dealing with stress. Many of our participants are happy that
their partner *isn't* present! It gives them the opportunity to deal
with issues without their partner's reactions. One woman,
Bridget, was married to a man who was devoted to her. Jim held
a very responsible position in a major government department
and by the time he had been diagnosed with liver cancer it was
very advanced. The thought of going to a cancer support group
was totally abhorrent to him. *She* found the groups gave her an
avenue in which she could express all the emotions, fears, and
concerns which she had been forced to hold tightly within herself. If she tried to broach any emotional issues with Jim, he
would immediately reply, "All the legal papers are in the hands
of our solicitors. There's nothing you need fear or worry about.
Your financial situation will be absolutely fine and I've made
sure you'll be comfortable." End of subject. He'd become agitated if she pressed for more.

Bridget desperately wanted to know how he was *feeling*. But
"feeling" represented a world quite remote, inconsequential, and
even inconceivable to him. He was very happy she went to "that
group" to get whatever she needed as "emotional support," so
long as it didn't involve him. Indeed, he actively encouraged her
to attend her support group.

In the group, through tearful exchanges, Bridget explored the
relationship that she and her husband had experienced in the
past. She acknowledged that Jim had always been emotionally
removed from her, not because of any lack in herself but because
that was his nature. They had toured the world extensively,

lived a wonderful life among high diplomatic officials, and had
the best of what the world had to offer, but they had never
shared deep emotional intimacy.

Her feelings were both happy and sad: happy that he'd
shared his ambitions, his achievements, his successes with her;
sad that they'd never had the opportunity or wherewithal to dig
deeper into the recesses of his mind. She felt she was a part of
his life, and yet removed from "what made him tick." She ached
to be a part of his world. Yet *his* concerns were for her future
support, both emotional and financial.

When Bridget was pressed to talk about Bridget, about what
was important for Bridget, about what made Bridget tick, about
what made her life of value, about her ambitions, her goals, her
dreams—she was silent. She had given her life to Jim, had given
her love to him; she felt she had given her soul to him.

In time, she began to heal. Before he died, she began to heal;
to recover from the mistaken notion we're here to provide the
next step for those we love. She could come to the group for *her*
needs and leave *his* at the door. This is the essence of true healing. We can only ever provide for our own healing. In healing
ourselves, we can set free the other person to do the necessary
healing for themselves.

Most support groups encourage the caregivers to attend
either a general support group or one designed to meet their
particular needs. Groups are generally flexible in content. No
two sessions are ever the same. Participants address whatever
issues arise out of each one.

Many of those people who are the least willing initially to
share find the most benefit from their new associations. The
empathy and love generated during the sharing is a powerful and
growing thing of itself, and a bond which strengthens us to go
on. We can gain great encouragement from someone who is further down the track than us and is comfortable and at peace
with their situation. People who come into the room dejected
and anxious always leave cheered and ready to face whatever lies
ahead. I have found there are many people in our groups who
are in remission after they'd been told this would be unlikely or

impossible. They provide great inspiration and encouragement to those who are just starting out on their journey. It is generally surprising to people to find these groups are full of laughter and good humor; there are tears, too, and these are freely expressed as the need arises. To have permission from others to have a good cry is invaluable. Very often families don't want to see us cry because it puts them in touch with their own distress.

On a Friday afternoon just before we were due to leave the city for one of our residential workshops, I received a phone call from a young man who said the doctors had just told him he was dying and he was frightened and needed help in order for him to live. He sounded very distressed and I suggested he come away for the weekend with us and that someone could pick him up in a couple of hours. Thus Craig came into our lives.

Craig was twenty-four years old, and an opal miner from Lightning Ridge, a small, very remote town twelve hours drive from Sydney. He told us he had a "life-*frightening* disease"; he referred to his tumors as tulips and said he had a bunch of public servants for an immune system and he wanted to sack the lot of them and get in some private enterprise. It was refreshing for Craig to be among people who were all in the same situation and who were all endeavoring to live their lives as fully as possible. There was such a lot of laughter and tears that weekend. Something magical happens during these weekends where we've gathered together twenty to forty people who all have a life-threatening disease. There's a feeling of camaraderie and compassion and the presence of great courage. People go beyond their habitual bounds because they're in the presence of others who are doing the same.

Craig gained greatly from that weekend and was present also at the following one three months later. His doctors were very pessimistic about him and at one stage told him he only had weeks to live. Craig never listened to such advice, knowing full well he'd die when *he* was good and ready, and that certainly wasn't going to be in the next few weeks. It was true that his body was not doing so well with his melanoma advancing painfully into his bones, but his spirit remained strong.

During Craig's participation in the support groups, he became friendly with several men his own age who had AIDS or
were infected with HIV. Up until then, Craig had viewed all
homosexuals (from the distance of Lightning Ridge) as "poofters
who deserved to die." His attitude changed as his heart began to
open more to the suffering he and they shared. Some of them
became his greatest supporters, not only helping Craig but also
his mother and sister who'd come down from the country and
who knew no one in Sydney.

Craig was finally admitted into a palliative care unit near my
home, and for several months his mother stayed with me, spending her days with her son. He was very dependent upon his
mother, Helen, and didn't like her to be out of his sight for very
long. They both came from the hospital to the support group
until it became too painful for Craig to move. He used to "let"
Helen come to the groups, knowing she needed support. It was
the only place where she could cry and talk about how she was
surviving this painful experience.

By this time, Craig could barely walk as his pelvis had disin-
tegrated into three separate pieces. Sitting for very long was also
a problem. Nonetheless one day Craig announced he had every
intention of coming to the next residential weekend in the country. The next one was scheduled for a date about six weeks from
this statement. He said the only thing which would keep him
away was death, and at that point death seemed very likely to
intervene. However, I'd long since given up attempting to pre-
dict how long a person might live.

In the week leading up to the weekend, Craig was very much
alive and still keen to come. We had to face the problem of *how*
to get him there. He was unable to move without enormous
pain. Stopping and starting in traffic and dealing with curves
and bumps in the road was out of the question.

We finally hit upon a solution. Perhaps we could get a helicopter! My assistant, Jennifer, telephoned all over Sydney trying
to track down someone who would be kind enough to fly our
intrepid Craig to his destination. The Natural Gas Company
came to our rescue, and Craig's flight was comfortable and rapid.

I'd told the pilot, "Take the highway out of Mittagong, and when you're over the Paddy's River bridge, take a right. One kilometer inland you'll see forty people standing around in a field." There wasn't a dry eye in our group as we listened for, heard, and waved at the approaching helicopter. To see Craig's very pale grinning face was wonderful and more than worth all the effort we'd put into making it possible. Craig couldn't participate in any of the activities of the weekend, and yet he was at the center of everything. He lay in bed in the main room where most of the activities were held and was joked with, massaged and hugged. The next day the helicopter returned for his journey back to the hospital. To save on bumps and jolts, his wheelchair was carried to the helicopter. One of those who carried his wheelchair had a life-threatening disease himself.

On his return journey, he and the pilot saw a very bright double rainbow stretched across the harbor. We work a lot with rainbows and I shall talk about them shortly. The pilot, Laurie, flew through the middle of the rainbow and Craig was ecstatic. The weekend provided Craig with a tremendous boost and he lived another two months (mostly on the strength of telling his '"helicopter story"!).

We can't always change the outcome of a disease, but we can change the way we experience that outcome.

We can retreat into a lonely, fear-filled world or we can join with others who are facing the same situation as ourselves and gain courage and spirit from them. Craig received much in his weekend with us, and the simple fact of his presence gave much to those attending also. He exemplified courage, humor, perseverance, and spirit.

We don't value a life by its length. It's not how long we live but the spirit with which we live which is of importance.

One apprehension newcomers have often expressed about participating in a support group is that they might meet people who are sicker than they are, or who are going to die. This certainly happens in support groups, yet facing death or serious illness *together* has been a great blessing and strength to many people. I don't believe it's a negative thing to look at and discuss death. In fact, looking at the prospect of my own death and the process of dying was the turning point for me. Once my fears were acknowledged and dealt with, my strength began to return. If we have a life-threatening disease, then one definite possibility is that we might die. *Not* to look at that possibility can sometimes take an enormous amount of energy which would be better spent in healing. Being open to life also means being open to death. Once death has been looked at fully, or as fully as we're able, we can really get on with living. Once I'd accepted the inevitability of my own death, I made a full commitment to life. If I was going to die, I'd do it with good grace, but while I had life and breath, I was going to be doing my utmost to live. And I set about finding ways in which I could affirm life.

Keith, a man in his mid-forties, uses the group as a forum to discuss and clarify his thoughts about life, relationships, and love. His honest explorations of these topics gives others the opportunity to investigate their own attitudes and beliefs. He enriches us all with his insights into life and we get a sense of joining together to explore our individual search for meaning and purpose.

To be in a group where people are exploring their feelings about dying can be invaluable as a way of gaining insight into our own feelings. Sometimes we're a little nervous about looking at our own feelings, and to hear someone else courageously exploring theirs can help us.

Several rituals have evolved with time and experience within our groups. Often if someone is too ill to come to a group, is in pain, or frightened, we will "send them a rainbow."

One evening I received a phone call from one of the participants in our groups. John was a member of our Tuesday evening meditation group. I barely recognized his voice because he was speaking through a haze of analgesia. He was in a hospital nearby with "undiagnosed pain" which didn't seem related to his disease. His pain was so intense he was on a high dosage of morphine, every four hours. He told me he was praying he would die because he couldn't cope with the pain any longer. He asked if would we please remember him in our prayers and send him a rainbow.

As it happened, he had telephoned just before the Tuesday evening group was due to begin. At the beginning of the meditation we imagined that the group was bathed in the light of one end of the rainbow. We imagined the iridescent colors surrounding and permeating each person present. We took some time to breathe in our favorite colors. Then we visualized the other end of the rainbow going up through the ceiling, across the sky, to John. We imagined him bathed in the light and colors of the rainbow—given strength, peace, comfort, and healing by the power of the rainbow. We extended our love, support, and blessings across the rainbow to him.

John telephoned the next day to let me know what had happened. Our rainbow had been sent at about 8:00 P.M. when John had a visitor with him in the hospital. In mid-sentence, John had fallen into a deep sleep and had not awakened until morning. When he awoke, he thought he'd died and gone to heaven because his pain had completely gone. Then, on opening his eyes, he realized he was still in the hospital. He was discharged later that morning and has never had a recurrence of the pain. I believe that just as you can have a vitamin A deficiency, so you can have a rainbow deficiency. Rainbows represent being remembered with *love*. I believe love has the power to heal all wounds. John's story is a dramatic one of healing. There are many others who've requested rainbows be sent to them. Their stories are every bit as dramatic as, though different from, John's.

Chris first came to one of our groups when she had a recurrence of her breast cancer. She was facing choices and decisions regarding her treatment and needed an environment where she could sort out for herself the best course of action, without pressure from anyone. She was very much against having the chemotherapy her doctors were advocating. Chris had been in a number of support groups over the years. She had gone to these groups in order to overcome her drug and alcohol addiction. She'd been very successful and had been "clean and sober" for eighteen months. She'd found the lump in her breast three days after she had admitted herself to a detoxifying unit. She had a mastectomy during her withdrawal from drugs and alcohol.

Chris is one of the most spirited people with whom I've ever had the privilege of working. She has a wonderful sense of humor which lightens up her most despairing moments. Her story is remarkable. As well as being in recovery from her drug and alcohol addiction, she has recovered from anorexia.

Because the cancer had spread into the bones, her doctors wanted to give her chemotherapy as soon as possible. As a compromise, she decided to take Tamoxifen, a drug used in the treatment of breast cancer. Several months after being on this drug her abdomen began to swell and many of us feared that she had developed ascites (fluid in the abdomen). When she became quite uncomfortable with the swelling she went back to her doctor. Imagine her (and our) surprise when she was told she was seventeen weeks pregnant with twins!

Here she was, forty years old, on a drug which interferes with a woman's hormonal cycle (making it "extremely unlikely" for her to conceive) with advanced breast cancer ... and twins! She had to make a decision quickly as to whether to keep or abort the twins. The ultrasound showed two healthy little girls. It didn't surprise any of us when Chris decided to continue her pregnancy. Considering her life so far, she felt that these children must really want to be born and have her as their mother. She continued to blossom and thrive until she was twenty-six weeks pregnant, when she entered a hospital to rest and "cook" the babies as long as possible before having them by Cesarean section. This meant she could no longer get to support groups. Each week, all of the group sent her, her partner, and the twins a rainbow.

At thirty weeks she gave birth to the two healthy, beautiful (and tiny) girls. She was ecstatic and, though not very well herself, still managed to look radiant.

On reflection, Chris was very grateful she had listened to the still small voice within about her decision *not* to have chemotherapy when it was first offered. If she had, it would certainly have resulted in the deformity of her babies. Once the babies were born, she decided she would have some chemotherapy.

Chris and the babies continue to do well. Chris has her ups and downs, of course, but her babies give her enormous joy and hope. She says she would never have gotten through the pregnancy as she did without the support she felt she received from her faith in a higher power and the rainbows. A year later, they are all thriving.

I believe that sending rainbows is really the essence of prayer. Through them we uphold and see the other person as healed now. We don't perceive the person as sick and miserable. We imagine the person as whole, at peace, and strengthened by the light and colors of the rainbow. We frequently send rainbows to our doctors. We see them bathed in the light of the rainbow, filled with peace, compassion, and understanding. Offices and waiting rooms are bathed in its light and colors, creating an oasis for all those who enter. We send rainbows to our homes to create an atmosphere of peace and joy. We see the people, plants, and pets who live there bathed in its light and colors, given strength and peace and healing by the power of its light. We've sent rainbows after earthquakes, to the Middle East, to presidents and prime ministers, to prisoners with AIDS, to our friends in hospitals and hospices, to the lonely, depressed, and despairing in our community. Sending a rainbow gives us a way of joining with others who are facing their own particular dilemmas and crises in life. It's a way of feeling linked with all humanity.

When you're first diagnosed with a life-threatening disease, it can feel as though you're out at sea on a little leaky raft. Even if you have support, this experience is happening just to you. If you look out and see another person on his leaky raft, you can call out, "Hi, George, how are you?" George might say, "Not too good. The pain's pretty bad." It gives you the opportunity to say, "I'm sorry to hear it, George. I'll send you a rainbow." You haven't changed George's situation but you may well have helped change the way George *feels* about his situation. You can be out in the big sea, on a leaky raft by yourself, or you can be on your leaky raft surrounded by fifty thousand other leaky rafts with everyone sending rainbows to each other. You haven't changed the fact you're still on your leaky raft, but it's the way you experience it which becomes important: alone or united by rainbows.

The sending of rainbows to each other might sound a little crazy or over the top to some people, and that's O.K. After all, rainbows aren't for everyone. However, many of us have found this simple ritual brings comfort, peace, and a tangible means of heart reaching out to heart. In fact, we've had calls from South Africa, Hong Kong, and America, where the caller has simply said, "I believe your group sends rainbows. My son [daughter/ mother/father, etc.] is about to have surgery/chemotherapy. Would your group please send him [or her] a rainbow?" Heaven knows how they hear of us, but then, heaven knows, rainbows reach to the ends of the earth!

When Someone Dies

We have another ritual we implement when someone dies. We usually join hands and allow our eyes to close gently. We take a moment to center ourselves and then we visualize the person who has died in the middle of the group. We extend a rainbow from our heart to the heart of that person. Then we acknowledge inwardly the qualities which endeared that person to us: perhaps the person's sense of humor, love of life, perseverance, compassion or courage, faith or ability to trust, supportiveness toward us, or whatever quality was of value to us. We spend some time in silence saying in our hearts the things we'd like to say to the person and we listen for his or her reply. Then we visualize the person surrounded in light, given strength and peace and healing of the spirit by the power of that light. We allow the qualities which endeared the person to us to flow back across the rainbow bridge into our hearts as his or her gift to us, and we extend our love and blessings to them as we release the person into the light.

This ritual gives us the opportunity to "complete" with the person. Yes, there's sadness at the loss of those people who have grown very dear to us. Sometimes they've shared more intimacy with the group than they have with their own families. We miss them. Yet their presence can always be felt in the group and we often talk about the gifts, the solutions they found which are valuable to us also. We remember them more with smiles and joy than with depression. When someone in the group dies, our tears aren't all for that person; there are always tears for ourselves. Perhaps this will be me in six months, or a year or two, or ten. Partly we grieve for our familiar loved ones, our familiar group environment; we feel our own uncertainty about letting go into the arms of the unknown.

While we're alive, we're living with a life-threatening disease, not dying with a terminal one. We need all the love, support, and encouragement due to any living being.

Anger

It's very common for people to express anger within the safe confines of the group. The group is often the only place where a participant feels free to explore, express, and resolve his or her anger without the judgment, criticism, or upset the anger may cause at home. Very often there are tears of frustration, resentment or sadness, behind the anger.

Guidelines for Running a Support Group

The guidelines which I've found essential for the smooth and effective running of the groups are very simple. I repeat them, in their entirety, for every group. If you are in, or currently looking for, a support group, these are four general guidelines you might consider. Often the healthiest groups respect these guidelines, and I believe that groups which follow these principles are the most effective. The four guidelines are:

1. *What transpires within the group is confidential; we don't discuss people or their experiences outside the group unless it is with their permission. If we already know the history, background, or profession of any person present, we make no reference to it during the time of the group.**

2. *We stay with our feelings rather than theorize about situations. This means we talk about how things actually are for us rather than how they could, should, or ought to be, or how our doctor, family, society, or anyone else thinks things ought to be.*

3. *We don't judge or criticize. If people are feeling negative, angry, joyful, peaceful, positive, suicidal, or depressed, we don't tell them they shouldn't feel that way. To do that would be to negate the person's present reality, which needs to be acknowledged before that person can change his or her perception.*

4. *We listen 100 percent when someone is talking, so that we don't dissolve into several chattering groups. It also means that we hear what the person's experience is rather than our own reactions to the person's experience. It is important to listen behind the words to the underlying feelings or issues.*

The form the group takes is as follows. We always begin by welcoming people to the group. We then go through the guidelines for the running of the group. We join hands and the facilitator then guides the group through a brief relaxation and centering exercise, and into a brief meditation.

After the guidelines are explained, we introduce ourselves to each other. This usually consists of giving a first name and any information we like. It can include our diagnosis, an update on the past week, what we receive or want to receive from the group, or mention of a particular problem we're experiencing. For some who are shy, a name can be sufficient. Some will say they're nervous and would prefer to just sit and listen, and of course their wish is respected. Once these people feel at ease, they might wish to share more of their feelings.

---

* We extended the parameters of confidentiality when well-known or easily recognizable people came to the groups. To have someone comment on a person's "public" side can be very unnerving for that person. Well-known people come to the groups to share their vulnerability, not their "high profile."

By the time we've completed introductions it's very clear where the needs of the participants are, and these are then addressed in a compassionate and supportive manner. The idea is not to outdo each other in the telling of our dramas, but to listen carefully to what each person is saying.

When we listen carefully to what people are saying, either directly or indirectly, it actually enables them to *hear* better themselves what they're saying and gives them courage to explore and discover their own solutions. *My* solutions are always *mine*. They may benefit someone else as well but ultimately we all need to find our own solutions to the problems which arise in our lives. It's not a case of, "Where there is *this* problem, there is *this* solution." A solution entirely appropriate to one person will be inappropriate, perhaps, for another.

Support group settings are opportunities to air our fears, angers, and apprehensions and perhaps gain another perspective. Nothing is more healing than to laugh at something which was once fearful to us but which now has no power over us. There's a silent permission that often permeates the group, which allows for free expression of whatever emotions are being experienced, be they grief, panic, anger, frustration, depression, regret, sadness, joy, love, fear, guilt, powerlessness, and so on.

There's no agenda for the group. It doesn't set out to talk about any particular subject. Each session is unique and special in its own way. All our groups are "open," so new members are always welcome. We find people cannot always commit themselves to being there every week because of treatments or other responsibilities. And, also, not everybody wants to come every week. Many of our participants have to travel great distances to experience this support.

Michael was a member of our Monday group. He used to travel down from the Blue Mountains outside Sydney each week to attend. One day he told us he needed to go for a particular treatment immediately after the group. This treatment always made him terribly sick for three days after and he wasn't looking forward to it at all, as he was already feeling frail. The group assured him they'd be sending lots of love and rainbows to him in the next few days. Just before he left he commented on how much he loved gardenias. There were half a dozen left in the garden and I picked them for him.

When he arrived at the hospital, he was given the same dosage of drugs as previously. However, he was sixteen kilos *lighter* this time and ended up, due to the hospital's failure to take this into account, receiving quite an overdose. He managed to get home, where he collapsed and in his words, "I lay on the floor and couldn't move. I thought I was dying and I felt so afraid; but there *was* the smell of gardenias. The pain was indescribable and I felt so alone but there were flashes of rainbows and moments of warmth when I knew I was being loved. In this way, remembering love, rainbows, and gardenias, I survived until help arrived."

Michael was so touched by the love and support he received in these groups that he bequeathed his home to the Quest for Life Foundation. The sale of this house came at a time of great financial need for the foundation, and the funds raised were instrumental in our being able to continue and expand the programs we offer.

Outreach

A lot of support flows outside the formal meeting of the group. It's common when members are going to the hospital for surgery, chemotherapy or some other procedure, that other members of the group will telephone or remember them in their own meditations. This feeling of being supported by others is tremendously valuable. It's often said by a participant that even in the darkest night of depression, fear, or pain, the remembrance of the group has brought light and comfort.

These outside activities have also extended to the bedside of someone who's hospitalized or sick at home, when two or more people from the regular support group will go and hold a group for that person. In this way, the person still feels connected to the main group. When we're beginning our groups, we spend some time visualizing anyone who's unable to attend that day

due to illness or hospitalization. We visualize the person surrounded by light, made whole, content, and at peace by the
power of that light. We also send the person a rainbow. Many
people have said they've felt an inflow of strength or support at
those precise times and have suddenly felt at peace!

When we have a life-threatening disease we can feel useless
as far as our capacity to be actively involved in the community
is concerned. Often we need to give up work, sports, or other
activities that we're used to being involved in and it can easily
lead to a feeling of being an observer of life, rather than a par-
ticipator. We can begin to question our value as a human being,
especially when an illness is protracted. Participating in a support group can allay those feelings entirely. Often those who
are sickest and weakest give more strength and the most valuable insights into another's dilemma, and it's only because of
their courage and awareness of their own plight that they're
able to do so. Support group members often say that they've
never felt so connected to other people as they have since their
illness. They say they've found a strength within themselves
which they've been able to share freely with others in a way
never before possible. When we're able to share deeply with
others it brings about a completion and healing within
ourselves.

My belief is that we're primarily spiritual beings who happen
to be in bodies, rather than bodies who happen to have spirits.
A support group allows people to experience spirit reaching out
to spirit in love and compassion—and frequently humor—to
bring insight, comfort, and perhaps a changed perception. The
depth and strength of the human spirit has the power to show us
the flimsy nature of fear. A situation first perceived as terrifying
can, when brought out into the open and looked at in the light,
be perceived quite differently—especially with the added
strength of others.

There are a few other practical suggestions for the running of
a support group. The facilitator will need to ensure that the
group stays within the framework of the guidelines. The groups
are not times for swapping recipes, discussing exercise programs,

or sharing other information about treatments. This can be done during the break at the end of the meeting. In this way, the group stays focused on the intended content of the group. It's equally essential that the group stay within the prescribed time. I've found a two-hour group to be the most effective. In this time participants are able to address fully their needs. A tea or coffee break at the end of the group provides the opportunity for more relaxed conversation. Support groups often lead to friendships outside the formal meetings and also to many shared activities. We've had picnics from time to time, and these occasions give the families an opportunity to mix in an easy social atmosphere. Much recipe swapping happens at these events! Wives of sick husbands have the opportunity to hear how others are coping. Children are able to share with each other the joys of kite flying or duck feeding.

When we're sick, we're often limited by our pain or energy level, and yet it's nourishing to the spirit to participate in these activities with others who have an understanding of our restrictions. Our residential weekends away in the country are very popular and are always a great success. During these weekends we focus on meditation, massage, hands-on healing, drawing, horse riding, tennis, kite flying, eating fantastic (healthy!) food, sitting around open fires, swimming, and so on. They provide an opportunity for the giving and receiving of love and support.

A support group can be made up of as few as two people who are committed to self-exploration and discovery, and indeed this is how our support group originally began. That first small group was extremely valuable and gave us an opportunity to find out just what *were* the essentials for such groups. Out of them arose the four guidelines for the groups. There are now dozens of such groups fashioned along these same guidelines.

Much of my time now is spent in giving seminars in various parts of Australia to help set up their support services. This work has also extended to support services for those who are working *with* people with life-threatening diseases. Often the doctors and nurses experience burn-out after failing to look after their own needs adequately.

When a support group was in its formative stage, even when no one came, I still spent the allotted time in reflection and in sending love and support to those unable to attend on that particular day. In this way an energy was built up. Mondays from 11:00 A.M.-1:00 P.M. are set aside solely for this purpose. This particular group has been running for seven years.

Our first group grew steadily until it became too big to be effective. As a group we discussed what would be the best solution to the problem of large numbers. The groups at that time usually consisted of between twenty and thirty people. We decided to have two groups each week. But because people gained so much from the groups, instead of the numbers being halved, many of the participants came twice a week! The ideal number for a group is somewhere between eight and twelve people, though this is flexible. We've had some of our most memorable groups with three participants, and also with thirty-six participating.

My preference is to hold the support groups in a private and homey setting, as most people find it less intimidating than a clinical environment. Most of the groups I facilitate each week are held in my home where there's an assortment of seating, including sofas and upright chairs, cushions, beanbags, and a fold-out bed. The atmosphere is anything but clinical.

Most groups are self-supporting, and operate on a donation basis.

After the group has completed its discussions and there are no further emotional loose ends, we have our joke session. This gives us a wonderful opportunity to discharge emotions through laughter. Often times the jokes contain the blackest humor. This seems to be something we can all relate to very easily!

At the end of each group, we close by joining hands and perhaps focus our thoughts and love on any person in the group (or at home or in a hospital) who's in particular need.

Sometimes we finish by sending love and healing through our hands or hearts to those participants who desire it. There's nothing mysterious about the laying-on of hands and people always gain greatly from the experience. The person either lies down or remains seated, if that's more comfortable, while the others in the group gather around and gently place hands on the person. Some prefer to remain in their seats and send loving thoughts or healing from there. Those who feel comfortable with prayer pray silently for the healing of that person. Others prefer to imagine or feel healing energy pouring through their hands into the body of the other, healing in whatever way is most appropriate. Others will channel love and support. The gentle touch of a loving friend can heal the spirit instantly, and a healed spirit has unlimited potential.

Breast Cancer

Marianne was a newcomer to the support group. She was pretty, looked healthy, and was in her mid-thirties. She looked slightly awkward coming to a support group for the first time, but that dissolved quickly as she felt the warmth and acceptance pervading the room.

The group began and shortly, after one or two others, Marianne shared her story. She began tentatively, then feeling she was in a safe place where she could express her feelings without criticism or judgment, her story tumbled out. Six weeks before, Marianne, who has three children, found a lump in her breast where she felt a slightly tender area. She put it at the back of her mind as she had many duties to perform that morning: school lunches to be organized, breakfast to be prepared and cleaned up, children to be dropped off at school, and the weekly shopping to be done.

The lump niggled at the back of her mind all morning as she shopped, put groceries away, and went to the school to perform her voluntary work in the school library. On the way home she popped into her local doctor who assured her that tender lumps were rarely anything to worry about. But because of her family history of breast cancer (her mother had died from it at seventy years of age), he advised her to have a mammogram as soon as possible. As soon as possible turned out to be the next day. The mammogram showed positive, her doctor referred her to a

surgeon who performed a needle biopsy, and within three days
of finding the lump she was scheduled for surgery. She awoke
from the surgery minus her breast and, though she knew to expect this, it came as a shock. Her doctor talked of further treatment including chemotherapy and radiotherapy because the
cancer had spread into the axillary lymph nodes in her armpit.
She recovered well and quickly and was back home with the
children whom she missed. They were equally pleased at her return. She was overwhelmed by the flowers, cards, and loving
responses of so many people, some of whom she hadn't seen for
years. Gradually the household returned to some sort of normal-
ity with Marianne back to preparing school lunches and break-
fasts, cleaning up afterward and dropping the children off to
school on her way to the hospital for radiotherapy. Her husband, Brian, who'd been extremely supportive and loving
throughout her ordeal, held the fort while she was in the hospital and was overjoyed to have her home once more. Everyone
said how well she looked. She felt like she was taking radiotherapy in stride with only a couple of days of feeling off-color
when she had her chemotherapy. Brian had long since returned
to work. The children thought Mom looked, and therefore must
be, fine, since she was back to all her motherly duties.

Now, six weeks later at our support group, Marianne was in
tears, thinking she would never be the same again, and that
there was something seriously wrong because she dissolved into
tears at the drop of a hat. She was trying to keep her despair
from her children and Brian because, "They've all been through
so much already." She felt isolated, alone in her experience, and
even wondered if perhaps the cancer had spread into her brain.
After sharing her story, she began to laugh a little at herself,
hearing how silly it sounded. She began to hear that she had
just been through a nightmare and that it was no wonder she
was feeling a bit down and depressed. By the time some of the
group members reminded her that she *was* still recovering from
the trauma of surgery and *was* having radiotherapy *and* chemotherapy *and* running a household *and* still grieving for an important part of her body, she was able to acknowledge she was

doing a splendid job up until now and that maybe she had been setting herself some unrealistically high standards. After hearing several of the other participants' stories, Marianne looked far more relaxed and at ease. She found others who shared in the ordeal of breast cancer and who could recount stories almost identical to her own.

It's not that the support group can change the outcome of any person's disease, but by joining together we remember the beauty and strength of our common human spirit and we're able to reestablish our commitment to life.

Marianne's story has been heard often in groups: it's about courageous people living under great pressures who are endeavoring to get on with life. Sometimes we need to stop in our climb up the mountain to enjoy the view; to acknowledge how well we're doing and to re-energize ourselves for the path ahead.

I spent much of my life looking for what was wrong rather than celebrating what was right. It took cancer to turn my attention to seeing the glass as half-full rather than half-empty.

Another woman, Rosemary, had extensive breast cancer seventeen years ago. The cancer had spread into her liver and bones and she was told she only had a matter of months to live. She sold her home, gave away her possessions, moved in with her sister, prepared for her departure—and went into complete remission! She attributes her healing to her positive attitude, prayer, and a sense of humor. She says, "I didn't pray to be free of cancer. I prayed to be free of fear; not just fear of dying but fear of living, too! It wasn't until I had cancer that I realized what a scaredy-cat I was. Always planning, controlling, worrying, organizing. Now I just love life and living!"

Many women whose cancer is completely removed have difficulty coping. Often women are told by male doctors that there's no follow-up treatment necessary and to put cancer out of their minds. They try to, but often don't succeed very well. What the doctor doesn't understand is that this woman has just been confronted with her mortality in a very unexpected and frightening way. She could feel mutilated, frightened, confused, out of control, depressed, abandoned, isolated, and rejected. And *he* says not to worry!

In this situation, the doctor is dealing only with the medical facts and failing to recognize that anyone who has been through such an experience is likely to feel emotionally traumatized—not to mention the fact that anyone who experiences the feelings just mentioned on a long-term basis is likely to draw ill health to herself. If you asked him, the doctor would probably say the woman should be happy that it was caught early: two different viewpoints, resulting from poor understanding rather than any intent to distress. The day might dawn when she feels happy it *was* found early but right now she needs support of a different kind. It's a bit like the story of the poor fellow who tried to commit suicide by leaping off a four-story building. He didn't die, but broke many bones in his body and became a quadriplegic. To tell him he's lucky to be alive might not gladden his heart. Many women in similar circumstances struggle to come to terms with their present situation. Do I have cancer? Did I have cancer? How do I know if it will return? How can I live my life with so much uncertainty? Who'll want me now I'm without a breast? Can I safely make plans for my future? Who should I tell? Do I change my diet? Do I change my lifestyle?

Sometimes these women are particularly reluctant to come to a support group or to talk to a health professional because they don't believe they really qualify. After all, "The doctor says I don't have cancer any more." Counseling should be offered to *everyone* regardless of the prognosis of the disease. We all need assistance to find our way through the confusion and bewilderment.

For some women, losing a breast is a major trauma, while for others it's not much different from losing an appendix. For some, it wasn't until they lost their breast that they even began to think about their body image. Some women feel completely comfortable with a prosthesis while others will arrange for an implant as soon as possible. In some cases surgeons actually insert the implant at the time of the mastectomy. Some women have been overjoyed at their implants and some have cursed them for having concealed a recurrence at a later date. Talking with other women who are facing the same kinds of issues, choices, and decisions can be very helpful in clarifying how you actually *do* feel. You don't have to feel alone in your situation. Though your choices will be your own, having a neutral environment in which to talk through your options can help crystallize your thinking. This might not be with a formalized support group. You could have a friend, relative, or partner with whom you feel you can share these private thoughts and who won't influence you in your choices and decisions.

You could choose to see this experience as a turning point in your life: a time when you reflect upon what has been, and what you would like to be in the future; a time to reassess, evaluate, choose anew, and step forward with a grander perspective and a joy in each day lived. Many of the stories and techniques in this book are about those who have done just that. The issues, choices, and decisions that women with breast cancer face will be explored in much greater detail in my next book.

Groups for Those Living with HIV

The issues that come up for discussion in a group where all the participants are HIV+ are similar to the ones mentioned throughout this chapter. However, there are some separate issues which are particular to this group and the following points need to be acknowledged.

- *Many of the participants have experienced multiple losses of friends, acquaintances, lovers, and, occasionally, siblings to the same disease from which they suffer.*

- *The social stigma still attached to infection with HIV stops some people from being able to access adequate emotional support.*

- *Hope is hard to come by because the medical and media sources of information are almost always depressing.*

- *Sometimes there are other complicating health factors which need to be addressed such as drug or alcohol addiction.*

- *There's frequently no family or "significant other" to care for or give support to the HIV+ person.*

- *Long-term chronic "unwellness" is extremely draining both emotionally and financially.*

Some HIV+ women feel completely comfortable within a group made up mostly of gay men, and have gained greatly from their attendance. Other women prefer an all-female group. No matter what the gender, participants often experience "battle fatigue" as a consequence of being among the vast numbers of people struggling to find meaning in a difficult and chronic health crisis. The group provides a safe place where all fears, angers, insights, hopelessness, inspirations, courage, and humor can be shared. Often there are discussions about death, dying, suicide and euthanasia. These issues are more fully covered in chapter 11, Living Well with HIV, and chapter 12, At What Point Do We Stop Living and Start Dying?

Some heterosexual men and women who are HIV+ prefer to attend a general, or non-gay, support group for people with a life-threatening illness. Some gay men feel uncomfortable in a "gay group" and prefer to be with others who are facing a life-threatening illness rather than a particular disease. I've never witnessed any difficulty in combining illnesses within a framework of one group. However, this might be quite different in other areas where more judgment and prejudice prevail.

There are also many groups that provide support for the parents of HIV+ sons and daughters and others for caregivers of people with life-threatening illness. If there's no support group in your area, you could approach the social worker or doctor at your local hospital and express the need for one. Most hospitals within major cities have such groups. Some of these groups are more educational in their function and these can be very beneficial also. However, they're quite different from the kind of group discussed in this chapter. You could begin a group yourself by adapting the guidelines set out here to your particular requirements. You could approach your doctor for the names of other people who might be interested in participating, or ask for the cooperation of the social worker attached to the hospital oncology or immunology department. The important thing is: don't be discouraged; a group of two is still a group. When two or more are gathered in the name of truth and understanding, the spirit and strength of love are always present.

The Quest for Life Foundation is planning to produce a video on the structure and function of support groups. This video will then be used as an educational tool to assist those interested in forming their own groups. For information please write to the Quest for Life Center (see page 368).

Chapter Five

MEDITATION—A KEY TO LIFE

. . . .

Jane

I first found out I was HIV+ in March of 1989. I'll never forget that day—the counselor said matter-of-factly, "It came back positive." I thought, "She's so calm, it must not be a big deal." Then I cried. I met my husband at a beautiful water fountain; he was stunned. I spent the next day or so in a wrenching state of anxiety, thinking of tombstones and epitaphs, trying to get my mind around the fact that my indomitable health (the worst illness I've ever had was the flu) was under threat.

I soon recovered and started going to a women's support group. I mean, my life changed permanently on that day, but the crisis was over. I've always been good at coping with stress and springing back. I found a book called AIDS: A Guide to Survival and started focusing on survival. I've always been a health food person and had good habits of living—exercise, no addictions, normal weight—so I didn't have a lot to change in my lifestyle. (I guess my only real vice was sex—too much of it or in the wrong places.) But I revved it all up, started taking megadoses of vitamin C and lots of other things as well; started learning a lot about holistic approaches to HIV. I immediately changed my attitude to stress and frustration—a luxury I couldn't afford. No more fuming at the traffic; I cultivated a calm, accepting attitude, which has been great as it's made me so much more able to let things be, to let people be, to relax and know that things will work out for the best.

I also started to meditate, about a year ago, to help with stress and because I kept hearing it's good for your immune system. Meditation has brought treasures into my life—peace of mind, great stress resistance, and a renewed sense of spirituality. I talk to God sometimes; I visualize marvelous healing waterfalls and oceans in which I swim, great shafts of light which penetrate my body and being. I feel more and more connected to a larger reality, the cosmos or whatever you want to call it, and it's immensely comforting. It's harder to feel all that if I'm struggling with my body or feeling down, but meditation is like a safe haven.

So while having the AIDS virus has brought things into my life I would never wish for—anxiety, eventual pain, suffering, even death, safe sex (just kidding—I'm getting used to it!), it's also brought great gifts. The first one was getting my family back together: my husband and I had separated while I went on the quest for the perfect man. Now we live together again with our two sons. I have a beautiful place to live, a wonderful job, and social life. All the things I was always chasing. When you're faced with a life-threatening illness, you stop worrying about whether there's something or someone better than you've got. I appreciate the people in my life, my home, the world and all its beauty, just being alive. Life becomes precious. HIV is a good life-threatening illness, if there is such a thing, because it gives you lots of time to learn, to change, to reorder your priorities, and start paying attention to the real things and to all the unfinished business in your life.

I don't know how I'll feel further down the track when I may be ill and struggling hard. I'm seven years into being positive (I think) and going strong, though I work hard at staying healthy every day. I don't assume that I'll get AIDS and die, though I may well. Meditation is helping me be less scared of dying, but I think we always have a choice about whether we focus on the positive.

In the meantime, I try to live life as fully as possible, though it's hard to know what that means sometimes. I feel lucky, really, because I've done so much already—I've traveled the world, been married, single, had two children, lots of lovers (one too many) and adventures. I'm not finished yet, but it's been a hell of a ride. The pace has slowed to more contemplation, more stability. My sexual adventuring is over, *the carefree days are gone, but I've found a more inward kind of adventure that gives me richer satisfaction.*

> *Truth is within ourselves;*
> *It takes no rise from outward things,*
> *Whate'er you may believe.*
> *There is an inmost center in us all,*
> *Where truth abides in fullness.*
> *And to know, rather consists in opening out a way*
> *Whence the imprisoned splendor may escape,*
> *Than in effecting entry for a light supposed to be without.*
> *from "Paracelsus" by Robert Browning*

This verse articulates beautifully the role which meditation can play in our lives. Meditation is indeed one of the golden keys to life. More than any other technique it opens up new vistas of experience and enrichment, awareness and joy. It's simple to practice and its benefits are readily available, even to the novice.

What is Meditation?

Meditation is the state of being fully aware of the present moment. The *practice* of meditation includes any activity which facilitates the experience of being fully aware in the present moment. It has no particular religious connection though it can be a profoundly moving spiritual experience. It depends on what *you* regard as spiritual.

Meditation is simple to learn and with regular practice brings a great sense of well-being. This can range from greater peace of mind to a relaxed body. Meditation also releases energy within the body which can be used for healing. Remember, a good day's worry is far more exhausting than a good day with an ax. After a day with an ax we fall into bed and sleep contentedly. After a day of worry we stumble off to bed and twitch all night.

Stress and Its Effect Upon the Body

We have already seen that when our minds are anxious or stressed our bodies secrete many chemicals and hormones into the bloodstream which inhibit the body's natural functions, decreasing the activities of some while increasing the activities of others. Stress itself isn't a negative thing. It's essential to have stress in our lives. Stress provides us with challenge. By overcoming challenging stresses, we gain satisfaction and fulfillment. However, stress over which we feel we have no control can be very detrimental to our peace of mind and our health. Many people will be able to identify some major stress which occurred in the six months to two years before they experienced any symptoms of their disease, though this time frame is not arbitrary. Sometimes the stress goes back much further, and it has been gradually accumulating until the body's defenses can no longer cope.

Meditation as a Basis for Healing

Meditation can give us the impetus to implement and maintain a program for our healing. It affirms our own inner healing power and it activates the wisdom of healing within our bodies. When you cut yourself, your body quite naturally sets all the necessary processes in action to enable healing to take place. You don't need to panic and think, "Oh goodness, I'd better send down some fibrin and collagen. Don't forget the leucocytes in case there's any bacteria!" It all just happens perfectly naturally. Your body has perfect wisdom within it and knows precisely what's necessary for your health and well-being. All *you* need do is provide the ideal healing environment and, for the rest, trust that healing is taking place.

More than anything else, meditation will give you the finest energy needed for healing. Remember, your mind isn't separate from your body, your emotions aren't separate from your body. As human beings, each of us is an integrated whole. The thoughts which we hold in our minds affect the functioning of

our bodies. The feelings we have, whether acknowledged or ignored, have an effect on our bodies. The thoughts, beliefs and
feelings we hold will dictate *our* experience of reality. Each
person's reality is his or her own. The mind has an extraordinary
capacity to change the thoughts which it holds dear. This gives
us a tremendous point of power in that we can change the
thoughts which cause us stress into those which lay down the
foundations for greater peace, fulfillment, and joy in our lives.
This choice is unique to humankind. All it takes is a little willingness to change our perceptions. To let go fear and experience
the presence of love can become our goal.

Using Meditation as a Tool for Change

There are many techniques of meditation and the best is the one
that works for you. There's no right technique, no higher or
lower technique—nor is there one teacher. There are as many
techniques as there are people. Allow yourself the freedom to
find a technique and a teacher that works for you.

Meditation reestablishes the body's own equilibrium. You'll
notice your breathing begins to slow down, your heart rate and
blood pressure drop. Your muscles relax and physiologically you
come to rest as the mind begins to settle and a sense of ease and
peace is experienced.

Meditation is like relaxation for the mind. It's very simple.
Just as we bring our awareness to the various muscles in our
bodies and allow them to soften and relax, so we observe the
thoughts and feelings which pass through our minds. Observe
and let go. An analogy I often use is that meditation is like sitting deep below the ocean, at rest on the ocean floor. The
thoughts are like waves on the distant surface, each wave dissolving back into stillness. They don't disturb our peace.

Another way to think of meditation is to imagine that your
awareness is the whole vast dome of the sky; thoughts, feelings,
beliefs, judgments, and sensations are like the clouds which drift
across this sky. Some clouds are easy to observe, the way some
thoughts are easy to observe. Others are far more difficult and

the mind wants to leap in and have a good "think." Sometimes the clouds (thoughts) are little white fluffy ones like, What's for dinner? and sometimes they're big steely gray ones like, I get my biopsy results tomorrow! The art and practice of meditation is to keep your awareness as if it were the *whole* sky. These thoughts (clouds) pass through your mind but you don't become lost in the cloud. The moment you forget your awareness and become absorbed in the thought, your vision and perspective become clouded. Observe and let go. If you find you've started being busy with the thoughts, just let them go again. Do the same with feelings which arise, not judging, not criticizing yourself for having them. Let them come, to pass. Observe and let go. Be an ocean of awareness, not focusing on any particular thought or feeling. Be patient with yourself throughout your practice sessions. Treat meditation like a new adventure into unexplored territory: a journey within yourself.

Another favorite image is that of sitting by a gentle river on which logs float continuously. You can choose to focus on each and every log as it drifts by, or you can keep your gaze soft, resting gently in the middle of the river, aware of, but not focusing on, any log in particular as it floats by.

When we physically relax our muscles, we let go of the body. We find that we can simply observe the body and its sensations. Who *is* this observer? Then, by observing the activity in our mind—its chatter, judgments, beliefs, attitudes, thoughts, feelings—we can also let go of the mind. Again, we experience a "witnessing" of the mind. And again, who *is* this observer? One who watches the body, but is *not* the body. One who watches the mind, but is *not* the mind. We realize that we are *not* our personality, *not* our mind. When we're at one with this witness of our body/mind then we experience a profound sense of being. In this simple state of being lies all peace, silence, and bliss.

Meditation and Intuition

One man, Richard, was loath to have radiotherapy and had struggled long and hard with his decision on whether to go

ahead and follow his oncologist's advice. He saw radiotherapy as
a damaging invasion of his body. In his work as a pharmacist, he
was on the periphery of medical treatment and had built up
some very powerful fears about it. In the weeks of indecision,
Richard put into practice many of the techniques mentioned in
this book and he was particularly enjoying his periods of meditation. After several weeks of discussion and looking at his alternatives, he was still trying to think it through. I suggested to him
that he follow the decision-making formula in chapter 3, Should
I or Shouldn't I? (see pages 67-73), and that his answer to
whether he should or shouldn't have radiotherapy would probably come to him when he least expected it. In his words:

"One morning, I woke very early and felt a strong urge to
meditate. I usually meditate on the verandah overlooking the
hills behind our house and quite quickly I fell into a deep state
of meditation. Suddenly I felt the presence of a 'being of light.'
Now, I'm not a particularly religious man, but the feeling that
accompanied this apparition was so wonderful and profoundly
peaceful that I didn't want to stop it. In its hands it had some
equipment, which I took to be a radiotherapy machine (though
I'd never seen one in my life before). This 'being' was offering it
to me and I *physically* felt all my fears drain out of my body.
After this experience, I felt entirely comfortable with the
thought of radiotherapy. The amazing thing was, when I went to
the hospital for my first treatment, the machine looked exactly
as I'd seen it in my meditation!" Meditation gives us the opportunity to heal our minds of their fears, anxieties, and apprehensions. It gives us the chance to *hear* the still small voice within.
Many people find their intuitive powers increase enormously
with the regular practice of meditation. Richard was able to
settle the chatter of his mind sufficiently for a deeper truth to be
heard. Often the mind will present these truths in a symbolic
form.

Frequently the benefits of meditation are not experienced
during the practice itself. Suddenly, while you're driving to work
or in the shower, you'll find you have an answer to something
which has been puzzling you, or you'll know the solution to a

problem you've had for a long time. Inspiration seems to flow more easily and a lightness of spirit seems to pervade your world.

Basic Requirements for Meditation

You'll need three things in order to learn to meditate. The first one is *motivation*. Those of us who have an illness, who feel stressed, panicky, or fearful have all the ingredients necessary to provide motivation! The goal of peace of mind is definitely achievable and you deserve to have it. Second, you'll need to make an *effort* in order to put into practice the techniques of meditation. While thinking about meditation, reading about it, and hearing others' experiences will likely inspire your levels of motivation, *you* will need to put in the effort in order to experience the benefits of its regular practice.

Third, to sustain motivation and effort you'll need *determination*. Sometimes the fire can go out of our practice and with it can go our motivation. There are often dry patches in our practice when our meditations don't seem to be producing any new or exciting information or experiences. At these times, we need to continue quietly with our practice without making judgments or evaluating our performance.

So, How Do I Begin?

There's nothing mysterious attached to learning techniques of meditation and at the end of this chapter you will find one I've used for myself and for many others. You could have a friend read it to you slowly or you might like to make a tape of it so you can play it back to yourself until you're quite familiar with the technique. Alternatively, you can order my own cassette recording of this technique from Dawn Publications (see Cassette Tapes, page 379). The benefit of having someone talk you through the process (as in a cassette tape) is that you're committed to the practice for a prescribed period of time. What often happens, unless our self-discipline is really strong, is that ten minutes or so into the practice we have thoughts like, Hmm, if I put the potatoes in the oven now, they'll be ready when I finish meditating...hmmm, while I'm up, I'll just put the hose on the petunias, and before we know it, we're up and off and we never quite find the time to get back to our meditation.

I suggest you practice these techniques regularly, preferably twice a day as a minimum. You'll need to find out what the ideal length of time is for you; also how frequently you need to meditate in order to feel a real benefit. Some people gain all the benefits in the first ten to fifteen minutes and for them to do a little and often might be best. Avoid falling into the trap of believing meditation is difficult or requires long practice to become effective. It's actually very simple; quite quickly you'll begin to experience the benefits of meditation. Allow your own pattern of meditation to emerge. I find most people can easily start off with two forty-minute sessions of relaxation and meditation per day. After a while it becomes so inviting and enjoyable you might find you need to rearrange your schedule so you can have longer sessions.

Emotions That Bubble to the Surface During Meditation

There are times when meditation brings to your awareness painful issues from the past, or it may allow emotions long held in to flow to the surface and be expressed. Many people find they have tears flowing down their cheeks and yet are unaware of their cause. Often we're in situations where it's inappropriate to express our emotions. Dissolving into tears in the supermarket isn't considered to be appropriate in Western society, and yet it's in just such places that we can be overwhelmed by emotional pain, grief, panic, or other powerful feelings. Meditation gives us the opportunity to release pain, sorrow, and fears from our past. Some people are tempted to stop their meditation at that point, but I encourage them to continue. By continuing the process of healing we're actually able to let go of the pain, which gives us a sense of resolution and tremendous peace.

A dear friend of mine writes:

I've never had any reason to doubt the power of meditation because all my experiences have been of a very powerful nature, with many benefits accruing from my practice.

However, at one point in my life, not my belief but my ability to practice meditation was severely threatened, and at a time when I needed it most. My concentration was at its lowest ebb and all peace was swallowed up by extraneous and damaging thoughts.

My son had died by his own hand—my gentle son had taken his life in a particularly violent manner, and although I could come to some sort of terms with his death, there was no way I could accept the manner of his going. It overshadowed the loss of his presence, the humor we'd shared, the closeness of our deep understanding of each other and left a gaping ache that nothing seemed to assuage.

I knew how desperately I needed to meditate, yet each time I settled myself it was as though a wall of crude colors blocked my mind, robbed me of peace and concentration and, I almost came to believe, my sanity also.

My faith aided me in my acceptance but nothing helped the negation of my heart to the manner of his death. One morning—a real 'end of the tether' morning, quite desperate for peace, I began to meditate. What followed was a terrifying swirl of frightening colors, murky greens, burnt oranges, forbidding gray and black—the power of the surging movement of these cloud-like forces held me in thrall. But suddenly, it began to change. The murky green, orange, gray, and black colors were lightening to palest blue, golden yellow, tranquil soft gray—the black all gone. All the gentle colors I think of as 'harmonious' took over, the movement gone, the peace and stillness tangible.

As I came out of this meditation, the peace and stillness remained and I felt totally free.

I've never experienced those feelings of dread since; I was totally cleansed of the horror. It was wonderful to get back to the wholesome working through of grief and to come out the other side with a 'uniting' and reidentification with my son.

Meditation and the Art of Living

Indeed, ultimately, meditation becomes a way of life, of living. We begin to live all parts of our life with awareness. In this way, we're aware of the patterns of the past, the habitual responses, the fears and apprehensions for the future and have the opportunity to release them as we live each unfolding moment. Meditation gives us the possibility of being fully present in each moment. The mind is always projecting into the future or chewing over the past. We must strive to be right here, right now, not regretting the past or anticipating the future. Just being here, now. Life is made up of many moments. In order to look back at life from our deathbed, whether we're 33 or 103, and be able to say, "What a fantastic life that was. I know I *really* lived and gave it my darnedest!" we have to actually *be* here!

Some of the benefits of meditation you'll notice include a certain calmness in your attitude, and the things which used to distress you will become inconsequential. Your memory will improve and so will your powers of concentration. You'll also find you're able to accomplish more in your day, you'll have more energy, and you might find you need less sleep. The sleep you do have will likely be deeper and more refreshing.

Where Should I Meditate?

It's a good idea to establish a place of meditation in your home. A room set aside for the purpose is great, and yet a corner of a room is ample also. Wear loose and comfortable clothing which doesn't restrict your breathing in any way. You could make this corner or room special by placing an uplifting picture of nature, or some fresh flowers there. For those who have any spiritual or religious leanings, an appropriate picture or symbol might help to instill a calm attitude. For some, a cross or rosary is appropriate. You'll probably find you're more comfortable in an upright chair which supports your head. Feel free to supplement your sitting position with cushions.

After a time you'll find you begin to relax and become calm

as soon as you enter that quiet and special place. If you share
your home with someone else you could ask for his or her cooperation at the times when you choose to meditate. Or you could
encourage your roommate to join with you in your practice. It
doesn't matter that there are sounds around you, though it's preferable to practice in a quiet environment. You might like to leave
a note on the door asking not to be disturbed, and take the telephone off the hook. Why not let your friends know that you
practice meditation at certain times each day? Tell them you
consider it to be really important in assisting you in your recovery and ask for their cooperation in not visiting or telephoning
you at those times. You could invite them to join you in your
practice. If you do need to break your meditation, it's not a problem. Just take a couple of long deep breaths, open your eyes,
stretch, get up slowly and attend to whatever you need, knowing
you'll easily resume the depth of meditation when you return.

The Hallmarks of Meditation

Some people worry about the technique, experience, or "pro-
foundness" of their meditation. You might wonder how you will
know if you're meditating.

- *The mind becomes much quieter than usual.*
- *Your breathing becomes very light.*

If that's happening, trust you *are* meditating. You'll find it
helpful to begin your sessions with some deep breathing. Begin
with some long slow deep breaths to release any tension and to
bring about a sense of calm and stillness. If you have any difficulty with breathing or coughing, work comfortably within your
particular limitations. Sometimes, when concentrating on their
breathing, people find that they begin to cough. For these
people, it's best to focus their attention on the rising and falling
of the abdomen, or right at the entrance of their nostrils, where
the air enters the body.

For How Long Should I Meditate?

Meditate for just as long as you enjoy it, and gently begin to stretch the *boundaries*. Don't give yourself negative messages about the length of time you "should" meditate. You're completely unique and only *you* will know the appropriate length of time for your meditation sessions. You might have read that you need to meditate for three hours a day for it to have any real healing benefit, and yet perhaps you know that's quite impossible or undesirable for you. *Trust* your own knowledge about yourself.

You'll probably need to plan a program for yourself when you first begin. For instance, you might want to begin with two twenty-minute sessions per day. You'll need to have the three requirements firmly in place to achieve the best results, that is, motivation, effort, and determination.

Most people are amazed at how quickly time passes when they're in a deep state of relaxation/meditation. Even people new to our groups find that a forty-five-minute session poses no difficulty at all for them. Treat meditation as a wonderful adventure into a new and unexplored world. If you can maintain a childlike curiosity about the process of meditation you'll experience all of its many benefits.

You're simply aiming to achieve a state of complete alertness while deeply relaxed.

The Use of Mantras

Eastern religions which are based on meditative practices have traditionally used focus words or phrases called mantras. The Sanskrit word or words which make up a mantra have a spiritual meaning. The benefit of practicing with a mantra is that it gives the mind something to focus on instead of being invaded by the idle chatter which the mind is usually heir to. The words can be "attached" to the breath so that they're silently repeated in the mind with each inward and outward breath. You might wish to experiment with a Sanskrit mantra, or you could choose something which has meaning to you. It isn't necessary to understand the meaning of the words used. In fact, not understanding the words can be beneficial because the mind has no association with them which might encourage mental activity. Here are a few common Sanskrit mantras.

- *Om Shanti.*
- *Sri Ram (pronounced Shree Rahm).*
- *Om Namah Shivaya.*
- *Ham Sah (pronounced Hum Sah).*

There are, of course, Christianity-based mantras also.

- *Lord, have mercy upon me.*
- *My soul doth magnify the Lord.*
- *Hail Mary, Mother of God.*
- *The Kingdom of Heaven is within.*
- *Lord have mercy, Christ have mercy.*
- *Gloria inexcelsior Deo.*
- *Let go and let God.*

You can use any word or phrase from the Bible, or prayer book, or a prayer of your own making. Mantras are used as a *technique* to enter into a state of meditation. The repetition of the manta is *not* the aim of your practice. It is a tool by which you enter into the realm of peace and stillness.

Yantras

Like a mantra, a yantra is a device which will help to focus the mind so that you can enter a state of meditation. A yantra is a symbol which represents spiritual laws. One which most people would recognize is the symbol drawn by Leonardo da Vinci of a man standing in the shape of a cross superimposed over the form of another man with legs and arms outstretched in triangles. That man stands within a circle which is surrounded by a square.

Highly intricate and decorated mandalas are designed for the same purpose. They give the mind something upon which to rest and in which to become absorbed.

The symbol of the cross can be used in a similar way. Many religious groups have symbols which utilize the cross: for instance, a square within which is a circle. Inside the circle is a triangle and, within that, a cross. These symbols can be drawn upon a piece of paper or a white board and then you simply allow the eyes to rest upon the shape and form, perhaps while practicing some breathing technique. Other objects which can be used in the same way are candles, religious medallions, flowers, scenes from nature, or even a spot on the wall—in fact any object upon which the eye can rest without creating a lot of activity in the mind. This is, by its very nature, an open-eye meditation.

Breath Meditations

Many meditation techniques focus on the breath. By simply focusing all of our awareness on observing the way the breath flows in and out of the body, we are brought into the present moment. You don't have to do anything to your breathing. Simply allow it to flow softly in, softly out.

Some people focus their awareness right at the entrance to their nostrils, others might wish to focus on the rising and falling of their abdomen. If you have a problem with constant coughing, it's better to focus upon the gentle movement of the abdomen. You might find that to focus on your breathing will cause you agitation; in which case, use another technique. After a short period of focusing on the breath, you'll notice that your breathing slows right down and becomes more shallow. This is because your body is beginning to relax deeply. This means you require less oxygen and that your metabolism is slowing down. You may get a sense of "the air breathing you" rather than you breathing the air.

If you are feeling agitated, you might like to practice the Quick Release Technique.

1. *Take a deep breath in and then breathe out with a long sigh. Drop your shoulders.*
2. *Relax your face and forehead, and release your jaw.*
3. *Keep your breathing calm and easy.*

Counting to the Breath

Another valuable way of stilling the mind is to count each breath. This can be done in a number of ways.

Technique 1

With this technique you count one on the inward breath, two on the outward breath, three on the next inward breath, four ... and so on until you reach ten and begin once more at one.

Technique 2

This is very similar to the previous technique. However, you start at one hundred, and count back to one. If the mind wanders, gently bring it back to one hundred and begin again. Don't fall into the trap of giving yourself a hard time because you lose count, become absorbed in other thoughts, forget completely what you were doing—that is entirely normal! That is why these techniques have been designed: to help to discipline and control the mind.

Technique 3

With this technique you count with each inward and outward breath. For instance, you might like to start by counting to four with each inward breath, hold for four and release to the count of four. This can gradually be extended to six, then eight and so on until you reach your comfortable limit.

One of my favorite times to use this technique is when I'm walking along the beach (or elsewhere). I breathe in to the count of four footsteps, hold for four steps, and breathe out to the count of four further steps. Again, I can gradually increase this so that I breathe in to the count of ten steps and so on.

Technique 4

Another old favorite, which works particularly well if there is a lot of agitation in the mind, is to imagine there's a small bowl of very fine ash just below your nostrils and that your breath should not disturb the ash. This technique quietens the breath rapidly and centers the mind.

You'll probably benefit by beginning with the Quick Release Technique before you practice any of these four exercises.

There are other suggestions about breathing in chapter 9, (see page 270-274).

Music

Many people find that relaxing music, played very quietly in the background, is an excellent way to enter into a state of deep meditation. Other people find music a distraction. Experiment until you find what works best for you. As with a mantra, music is a tool or an addition to another technique, used in order to enter a state of meditation. Some people find listening to a piece of classical music leads them to a state of stillness. The sole purpose of the music should be to lead you to that place of stillness. To *listen* to the music is not the aim of meditation. To go beyond the music to the stillness from which it arises *is* the aim.

There are shops which specialize in relaxation music while most New Age bookstores or health food stores have a smaller selection.

Group Meditation

Most people find they have a much deeper experience of meditation when they practice with a group. I would highly recommend you attend several sessions with a group until you have the feel for what meditation is. If there are no groups in your area, you'll probably find the use of a cassette tape with a guided meditation invaluable in helping you to establish your practice. Remember, also, that at *any* time you sit down to meditate, you're joining with thousands of others around the world who likewise are entering their inner sanctuary. This joining with others can be both comforting and empowering, especially at those times when you feel isolated and alone.

Meditation in the Midst of Crisis

Many people have used their meditation technique at traumatic times. For example, they've meditated and been able to remain completely relaxed during bronchoscopies, lumbar punctures, colonoscopies, endoscopies. Some have taken their tapes and headphones into operating rooms in hospitals. The sound of a familiar voice and technique can bring comfort and reassurance when we're in unfamiliar surroundings. Remember, it is easier to practice with the *little* crises in life before embarking on the major ones.

Falling Asleep When Meditating

Our bodies are conditioned to fall asleep when we close our eyes and concentrate on letting go, so it might take a little time before we overcome this reaction. It's therefore preferable to learn these techniques sitting comfortably upright in a chair with arms and legs uncrossed, or cross-legged on a cushion on the floor. For those who are particularly unwell or who are on medication that makes it more difficult to remain alert and awake, this can be a problem. But remember, your body could very well need this deep and relaxed sleep and you'll still be benefiting for your practice. Normally when we go to sleep, it takes five hours to drift through our various sleep levels and to reach our deep sleep stage. We stay in this deep sleep stage for a relatively short period of time and then begin to ascend through the levels once more. In your deep sleep stage, your brain waves are in the alpha wave pattern. At night, those who are unwell, in pain, restless, or need to get up frequently to go to the bathroom, might never get five continuous hours of sleep, thereby missing out on their deep sleep. Within five minutes' practice of meditation or relaxation, your brain wave is in the alpha wave pattern and, if you fall asleep during that time, you immediately enter your deep sleep level. This is, of course, tremendously beneficial. Many people find that by going to bed with the intention of falling asleep and with a relaxation tape playing, they are able to find deep and restful sleep immediately.

Some people become very frustrated when they fall asleep regularly during their meditation practice, but all is not lost. You're still receiving something which is of tremendous value to you. You might find you're better able to schedule your meditation times when you are refreshed. For instance, meditate when you've freshened up after a sleep or rest, or first thing in the morning.

For Those Who Need to Wake Up!

For those who aren't in pain or on medication and who still fall asleep, the situation is different! *You* might need to change your position or your attitude, sit more upright, or put your feet in an ice bucket! Find a way to discipline your mind to be alert during your practice. This kind of chronic falling asleep usually has something behind it, perhaps not wanting to let go, perhaps a reluctance to wake up and live. Explore and experiment. It's preferable to make your regular practice at times when you're feeling refreshed and *before* you've eaten rather than after. Trying to meditate after a big meal, when you're very tired, while sitting on the edge of the bed in your pajamas, with the electric blanket sending out waves of welcome, is courting disaster. If meditation is to be a valuable tool in your healing then give it the priority it deserves. You will never *find* the time to meditate. You will definitely have to *make* the time.

Meditating When in Pain

For those who are uncomfortable or in pain, it might be preferable to lie down. Use cushions to support your body in a position as pain free as possible. Many people find these techniques tremendously valuable in dealing with their pain. There's much more on pain and its management in chapter 9, Beyond Pain (see pages 252-279).

Physical Considerations

For others, I suggest settling comfortably into your chair and allowing your feet to rest flat upon the floor. You could place a cushion beneath your feet if they only just reach the floor. Remove your shoes if you wish. Allow your spine to be as comfortably erect as possible so that you're not slouching in the chair. Loosen your belt or any tight or restrictive clothing. Let your hands rest comfortably in your lap in a position where they won't slide off and distract you.

Many people experience "strange" sensations within their bodies when they practice techniques of meditation. Some people find that their arms, legs, or other body parts feel like they've become enormous, numb, itchy, or that they've lost touch with their bodies altogether. Others find they have a "spinning" sensation or a "tilt" to one side. Some experience waves of warmth, temperature changes, or sweats. All of these sensations are quite normal. Some people find they become frightened of letting go of control. You'll likely experience a sense of letting go of the body, then a letting go of the mind, its activity, and chatter. This is the beginning of deep meditation. This happens when we let go of who we think we are, and we simply experience a sense of awareness or consciousness which is beyond personality, body, thoughts, beliefs, or desires.

Light-Headedness

Some people whose hemoglobin or blood pressure is low might experience a sense of light-headedness or nausea. It's recommended that these people lie down for their meditation practice. Meditation is known to lower your blood pressure. If, after the completion of your meditation, you feel a little light-headed, give yourself plenty of time to stretch and arise from your practice in a leisurely manner. Don't go suddenly from lying down to standing up. Slowly sit up, dangle and rotate your feet, stretch, breathe deeply, and gradually return to your activities. If you find that you experience nausea during your practice, then take the precautions mentioned under nausea in chapter 8, Burps, Burning, and the Dreaded Bloats (see pages 230-242), before you begin your practice.

Those who have been taking medication for elevated blood pressure often find that within weeks of commencing a meditation program they become dizzy and light-headed either during, or immediately after, their practice. If this happens, return to your prescribing physician, as it's very likely you no longer require the same level of medication.

Restlessness and Agitation

Some people become very agitated or restless and find it difficult to remain still throughout their practice. For these people, it's worth exploring *why* they're restless. The most common cause is a fear of letting go of control. Many of us are frightened of letting go into the unknown. We often feel safer if we can tell ourselves we're in control. I encourage you to experiment, be adventurous, take risks, and trust in the spirit within yourself, rather than trust in your mind.

Sometimes, we discover who we *are* by discovering who we are *not*.

If, when doing the practice included at the end of this chapter, you need to lie down because you have a problem which makes it too difficult to remain in a sitting position, then do so. If you need to scratch, cough, stretch, or shift position during your practice, then do so and return to your practice. If you need to have a glass of water nearby, have it! Don't turn your practice into a battle!

It's better to meditate with an empty stomach, since much of your energy goes into digesting its contents if you've recently eaten.

Making Comparisons

Avoid comparing one meditation session with another. You might have a truly profound experience one time and then make the mistake of comparing all subsequent meditation practices with *that* one. Allow each meditation session to be whole and complete in itself. Don't fall into the trap of evaluating each meditation practice.

Deep Meditation

It isn't unusual for people to feel a deep reluctance to leave their meditative state. Sometimes coming back into an awareness of one's body feels like putting on a very heavy overcoat. We need to bring ourselves out of meditation very gently and respectfully.

Twice during my recovery, I received hands-on healing from a group of charismatic Catholics in Italy. On each occasion I went into a profound state of meditation. The first time lasted for four and a half hours, the second time longer still. I was sitting in a chapel which formed the basement of a large home outside the town of Sorrento. I was intensely aware of everything which was happening in the rooms above where I was sitting: aware of people, conversations, laughter, the weather and, at the same time, was riveted to the spot by pure bliss. I didn't feel like ever returning to my previous existence and it took quite some time before I was fully able to "reenter" my body. These experiences provided a solid platform from which I was able to see the truth about myself. Through this knowledge I could more clearly see the fears that I needed to relinquish in order for that truth to be more fully present. During the years since these "healings," I've been able to experience similar states each time I meditate deeply.

The Trap of Expectations

Having said all of that, I suggest that you endeavor to let go of any expectations you might have of meditation. Don't evaluate your practice. Some people expect to hear the Hallelujah chorus with a choir of ten thousand angels! Sometimes we *have* such experiences, but the surest way to sabotage an openness to each unfolding moment is to hold an expectation of what it *should* contain.

Above all else, be compassionate toward yourself in your practice of meditation. Don't fall into the trap of unrealistic standards, lengths of time, or depth of practice.

The practice of meditation is not sitting there with a still mind. It's not the nature of the mind to be still. Meditation is the state of being fully alive in the present moment, fully aware, fully conscious in each unfolding moment, not projecting into the future nor chewing over the past, nor holding any expectations. Being here, now. When that is your experience, you will witness the thoughts dissolving into stillness. In this stillness resides profound peace.

There is no more worthwhile or rewarding adventure than to discover who you are. Allow yourself the pleasure of the experience.

The following technique is the one I've used with many people who are learning the simple skills of meditation. Although the skill is a simple one, it does take consistent practice to achieve all of its benefits. Remember, the following meditation can be read very slowly by a friend, put on to a cassette tape, or it's available on tape from Dawn Publications (see Cassette Tapes, page 379).

Find a position that's comfortable for you, preferably sitting or lying down. Begin by taking some long, slow, deep breaths as you allow your eyes to close over gently. Breathing in relaxation, breathing out all tension in your body and in your mind. Soft, open, deep breaths that help you settle in to your body.

Set aside all the roles that you normally play among your family, friends, and at work. Devote this next little while just to yourself. Really being in touch with yourself ... to create an environment for peace. And allow your breathing to return to its own natural rhythm. Bring your awareness to your feet. To the soles of your feet. Feeling the sensations which arise. Where there's pressure, where there's space. And to the tops of your feet. The touch of the air. The texture or pressure of anything touching the skin on the tops of your feet.

Then bring your awareness to your toes. Beginning with the big toes. And to the next. And next and so on down to the little toes. Letting the muscles soften and relax. Take your mind deep within your feet. To all the muscles, tendons, and ligaments. Each strand of muscle softening. Becoming warm and comfortable. Allow your ankles to be loose. And the muscles of your calves to soften. Just hanging from the bones. Let your knees be relaxed. And the muscles of your thighs, let them soften and spread.

Feel the chair or the floor against the backs of your legs. The touch of your clothing against your thighs.

Relax your buttocks. Just let them spread. Cushioning and supporting you without any tension.

Let your abdomen gently rise and fall at your own rhythm. Take your awareness deep within your abdomen. Let each organ float in its own soft warm space. Let that warmth flow deep within your pelvis. Let it spread up into your solar plexus and tummy. If you notice any tightness in your solar plexus, visualize it as a pond and see a pebble dropped right into its center. And see those ripples of relaxation flowing out from its center, softening and soothing. And on into your chest. Feel each small movement as your rib cage expands and contracts with each breath. Let the air do the breathing for you. Allow your heart to be open and warm and soft.

Let go of all unnecessary tension in your shoulders. Perhaps visualize two gentle hands resting on your shoulders that absorb any tension there and that send waves of relaxation down and across your back. Down through your upper arms into the elbows and forearms.

Let your hands rest quietly in your lap. You might find they become very heavy or very light as you relax even more deeply. Whichever feels right for you. Let your wrists be relaxed. And your hands at rest. Each of the muscles softening, releasing all tension. Right down into your fingertips. Perhaps you find they begin to pulsate or tingle with the soft presence of relaxation.

Allow your throat to be open and relaxed. Letting go all unnecessary tension in your neck. If you're sitting visualize your head floating like a balloon at the top of a string. As if your spine were the string. Letting it float up toward the ceiling till it finds its own perfect balance.

Let your lower jaw drop just a little. Enough to let your teeth part. Allow your tongue to be soft in your mouth. Soft lips. Cheeks. All the little muscles around your eyes smoothing out and softening. Smoothing away all tension. And deep behind your eyes, let go any straining, any trying to see. Allow the space between your eyebrows to widen as your forehead relaxes. Your temples and ears. The whole of your scalp. So that the whole of your body becomes deeply calm and relaxed. Every breath you take helps you to relax even more deeply. Any sounds around you are familiar and there's no need to judge or criticize or even to label the sounds. Let the sounds share each moment with you. A soft openness. Now bring your awareness back to the toes, the feet, and ankles. Allow the feet to fill with a soft silence. Filling silently with space. Breathing in space. The stillness expanding.

Flowing softly up through the calves of the legs. The knees filling with stillness. The thighs. Soaking in spaciousness. Softness. Let that silence flow into the hips and buttocks. A deep silence. A spaciousness. Soft openness. The abdomen filling with space and silence. Each organ resting in great quietness. Feel it spreading into the solar plexus. The stomach softly opening to stillness. Each breath bringing stillness into the body. As if the air breathes for you. The lungs full of a vast silence. The heart resting softly, cradled in peace. The spine dissolving into stillness. No holding. Only peace. Space. Shoulders filled with soft openness. Let that softness flow down through the arms into the hands and fingers. Filling with a soft awareness. A vast stillness. Silence filling the body. The mind full of ease and peace. Allow the throat to fill with space. The neck relaxing into stillness. Sensations floating through stillness. Each sensation coming to pass. The jaw softening and opening. The muscles of the face slowly dissolving into great stillness. Behind the face. Letting go into silence. Soft openness. The body melting into silence. Dissolving into spaciousness. Boundaries dissolving. No resistance. Mind and thought melting into peace. Mind and body, floating in peace and stillness. Each cell, cradled in warmth and peace. The awareness floating free in this great stillness. Softly opening to each unfolding moment. Resting gently in this vast silence. Surrender into soft silence. No holding. No resistance. Letting go of the particular. Each thought dissolving into spaciousness. Soft silence.

Take a long pause.

Become aware of your breathing again. Allow it to deepen. Each breath drawing energy into your body. Bring your awareness back in to your body. Feel the muscle tone returning to your arms and legs. Begin moving your hands and feet just a little. And as you continue to breathe deeply, feel all of the energy coming back into your body. And begin to stretch. Using every muscle in your body. Enjoying the refreshment and relaxation in every muscle of your body. And in your own time, bring all of your awareness back into your body, back into the room. And just as you're ready, gently allow the eyes to open again. Bringing that calm, that peace with you. Spend some time just sitting quietly, until you're ready to go about your activities.

The Quest for Life Foundation is planning to produce a video which will give clear guidance in learning techniques of meditation. For more information, please write to the Quest for Life Center (see page 368).

Chapter Six

IN MY MIND'S EYE

. . . .

Jeanette

The diagnosis of secondary melanoma tumors in my lungs and liver was devastating. How could this be? They told me if all was clear for five years after the primary melanoma was removed, I'd be fine. They didn't tell me that in ten years my whole world would be shattered and I'd fall apart.

What a dreadful time it was for me and my family. The feeling we all had at first was only doom and gloom but with the love and support of my grown-up children and my wonderful husband, and the incredible attitude of my doctors that where there's life there's always hope, I came to believe that cancer isn't necessarily a death sentence— only if you want it to be.

I'm very fortunate to have an oncology specialist who has a remarkable outlook on the powers of positive thinking, meditation, diet and vitamins, so I embarked on a complete change of lifestyle and introduced all of the above into my daily routine.

How could I let this life-threatening disease get the better of me. I'm forty-six years old with the most wonderful husband in the world—how could I leave him and my beautiful loving children? At first all I could think of was that it was all over for me. When would it happen, and how on earth could they survive without me? I don't know if my tears were for myself or for them, and I cried day and night for weeks with this horrible feeling in the pit of my stomach.

After the first three months, I had further scans, and the news was a miracle—the tumors in my liver had completely disappeared and the other was possibly shrinking. We were all crying again and this time for this wondrous miracle! This was the first time that I realized I must get on with my life and live it to the fullest. Of course there was hope—there has to be, and there was!

I continued with my program for maintaining my good health and three months later the scans showed once again a miracle—the small tumors in both lungs had disappeared, leaving only two, one of which was much smaller. I feel so good and positive about myself when the news is good, and then I get a small tumor which appears under the skin and has to be removed and I go down in a heap again. This has happened twice in the last twelve months and no matter how positive I am, I get very distressed and it takes some time for me to become motivated again.

My life has changed, I know, for the better. I take each day as it comes, make the most of every day and spend as much time with my family as possible, I don't know what's in store for me for the future, but does anyone? My life is more calm and peaceful than before and I only do what I want, not what is expected of me. It's important to become No. 1, even if it means being selfish. I have to be on my toes constantly with my positive thinking, diet, meditation, and it isn't always easy. My doctor says "You're only human," and a little splurge now and then doesn't hurt—it's better to give in than to be miserable!

Since diagnosis, I've had friends who haven't been able to communicate with me and I find these are negative people and I don't need them in my life. Being around positive people gives me a boost and makes me feel confident and more like my old self again. So now I pick and choose whom I want to see. In twelve months I've come a long way—I lead a completely normal life and my program for good health and fighting disease is routine.

I have days when I don't feel so good about myself, but I only have to look at my family and my strength seems to regenerate. My aim is to feel happy and good about myself every day, and I know that day will come. In the meantime, I thank God for the blessing of each new day.

As human beings we have a truly remarkable ability in that we can change whatever thoughts we hold in our minds. We can be the masters of our own minds by changing our thoughts, attitudes, and beliefs. Thoughts are powerful and we have countless thousands of them every day. Even though we think we're in control of our lives, we're often plagued by the incessant activity of the mind. We can't remember a time in our lives when we didn't have thoughts. They drift through in a constant stream. We underestimate the power these thoughts have over our lives.

If we've programmed our mind with negative images and thoughts then the mind will accept those thoughts as being true. With understanding and patience those thoughts and images can be altered and a more healthy way of looking at things developed.

The key to thought control is *habit*. Are you aware of the thoughts you most frequently hold? Do you habitually expect the best or worst in any situation? Do you hold judgment or criticisms of your family, friends, and associates—see them through an habitual veil of judgment?

Begin to observe the thoughts which you hold in your mind. Sometimes you'll have to be very quick to catch them. The Indian teachers have long described the mind as "a wild drunk monkey swinging through tree tops." To tame the monkey and keep it on a leash can become our aim. Anyone who sets out to tame the mind will be rewarded.

Some people are worriers. They weren't born that way, they gradually developed—probably through childhood or adolescence. If there isn't something going on in their lives to worry about, they feel insecure and will often create a worry, just so they can be comfortable with their usual thinking patterns.

Some people expect to be successful at whatever they attempt. And, not surprisingly, they are. The only thing the worriers are usually successful at is—you guessed it—worrying! What's more, when their worries are well founded, they almost celebrate because the premise by which they live their lives has been proven right.

There are others who always expect to fail. And they do. If

you have an expectation of failure, then it's very likely you won't put all your enthusiasm and effort into whatever project is at hand. It's a self-perpetuating mechanism which ensures your thinking is "true." This truth you hold about yourself is not a fixed law for you unless you choose to make it so. It's entirely up to you whether you're willing to make the effort to change. No one else can do it for you. Only you can create the reality which you choose to experience.

Nature abhors a vacuum. So if we're unhappy about the way we feel and we choose to eliminate certain behavior patterns which cause us distress, it's imperative we have something strong and positive to put in the place of those thoughts which we choose to discard. We need to *want* to change our negative and constricting ideas to ones of positive receptivity, vitality, abundant health, or whatever it is we desire.

Imagination is a powerful tool we can use for this purpose. It's not enough for us to say we wish we weren't so negative about something. Often the negative program by which we're living has been in our subconscious since infancy, so to eradicate such deeply held notions requires real dedication.

For many people, change is a frightening thing. The familiar is comfortable. Our negative thoughts are "ours" and sometimes we'll go to great lengths to protect them, even when they're damaging to us or, at the very least, causing us stress. Sometimes we hold on to these old patterns of thinking because that was the way our mother or father always thought.

Sometimes there's no good reason for our actions. The thoughts which empower them just happen to be habitual. Likewise, we can find an appropriate solution to one situation but then foist that same solution on to a totally different circumstance where it could be entirely inappropriate. Perhaps you were shut in your bedroom for an extended period of time as a young child, and now in adulthood you find enclosed spaces confining or stressful. Or perhaps when eating fish one time, a bone became stuck in your throat and frightened you, so that was the last fish meal! Each of us has our own collection of "truths." The situation which first prompted our truth might no

longer even be remembered, but we live out our lives according
to the decisions we made at that time. These decisions can be
far more crippling than the choice never to eat fish again. If we
failed once we might hold the subtle programming in our mind
which says, "I'll never make it," or "My life is a mess," or simply,
"I'm a failure." Other subtle negative programs might chant into
our minds thoughts like:

- *"No one really understands me."*
- *"I'm so disappointed in myself."*
- *"I wish I was someone else."*
- *"I'll never get it right."*
- *"I don't deserve to be happy."*
- *"I can't finish anything."*
- *"I don't deserve a good relationship."*
- *"I'm worthless."*
- *"I don't deserve love."*
- *"I don't deserve to live."*
- *"My life is useless."*

Michael was brought up in a small country town and attended the local school which had only one teacher in charge of
kindergarten class through year six. He was a quiet, sensitive
boy who loved music but who wasn't much interested in foot-
ball. His teacher seemed to take a dislike to him from the start,
and for the seven years he was at that school his teacher regularly told him, "You'll never amount to anything!"

Such damage is difficult to heal. In fact, it wasn't until he
was sick and in his thirties that he even began to deal with the
impact those words had had on his life. Up until his illness, he
lived those words twenty-four hours a day. *Then*, he began to
fight for his life. Not just against the disease but against the
long history of only partly living.

Perhaps, in some cases, sickness is the body's cry of distress over self-imposed emotional suffering? These negative thoughts and the feelings they generate will dictate how we *see* that disease and other aspects of life. I haven't seen much benefit experienced from claiming responsibility for *creating* disease, although some people feel that if they created their disease then they're in a position to "recreate" health.

I believe we can always take responsibility for our response to having an illness.

Visualization techniques or guided imagery provide one of the most powerful tools for changing the negative programming in our minds. They use our imagination in a powerful way which can actually bring about physiological changes in our bodies. This approach is a means of communicating with the autonomic processes which occur without our conscious awareness. We have no consciousness of the functioning of our immune system, yet it's still busy about its work without our active participation. Although you might be unaware of it, you're already familiar with the techniques of visualization. Throughout your life, whenever thoughts of an ice cream, going for a swim, taking a shower, or any of the many activities of a lifetime come into your mind, a brief picture of that event flashes through. You need to be quick sometimes to catch it, but sure enough it's happened.

Some people are more visually oriented than others. Some spend hours fantasizing or daydreaming; some claim it's better than the real thing! Spend a moment thinking about a holiday on a beautiful tropical island. Think of the golden sands, the vibrant colors in the waters surrounding the island, the vast clear blue dome of the sky above, the palms swaying in a soft, cooling breeze, the sound of the waves flowing gently in gently out. Probably, at the very least, you experienced flashes of colors and isolated images even while just reading the words. Our more visual readers would perhaps have experienced much more. Some probably even smelt the sea air, heard the gentle ebb and flow of the waves, and felt the sand beneath their feet! There will be others who found that while reading even these few sentences they gave a long sigh and became slightly more relaxed.

Try another one. Let the image of a lemon, cut into quarters, come into your mind. Now, in your mind's eye, see yourself biting deeply into one of the quarters. You can feel the cool juice running through your mouth. Its astringent freshness waking up your taste buds. What happened? Did you produce a lot of saliva in your mouth? Here's another. A blackboard with a teacher standing beside it. She looks at you with a mischievous gleam in her eye as she scrapes her long fingernails down the board from top to bottom. What happened that time? This last example probably produced strongly felt but less tangible sensations in your body. An overall shiver perhaps?

These examples demonstrate in a very simple way the connection between your mind and your body. When we hold positive, healing thoughts in our mind every cell "feels" the confidence and caring that such thoughts bring. Science has now identified many of the chemicals and hormones secreted by the brain that are produced in direct response to these thoughts and feelings. You can send soothing and comforting thoughts and feelings out to needy areas of your body by holding in your mind some suitable image that's calming, and letting the effects of that image flow out. So, also, you can create a dynamic and vibrant feeling throughout your body by holding a more powerful image. The development of skills in this area is a major strength in our ability to heal ourselves.

Bernie Siegel, an American cancer surgeon, has written extensively on the research into the mind/body connection. His two books, *Love, Medicine and Miracles* and *Peace, Love and Healing* are brimful of case histories and are valuable reading for people with any disease.

In Western society, we tend to look for and believe the bad news rather than the good. When we visit the doctor, we put on our supersensitive ears so we don't miss a thing he or she says. We strain to hear the intonation, the emphasis, the choice of words. Usually by the time we leave, we can't remember much of what the doctor did say, and yet we'll certainly remember any negative intonation. Some doctors will still talk about a "time limit" for their patients. To be told, "You won't see Christmas," or "You've got three to six months" is a great shock to your whole being. We have so many people in our groups who are running late for their own funerals that it's convinced me we should never presuppose how long a patient will live. In one group of eighteen people with life-threatening diseases, from newly diagnosed onward, I asked how many were running late for their funerals. Twelve of them responded positively (and enthusiastically!); the rest were diagnosed fairly recently and either hadn't been given a time limit or hadn't yet reached it. It always amazes me when people say their doctor has given them three months. In reality, the doctor hasn't given them anything at all. The doctor's taken away the possibility of the rest of their life!

A doctor can still explain to us that we're very ill—without giving a specific time frame. He or she could even say, "Tom, the kind of illness you have is very serious. Many people with your kind of cancer die. It's very difficult to put a time frame on it because it will depend on your own constitution, your response to treatment, and a whole host of other factors. Some people who have this kind of cancer die quite quickly. However, there are others who seem to survive a long time, and still others who attain a remission. Often we don't understand why that is so but we want to do everything we can to help you become one of the ones who attains a remission. We won't know how *you* will do until we start treatment." *This* answer is truthful. Another doctor could have said, "Tom, the kind of cancer you have is incurable. We don't expect you to be here for Christmas." Don't laugh! This has frequently been said to people. Which doctor would you prefer? Dr. Possibility or Dr. Death?

A fifteen-year-old girl was doing her best to withstand the cancer she'd been fighting for two years. She told her doctor she was keeping a positive attitude, eating as well as she could, and meditating. His response? "None of those things are going to make the slightest bit of difference!" *Why* is it necessary to say such things? Most kids would have thrown in the towel, but not Michelle. She was tearful and would have loved him to encourage her with her efforts but she continued with her determination to give life her best shot despite his wet-blanket approach.

Dr. Possibility could refer us to a support group of people who are in a similar situation and who are doing their darnedest to live. He or she could suggest we learn some techniques of meditation and encourage us to have a look at the stresses in our lives to see if we can resolve or dispense with them. He or she could encourage us to optimize our nutrition and take some supplements to help us over the time when the treatment will knock us around. He or she could even put us in touch with someone with the same kind of cancer who *is* in remission. Then we'd feel this person *really* wanted to help us to live. As patients, we'd feel important to our doctor and know that he or she respected the fact that we have a part to play in our healing. I'd certainly want *that doctor* on my healing team! We need to move away from the statistical approach and be more concerned with the individual. Every doctor knows of the exceptional patient who didn't slot into the statistical framework he or she was "meant to." It requires a lot of courage to put aside the medical predictions and put all efforts into living and healing. I believe sometimes the doctor's words cut so deeply into their patients that they're unable to muster any positivity within themselves. All hopes are dashed and often these people die exactly when the doctor said they would. The truth is there's *always* hope, no matter what the statistics show.

AIDS is teaching us much about this. A few years ago, doctors predicted that once a patient had developed full AIDS he or she wouldn't survive more than eighteen months to two years. Now we have hundreds of long-term survivors. These are people who developed full AIDS more than five years ago. Surely doctors must feel encouraged to see these people making the most of their lives and being rewarded for their efforts?

The reason I've spent quite a time on the effect of the diagnosis is because most of us will believe what we're told, especially when told by a "specialist." It's difficult to conjure up a picture of hope and possibility when all the news seems to be depressing. The mind seems to be numbed. It takes a real effort to evoke an image of ourselves as whole and healthy. Yet it can be done.

We need to dream courageously. No great achievement is accomplished without a great dream preceding it. Give yourself permission to dream about a glorious future. Allow all the trimmings to be present in your dreaming. Be specific about what it is you wish to acquire, and then have the courage to focus on it as if it were already on its way to you.

If, in our mind's eye, we're projecting positive, vibrant images then they become our expectation of the future. Some could say it's not realistic to project a positive image when we've been told we're dying. Surely what matters is how we live every moment. Believe me, to practice dying all the time gets really boring! People sometimes forget that even though we might have a shortened life span, right now we're living—not dying. This is often brought home to me when I see a self-sown plant growing in a most precarious position, perhaps out of a crack in the road, or out of a tiny space between the bricks on a stairwell. The plant didn't think, "This isn't a good place to grow; I might get stepped on or run over by a truck. There's no one to water me and there's next to no soil. Not a good idea at all."

The plant just lives. It has an inbuilt urge to survive. So do we. While there's life, live it. Not just by existing but by giving it every affirmation possible.

To be surrounded by beauty uplifts the spirit. A bowl of flowers, a sunset, a child's smile, leaves in the sunshine, clouds, sunlight on water—all these things act as powerful and uplifting images.

We need to be diligent in watching the images which come into our minds. It's useful to have a powerful and positive image to place there whenever we detect a depressing or pessimistic attitude arising.

A very practical way of mastering this exercise is to spend several sessions each day implanting these images into the mind. First, you must find an image which seems appropriate to you. Many people don't really know what they want. They only know what they *don't* want. They know they don't want to die, for instance. Yet they have no clear image in their minds of how they really want to live. For many people life just happens. We experience a richness in our lives when we actually have a goal to aim for and then work toward it.

Shirley gave herself great hope and encouragement by making a collage of all the pictures and affirmations which represented what she wanted to achieve. She cut pictures and positive statements out of magazines, stuck them on cardboard backing, and wrote affirmations to match the images. She hung this collage above her bed, and each night on retiring and in the morning on awakening, she would spend time looking at the images and repeating the affirmations. This practice gave her the hope and encouragement she needed when her health news seemed so bleak. It's healthy to live with hope in our hearts. To exist without hope leads to depression and despair which is no fun for us and certainly no fun for those who extend support or care to us.

Making Goals

People sometimes experience conflict between living in the present moment and working toward future goals. It's healthy to have short-term, mid-term, and long-term goals. Short-term goals might include finishing a particular project, cleaning the house, planting bulbs for the spring, painting the back porch, learning to meditate, and so on. Mid-term goals might include planning a holiday to take after treatment, studying a course or subject which interests you, completing projects which have been stagnant for too long. Long-term goals might include buying your dream home, planning an overseas holiday, moving to the country, holding your first exhibition of craft work, attending your son's graduation, and so on. Once we've established what we'd like our future to contain, we can then live each moment fully while moving in the direction of our goals. We need to be flexible in achieving our goals and not be disappointed if they take longer to accomplish than we planned. Visualizing your goal is of immense value and can be done in both "formalized" sessions as well as being "held" in your awareness.

In these more formalized sessions we sit down and focus on the images or goals we've selected. We project them powerfully on to the screen of our mind. Tune out any other thoughts or impressions and let your mind be completely full of the image. Allow the feelings belonging with that image to surface and let yourself indulge in those feelings. Let them come alive in you now, as if that *is* your present reality. Trust that the image you have projected is already on its way to you in its fullness and you can even now feel its effect.

When I was unwell I worked with two images in particular. The first one came about naturally as I sat in the early morning sun. I'd focus on my breathing, let my body relax, and then concentrate on feeling the sunshine on my skin. After a while I'd begin to breathe in the sunshine, visualizing its warmth as a soft golden light gently filling my chest. I could feel it flowing down into my tummy and abdomen, down into the hips and buttocks, down through the thighs, into the knees, calves, feet, and toes. A soft billowy cloud of golden sparkling light. Down through my arms into the elbows and forearms, wrists, hands, and fingertips. Finally I'd fill my throat, neck, and the inside of my head with the golden glow of the sun. I'd concentrate all my thoughts and attention on breathing in this golden sparkling light, until every cell felt it was surrounded by a halo of light. After some minutes concentrating on filling my body with light, I'd visualize the borders of my body dissolving so the sunshine outside, and the sunshine inside, became one light. I became the sun. I'd then experience "being" the sun for however long it felt wonderful. It usually extended to at least half an hour, sometimes much longer.

This is a lovely image to work with and very simple. We're all familiar with the gentle touch of sunshine on our skin. It's an easy step to visualize it as light and draw it into our bodies. It only takes concentration. It leads easily into the meditation aspect where one just experiences a feeling of "being."

The other visualization which I developed was more concentrated and active in its implementation. Again, I'd begin with breathing and relaxation. Then I'd begin to breathe in angels. I've always been rather partial to angels and they were an image with which I felt comfortable. My little angels were exquisitely beautiful, each one different from the other. I don't know how many there were but I placed them about every eight centimeters around my body. I always started at my right thumb and put an angel just inside the tip, the next angel at the base, index fingertip, base of finger, and so on—right throughout my body. When I could "see" and feel every angel in place, I would get them to start sounding the word "Om" to each other. This is an ancient Sanskrit mantra, rather like "Amen." I'd been studying Sanskrit for some years and the way in which I'd learned its fundamentals was by sounding the very simplest of its components. It had always been an incredibly powerful exercise and was very effective in stilling the mind. So, choosing the sound of Om was born entirely out of my previous experience.

When the angels sang this sound to each other, I'd experience it as a feeling as well as seeing: imagining the sound as a vibration traveling through the bloodstream, through the muscles, tendons, and ligaments. I'd see it flow right through the bones into the bone marrow. And I'd feel the power of that sound setting all the cells dancing to its vibration. As the vibration from one angel met up with the vibration from the next, a network would be formed throughout the body. This network became more and more complex until every cell in the body was "touched" and encompassed by it, and then it would dissolve into the overall experience of sound and feeling. If thoughts or distractions entered my mind, I had a little volume control knob down in the left-hand corner of the screen in my mind and I'd simply turn up the volume until no other experience was possible. In this way, I dealt with the bone pain I experienced. It also shifted my perception from one of despair to one of peace as I found ways of positively working with the situation I was in.

As can be seen from both of these peaceful visualizations, my preference was to work with images which had a sense of increasing a positive experience within my body. I still work this way, choosing images which are powerful yet peaceful. Other people might find it more positive to work with a more aggressive approach to their disease.

Charlie, a ten-year-old boy, would visualize his cancer as weeds; his chemotherapy was carried in backpacks with handsprayers by men on patrol. Wherever they saw a "weed," they'd spray "weed killer" on it. The weeds would wither and die. His immune system, represented as little folk in white overalls, would arrive in trucks, cars, jeeps, motorbikes, and helicopters to pick up the dead weeds, putting them into wheelbarrows and dumping them over the cliff into the sea.

In this way Charlie was able to add his positive thoughts and efforts to his chemotherapy. It also helped to minimize the side effects because he chose to "see" it as a positive help to him.

The most important thing to remember when working out an appropriate visualization for your own situation is to choose something which comes easily from your own background or experience.

Many people have difficulty in accepting chemotherapy or AZT as a positive help to themselves. Often it's looked upon as a necessary evil. It's really important to rectify this attitude. If you experience the treatment as a toxic, poisonous substance going into your body, it's very likely to cause you more side effects than if you believe, and can "see," this substance as liquid gold pouring its healing power into your body. We *do* have the power to choose what we hold in our minds. If we've chosen to have drug therapy then we can follow up that choice with positive feelings and images about the outcome of the treatment. The same principle applies to radiotherapy. Those rays can be powerful forces of destruction or they can be powerful, shining images of healing light.

Kerry-Anne was diagnosed ten years ago with breast cancer which had spread extensively into the lymph nodes in her armpit. She was very fearful of the radiotherapy which was recommended after she had her mastectomy. She recognized this attitude wasn't to her benefit and she consciously determined to view the experience in a more positive light. The image she came up with was a beautiful one. When she lay on the table for radiotherapy she visualized that she was lying "inside" the body of an angel. The angel protected her from any harm and made sure the radiotherapy rays went directly to the area where they were needed. She suffered no side effects from her treatment and has not had a recurrence of her cancer since. She's gone for checkups over the years and her doctors are mystified as to why she's remained well. Kerry-Anne's faith is very strong and *she's* not the least bit surprised.

As mentioned earlier, drawing can be very useful in helping to clarify how we really feel about our disease, its treatment, and the response of our immune system. Sometimes we can *think* we're being positive, and yet when we draw our disease, our therapy, or immune system, another image might well emerge. Our subconscious attitudes and feelings are easily visible in our drawings. I often use drawings to help people understand what's really going on in their minds. On one sheet of paper I ask the person to draw his or her disease; on another sheet the recommended treatment; and on the third sheet to draw the immune system. These drawings can then be discussed and the fears or anxieties evident in the drawings can be aired. Its often valuable to have a three-way dialogue between disease, treatment, and immune system. This involves the person speaking in the first person and beginning a conversation between disease and treatment and vice versa, disease and immune system and vice versa, then treatment and immune system and vice versa, always speaking in the first person. These questions need to be asked by someone who can get behind the issues. There are several therapists who work in this way. Once you get the hang of it, you might find you can learn much about yourself through your drawings, without the assistance of a therapist.

I visited Clare in her home and she did some drawings. During the session she was quite shocked to hear the answers her disease, treatment, and immune system gave. Here are some excerpts.

I asked her disease, "Why have you come?"

Without hesitation she answered, "To punish my husband!"

"Why do you wish to punish him?"

"Because I hate his mother."

A long tirade about her husband's mother ensued in which she expressed her rage at his always putting his mother and her needs first.

"How do you feel about the treatment?"

"It won't work."

"Why is that?"

"I don't want it to work. I don't want to let him off the hook so easily. I want him to suffer the way I've suffered."

There was considerable anger and pent-up emotion in this woman (needless to say!). Her husband was present as this tirade came forth and was utterly shocked at the anger and intent her words conveyed. He had no idea she'd harbored these feelings for the twenty-nine years of their marriage. He was deeply wounded by the hatred with which his wife spoke of his mother. When Clare heard herself utter those words, she too was surprised. She said she felt as though a seething mass of snakes had been released in her belly (She had widespread bowel cancer). She was a very tightly "held in" woman, and her husband said this was the first time he'd ever heard her express any anger aloud. After considerable discussion which was often heated, the two of them decided to have counseling to rectify their differences and to reestablish healthier communication. It took a while for her husband to forgive Clare and vice versa, and for him to be willing to participate in such a program. After a time, he found Clare became much more alive and vital, with the sparkle and excitement returning to their communication and, therefore, to their marriage. It was not a smooth path they'd chosen and there were (and occasionally still *are*) many potholes. They both say they genuinely love each other and they no longer take each other for granted. A healed relationship might well create the foundation for healing within the body. Anyone would agree that a bellyful of snakes is hardly conducive to physical well-being. Once that pent-up energy was released, *then* it could be used for healing.

Over subsequent months Clare's drawings became lighter, more colorful, and less chaotic. Her drawings clearly reflected her life.

All that is necessary is a willingness to explore. Remember, the people in the picture can be very simply drawn though it's better not to make them stick figures. It's preferable to work with white paper and colored pencils or crayons. Felt tip pens aren't suitable as no gradation is possible in shading.

Some people have difficulty in actually "seeing" any images at all when they attempt to visualize. Drawing the visualization can often be helpful in focusing the mind upon the chosen image.

Another suggestion for those who find it difficult to visualize an image is to work only with light or color. If you're using a tape which embodies a visualization, then perhaps just go with the sound of the voice or music or the atmosphere of what's being said, rather than judging yourself harshly for not being able to "see" the picture created on the tape. Self-judgment or criticism is the antithesis of what the visualization is designed for, so avoid the temptation. For most people it only requires consistent practice before the images begin to flow easily.

The following visualization technique is the one I mentioned earlier, where we work with sunshine or light. It's a very simple and easily learned technique, although, like meditation, while the skill is easily learned it does take consistent practice to achieve all of its benefits. Let a friend read, very slowly, the following technique aloud to you, or read it slowly yourself on to a tape and play it back frequently until you're adept at the technique. Alternatively, I've produced a cassette which has an explanation of visualization on one side and the technique detailed below on the other. Cassettes are available from the Quest for Life Center (see Cassette Tapes, page 379).

Allow your eyes to close over lightly. Let your body settle into a position in which you feel comfortable. If you're sitting, allow your spine to be as comfortably erect as possible. Begin by taking some long, slow, soft breaths. Feel yourself settling in to your body. Breathing out all tension, all mental activity quietening down. Just long, slow, soft breaths that let you relax deeply.

As you breathe in this way, feel your body beginning to soften. Letting go of all rigidity. Your body open and soft and flexible. Let your feet soften and become warm. Bringing your attention to the soft warmth in your feet. Each toe full of softness. The muscles within your feet relaxing, loosening.

The ankles softening. Let them be loose. The muscles of the calves, relaxing and softening. Let your knees be loose. Let your thighs soften and spread against the chair or mattress. Feel the texture of your clothing against the skin of your thighs. Even the bones seeming to soften. Let your buttocks cushion and support you without any tension. Feel them spread against the chair or mattress.

Let your abdomen gently rise and fall with each breath at your own rhythm. Deep within your abdomen, allow each of the organs to soften. Their borders smoothing out, relaxing deeply. Allow the warmth and comfort within the abdomen to flow deep within the pelvis.

Feel it spreading gently up into the tummy and solar plexus. If there's any tightness in the solar plexus, just above your navel, then breathe into that area and allow it to soften and open.

Warmth and relaxation flowing on into the chest. Notice the movements of your chest as you breathe. The way your clothes move against the skin as you breathe.

Focus on your heart and allow it to soften and open. Relax your shoulders. Feel all the tension draining out of your shoulders. Feel ripples of relaxation flowing down and across your back. Over your shoulder blades, over your waist. Let the relaxation flow down through your arms, into the elbows and forearms. Let the muscles drift away from the bones. Dissolving into stillness. Your wrists soft, yielding. The muscles, tendons, and ligaments within your hands softening, becoming like loose elastic. Right down into your fingertips, letting go.

Muscles softening throughout the whole body. Each breath drawing in deeper relaxation.

Allow your throat to be open and relaxed and let go of all unnecessary tension in your neck. If you're sitting, let your head float very lightly at the top of your spine. As it floats, feel your spine lengthening and stretching, lifting your diaphragm.

Let your lower jaw drop just enough to let your teeth part. Allow your tongue to soften in your mouth. Soften the lips and cheeks. All the muscles around the eyes, softening and spreading as your relaxation deepens. Let the space between your eyebrows widen as your forehead relaxes. Soft temples, ears, and scalp.

The whole of your body relaxing more deeply with each breath. Breathing in peace and calm. Feel all tension in body and mind draining out with each outward breath. Gently in. Gently out. Each breath takes you deeper into relaxation.

Now imagine a light just above your head. You might see it as a brilliant ball of light. Or perhaps you can see a radiant sun. See its golden healing light radiating out from its center. You might begin to feel the warmth of the light gently showering down on to the top of your head. A soft golden light, full of warmth and healing.

Let that light gently penetrate through the top of your head, until the whole of the inside of your head is filled with a soft golden glowing light. Behind your eyes, through all the muscles of your face, a soft flowing golden light. Filling your mouth, cradling your tongue in soft light.

Feel the light slowly moving down through your throat and neck. Filling them with soft sparkling light. Dissolving all tension. And on into your shoulders. Light pouring from its unending source. A soft healing golden light soothing all the cells as it flows down and across your back. Flowing over and through the shoulder blades. On over the waist. Soothing, healing light.

Let it flow into the cavity of your chest, filling it with a sparkling cloud of golden light. Every cell healed, comforted, soothed by the presence of this sparkling light. The heart cradled in light.

Feel the healing presence of this golden light flowing freely down through the arms. Bringing rest and peace and light. You may find your fingers begin to tingle or pulsate with the presence of this golden, healing energy. Let the light flow right on out through the fingertips. Flowing from its unending source. Light and peace filling the body.

Soft billowy clouds of light flowing down through the tummy. Softening and soothing. Each cell surrounded and healed by the presence of light. Tiny little sparkles of golden light flooding into the abdomen. Filling the abdomen with light and peace.

Each inward breath drawing more of this healing light into the body. The pelvis cradled in a golden radiance.

Soft sparkling light filling the buttocks and hips. Feel it flowing down through the thighs. The bones melting into light and peace. The knees softening, dissolving into light. The lower legs filled with golden clouds of light. Flowing right into the feet. The toes filling with light, dissolving into light. The light flowing on out through the end of the toes. An unending source of light pouring through the body.

Let the tissues, the muscles, dissolve into the golden, healing light. The borders of your organs melting away. Soothed and comforted by the soft presence of light. Feel the warmth throughout your body. Each breath drawing more light, more healing into your body. The heart melting into light. All tension softening, dissolving into light.

Bones softening, dissolving into light. Floating in an ocean of light. A vast ocean, without limit or border. Only light, only peace. Floating in this ocean, without limit or border. Only light, only peace. Floating in this ocean of peace and light. Effortlessly drifting through light.

Now, with each inward breath, draw in light. With each outward breath let the borders of your body dissolve. Melting into an ocean of light. Becoming the ocean of light without border or limit. At one with the ocean of light. Each outward breath dissolving more into light. Only light, only peace. An ocean of light and peace.

Thoughts, feelings, drifting in this vast ocean of light and peace. Sensations floating in awareness. Each thought, each feeling, each sensation melting back into the ocean. Each sound melting back into vast awareness. Without border or limit. Only light and peace.

Take a long pause.

Gently begin to bring your awareness back into your body. Begin to take some long, soft, deeper breaths. Breathing in light and energy. Feel the muscle tone beginning to return to your body as your awareness comes fully back into your body. The muscle tone returning to arms and legs.

Begin moving your hands and feet just a little. Staying with the peace, bringing it back with you.

Begin to stretch the rest of your body. Enjoying the refreshment, the relaxation in all the muscles of your body.

Taking your time to bring all your awareness back into your body. Enjoy the peace and calm within your body.

In your own time, just as you're ready, allow the eyes to open.

You may wish to close them for a little longer, opening them in your own time.

To experience deep peace and love in our lives is healing. When minds and spirits are healed we're creating the very best environment for physical healing. It's up to us how we're going to create peace in our lives. The peace is always there and yet we need to make a conscious decision for peace. Even on the windiest, wettest, grayest day, you'll find the sun shining brightly in a clear blue sky if you can get above the clouds.

Several of the tapes I've produced rely on the use of images of nature to instill a sense of peace and profound relaxation. In this state of deep relaxation, your body, mind, and spirit know what needs to be done for your healing at each of these levels. These guided imagery tapes are used extensively within homes and hospitals throughout Australia, and there are further details about them at the back of this book.

For those who have definite spiritual beliefs, use visualization skills to call up your faith and give it new power to heal and establish peace in your life. I've been greatly helped by many religions and I believe every one has been inspired at its roots by love. The Christ-visualization described earlier is a very powerful means by which we can change our consciousness.

In the groups where I teach visualization techniques I usually structure the visualization around familiar natural images, as with the tapes. Perhaps working with the image of a garden, a beautiful waterfall, or pool. Or with a rain forest, or an ocean or river. Or working with sunshine, letting its light radiate on to our bodies, filling them with its light; visualizing the sun becoming small enough to place right inside our hearts, or inside an area of our bodies which is in need of healing, comfort, or energizing. People's experiences with these images are often profoundly moving, and they describe what they've experienced in very spiritual terms. We can use these images to work with forgiveness, increasing self-esteem, improving communication, healing, and letting go of the stresses we have in our lives.

When the heart is touched, the mind becomes peaceful. Our experience of God, of a higher power, or of love is always heartfelt. The greatest struggle in life for each human being is the war between the heart and the mind. The heart "knows" something and yet the mind replies it cannot understand this "some-thing" and therefore doesn't believe in it.

The mind is forever questioning and is often satisfied with superficial answers. When your heart asks "Why?" it wants only the truth.

The following Irish blessing is full of images which instill peace in the mind and nourish and uplift the heart.

> *May the road rise to meet you,*
> *May the winds be always at your back,*
> *May the sun shine warm upon your face,*
> *The rains fall softly upon your fields,*
> *And until we meet again*
> *May God hold you in the hollow of his hand.*

Chapter Seven

RECIPE FOR LIFE

. . . .

Desmond

Early in 1988 I began, for the first time in my life, to suspect that all wasn't well with my body. Initial, and as it proved, rather superficial tests, were inconclusive. I was, of course, hoping for a negative result. But things didn't improve, and later that year a colonoscopy revealed I had bowel cancer. My immediate reaction was a mixture of disbelief (not me!) and what my death might mean to my family. For two days I didn't want to talk to anyone until I'd come to terms with it and how I would communicate the news to those who needed to know. I might add that in the meantime additional tests revealed a secondary growth in the liver. My surgeon said, my heart permitting, he'd like to do both operations at the same time. I said, "Sure, let's get it over with."

My phone calls to those near and dear felt like final farewells—and rather tearful ones. They become so emotionally draining, I kept the list as short as possible. "Think positively" seemed to be the phrase on everyone's lips. Yet how difficult when all appears so negative!

Ten days after the operation I was home. Ten days after that I was back at work and, soon after, overseas on a business trip. I endeavored through whatever mix of conscious or subconscious determination to return as quickly and fully to my pre-operation life—both at work and at home. This I achieved in remarkably less time than was thought possible.

Nevertheless, I had to accept the fact that I'd undergone major surgery for a life-threatening disease. How did I get it and what could I do to prevent its recurrence?

I'd always enjoyed a better than average level of fitness for my fifty-five years and, having shed five kilograms as a consequence of the operation, I was determined to maintain as high a level of fitness as practicable.

While recuperating I read a wide range of books on cancer in particular and healthier life styles in general. I was amazed at the range. Some diets required a full-time staff merely for preparation. Many demanded that I retire on a substantial income! All were incompatible with my return to a fifty- or sixty-hour working week. Those books instructing me how to die with dignity were quickly rejected. I wasn't ready to die. I had no intention of dying but I wanted to do as much as possible—short of making my life miserable—to maintain a healthier lifestyle. Diet became an important consideration.

Although I'd never been a fatty food lover, I reduced substantially or ceased completely consumption of fried foods, butter, cheese, and avoided salt, sweets, sugar, and red meats. Early forays into organically grown fruit and vegetables were largely abandoned, mainly on the grounds of poor standards of freshness and taste. I increased, however, my intake of fruit and vegetables both in natural and juice form, supplemented with vitamin C, and raw nuts, mostly almonds. I increased my intake of fish, both deep sea and selected tinned, including tuna and sardines. Whole meal bread became a must. Chicken also now appears on my diet, as does rice and pasta. Fear of being destined to a life of organically grown boredom has given way to a wide and enjoyable range of alternatives. Business lunches are no longer out of bounds. Life is O.K. after all.

Therein, I suppose, lies the whole point. We are responsible for our own bodies and our own lives. Few things can make us realize that more than having cancer. It stimulates a need to reassess so many aspects and to place new values on things we never thought about or merely took for granted. I'm now, in many ways, a different but, I believe, a more complete and contented person. I experience less anger, resentment, and guilt. Life has more purpose and I'm able, as I was even during the immediate postoperative period, to find humor in so many aspects of what has proved to be a life-shattering experience. I have known those who, after a cancer operation no more serious than mine, went home only to die. This doesn't have to be the case.

Apart from my own healthier lifestyle and outlook, there've been other benefits. Some of my friends have taken greater interest in and responsibility for their own lifestyles. My family has adopted a healthier attitude to diet, and my wife has embraced concepts of meditation and other techniques.

I confess that, most of the time, I never think about cancer. It is, I hope, a thing of the past.

People often place a large emphasis on what should and shouldn't be eaten when they have a life-threatening illness. You can read books which advocate garlic until it's coming out your ears, only to pick up another which strongly advises against its use. One dietary regime prohibits the use of celery while another suggests you should have it juiced every day. Should you have a macrobiotic or a raw food diet, and so on? In fact, no subject is more open to debate, and very often the person becomes completely bewildered and frustrated by all the conflicting advice.

People trying to find the right diet can become so confused as to be paralyzed in their endeavors to whip up a quick snack! The premise on which the whole approach of this book is based is that peace of mind is our greatest healer and, therefore, our primary goal. Our choice of an appropriate nutritional program must be in accord with this aim. Many people will practice meditation, visualization, and relaxation techniques in order to help themselves establish a calm and peaceful attitude, only to be thrown into a flap because they're half an hour late with their carrot juice. We need to bring the peace and calmness we experience in our meditations into every other aspect of our lives. Some people put their lives, and their healing, into compartments—"I'm meditating for my mind and spirit and I'm sticking to this special dietary program for my body"—instead of having an overall sense of trust and wholeness in their healing process.

From my experience and having worked on a one-to-one basis with over five thousand individuals with life-threatening diseases, I can confidently say I don't believe that diet is the *most* important factor. I've seen people do well on many different kinds of diets. In each case the person chose the diet that appealed to him or her most. It's the attitude behind your eating which is of importance. Most people get caught up in the dietary dilemma because they feel this is one area over which they can readily take control. It gives a sense of "doing something" which can be evidenced and measured. I'm not by any means saying your diet isn't important, but don't turn it into a nightmare. Enjoy your food. Research what you feel might be appropriate for you, and *gently* move in the desired direction at *your* speed. It's the attitude for long-term survivors rather than their dietary approach that's most apparent. They're people who've decided to live each day to its full potential with peace in their hearts and joy in each moment. You can't experience peace of mind while you're feeling frazzled over which diet to adopt. Keep your sense of humor; it will get you through many a confusing or potentially panicky moment.

To experience peace of mind, with regard to nutrition, it's essential you have a program which:

- *You believe is of the utmost benefit to you*
- *Is well within your capabilities to prepare*

To decide that your healing lies in personally grown (and planted by the moon) produce, picked fresh from your own organically mulched garden; plus wheat grass, freshly prepared vegetable juices six times a day, and homemade organically grown wheat bread (kneaded when you were feeling joyous) when you live in a high-rise unit in the inner city is unrealistic, to say the least.

I believe it's essential that anyone who wishes to adhere to a cleansing yet nourishing diet to assist in the healing process should be under the guidance of a qualified and experienced doctor or naturopath. Choose someone whom you trust and who's accustomed to working with people who have life-threatening diseases. When tailoring this nutritional program, it's essential to take into account the emotional and psychological state, cultural background, religious restrictions, physical condition, and personal wishes of the patient—*and* the amount of support that person has at home to assist in the preparation of a special diet. It's important you find a diet which will work for *you*, as opposed to a diet in which your therapist believes but which turns your entire household upside-down in order to accommodate *it!*

If your therapist doesn't ask you lots of questions about the issues mentioned above (that is, doesn't tailor the dietary program to fit *your* particular needs), then you're probably with the wrong therapist. Don't fall into the trap of doing contortions to fit into the program your therapist has devised. He or she should be able to devise a program which is tailored for you.

Remember, diet is only one aspect of an overall approach to healing. Unless wisely guided, people will often put more effort than is really necessary into their dietary preparation and the other therapies which they've chosen to incorporate, simply because it's something tangible they can "do" to help themselves.

Western society is based on "doing" rather than the exploration of "being." When we're newly diagnosed with a disease, our tendency, after the initial panic has dispersed a little, is to find the things which we can actively do to help ourselves. It's very easy to get lost in the doing and thus overlook the importance of being. A new diet adopted out of fear of the disease and its consequences won't be nearly as beneficial as one calmly chosen to assist in our healing. Often members of the patient's family see their most useful role as the gatherers of information with regard to diets and other therapies. This is a valuable and necessary role. However, it can still be carried out with calmness. There *is* time: time to assimilate, to talk, discuss, share feelings, evaluate information, and consolidate your combined strengths.

Once all the factors mentioned before have been taken into account, a program can be designed which allows for healthy cleansing of the body while also providing optimum nourishment of a kind which can be assimilated by this *particular* person. Two people of the same age with the same disease might require two very different nutritional programs, based on the considerations mentioned earlier. These nutritional programs aren't curative of themselves. All healing power lies within the person.

We're endeavoring to provide first-class nourishment of a kind which can be assimilated by the body, so it will be in a position to cleanse and heal itself.

Remember, if we're primarily spiritual beings within bodies, rather than bodies who happen to have spirits, then our approach to healing *must* encompass more than dietary considerations. As long as there are unrecognized and unresolved fears, angers, guilts, issues from the past, resentments, and an unhealthy grasping at life, all the carrot juice and diets in the world will be of no avail.

It's of paramount importance that the person has faith in the chosen diet and *enjoys* the food he or she is eating. Many people make themselves miserable and create far more stress by adopting a rigid and unpalatable diet. Others may well thrive on exactly the same foods. This highlights the crux of the matter—finding the nutritional program which tastes good to you and which will provide the ideal environment for healing within your body. The first and most important aspect of healing is the loving gentleness and regard with which you hold yourself. All healing flows from this.

At the time of my diagnosis, I'd been a vegetarian and a meditator for fifteen years. I hadn't drunk coffee, tea, or alcohol nor consumed any "suspect substance" in that time, and had sustained several long fasts. Though my body was not full of toxicity through the ingestion of impure or chemicalized foods, my mind was certainly suspect! Much of my thinking was extremely rigid and inflexible. Indeed, my diet very much reflected my thinking: I was unbending in sticking to a rigid program because I believed it to be to my benefit.

At one stage during my recovery I was teaching meditation in some of the most ancient and beautiful monasteries in Italy. For a while I secluded myself in a monastery high above the town of Assisi. I'd actually planned to fast for several days at this monastery, but there was no way the monks would hear of it. They didn't speak English, I didn't speak much Italian, but they were convinced I was trying to follow in the footsteps of St. Francis by depriving myself of food. These monks were all of the

very round Franciscan variety and they insisted that while fast-
ing had been good for St. Francis, I most surely would eat. I
don't like to argue with a monk, and wouldn't have, even had I
known the language in which to do it!

The meals they'd lovingly prepared for me contained an array of foods which I hadn't eaten for fifteen years. Meat, sea-
food, chunks of white bread ("the whiter the bread, the sooner
you're dead" had been my creed for years), salt, and (delicious!)
sauces ... always accompanied by a large goblet of wine. These
foods, although lovingly prepared, were quite foreign to everything I had believed in. I wrestled with my confusion and realized that all my life I'd been struggling to get things under
control, to get it right, to be perfect and that this was a "disease"
every bit as lethal as leukemia. I humbly and gratefully accepted
the food life had lovingly prepared for me through these monks.
Sometimes they'd stand around in a semicircle with their hands
clasped across their contented corpulences, smiling beatifically
while I consumed the repast they'd prepared.

All the years of rigid thinking hadn't helped me a great deal.
I had excellent powers of concentration and was accustomed to
many hours of meditation without a break—sometimes six hours
in the one position. However, what I was now discovering was
the need for simple loving kindness and less bother with the
externals of *how* I should live: more openness to life; an acceptance of whatever came; allowing for more trust in each moment
with less of a need to control. An internal "yes" to life; even an
internal "yes" to leukemia and death, if that was to be the outcome. A letting go of having to have it *my* way. So, was it important to maintain the healthy habits of fifteen years?

It wasn't so much the diet I'd chosen which was at fault, it
was more the attitude with which I implemented it. One might
say, in the midst of leukemia, that surely a strict diet would be
essential. Or was it preferable to let go the rigidity behind these
beliefs and trust that the universe (life, love, or God, if you prefer) was caring for me and to believe I was loved and supported
in whatever I *did?* I chose this latter course of action and cultivated a gratefulness for whatever life lovingly presented upon

my plate. At home, I very rarely eat meat, but when I'm away I eat with gratitude what's been prepared.

This attitude in no way endorses a liberal diet of meat and wine! It's only to illustrate the importance of the *spirit* behind whatever diet one adopts. If my attitude had been, "Oh, what the heck, I've been eating strictly all these years and now I'm dying, I don't care what I eat; it's not going to make any difference anyway!" then that would be the absolute antithesis of a healthy attitude. I believe, for me, it was far more important to cleanse my mind of its negativity than to be overly preoccupied with nutrition.

For others, it might be advisable to have the strictest guidelines to follow as far as their nutritional program is concerned. Some people will only experience peace of mind if they feel their diet is a tried and true healing diet. For others, peace of mind will be experienced by taking gentle and gradual steps towards a more nutritious program. For those who have any kind of digestive problem, please refer to chapter 8, Burps, Burning, and the Dreaded Bloats (see pages 181-251), for a comprehensive approach to all digestive dilemmas.

Many people equate adhering to a difficult or rigid diet with their degree of determination to live. This often reflects their lifelong habit of setting standards so high that they are almost impossible to achieve. Then they can be self-critical if they don't measure up. Often the underlying thought behind this is, "If I really want to live, I should be doing everything 100 percent. There I am, failing again!" It's so sad to see this thinking in people. They can become so depressed by a seemingly insurmountable obstacle, and yet it's an obstacle entirely of their own creation. If this is *your* attitude, it's worth looking at other areas in your life to see if this is a common approach you have. Pick your diet, do your utmost, and *trust*.

Another common attitude behind the dietary dilemma is one of bargaining. "If I adhere to a really difficult diet, if I meditate for three hours every day, if I take my supplements and treatments, then maybe I will 'earn' my recovery." It usually stems from "If I'm good enough, I'll succeed."

Often when we're sick there are people—such as neighbors, friends, and relatives—who offer assistance. We're sometimes reluctant to avail ourselves of their offers as we like to be independent. The spouse or support person might well feel they want to do *all* the caring for the person who's sick—again, as a way of showing their love. If we can avail ourselves of offers to cook, pick up the children or groceries, take care of the washing or ironing, or whatever seems to be most helpful, it leaves the support person more available to spend time with his or her loved one.

Some of the diets advocated for the "cure" of cancer and other diseases almost require a full-time cook to keep up with the endless preparation of foods and juices. If you have the resources and want to be on such a program, and if it doesn't create a stressful home environment, then it could well be suitable and beneficial. However, if your entire day is dominated by a rigid program of juices and food preparation, and the atmosphere in the home is permeated by stress, then something needs to be changed. Again, it's not the juices or the foods that are at fault, but the attitude *behind* their use.

So, by all means enlist the assistance of those who have willingly offered their services. They wouldn't have offered if they hadn't sincerely meant what they'd said. When our priorities are right, we can relax and trust healing is taking place.

This principle applies in exactly the same way to the various other modalities that you might have encountered—vitamins, herbals, homeopathics, tissue salts, acupuncture, nutritional supplements, minerals, laetrile, iskador, cancell, Vitamin B12, to name but a few of the more popular therapies which are available. As well as these substances which can be *taken* (into the body), there are a host of other modalities which can be utilized: reiki, shiatsu, rebirthing, regression therapy, psychotherapy, float tanks, yoga, Chi Qong, spiritual or psychic healing—the list goes on and on. Don't forget, peace is your one goal. Choose from the modalities and therapies which come easily into your orbit. Again, it comes back to trusting that the things which you need for your healing are at hand.

In my practice, I rely on sound nutrition of a kind which can be readily assimilated by the client. This nutritional program is tailored to the individual, bearing in mind the essentials mentioned earlier in this chapter. In addition to this, I recommend vitamins, minerals, and other nutritional supplements designed to improve overall health and well-being. I use herbals and homeopathics which I find particularly valuable in alleviating the side effects of the necessary medical treatments the client might be undergoing, and to relieve the unpleasant symptoms of the disease process.

None of the therapeutic substances which I use are designed to cure the disease. All of them are intended to assist the person in creating an ideal internal environment in which healing might take place. If we have a diet which is nourishing and which minimizes the stress to our bodies, we're cooperating with our own healing process. For instance, your body could well make excellent use of fish and potatoes. However, if you eat fish and chips—that is, fried in batter and oil—you're creating an unnecessary stress for your liver. It's not only impossible for your body to digest oils which have been heated to a high temperature, but they're positively detrimental to your liver. If you have cancer or any other serious disease, it's advisable to assist the liver in its mammoth job of detoxifying the bloodstream. It certainly isn't helpful to increase the stress on an organ which is already overloaded. It's simple common sense to work in accord with your body, which is under stress at the outset.

Just as we need assistance in choosing an appropriate nutritional program, so we need to have any other chosen therapy tailored to meet needs. To find someone qualified to help you in this area, seek out help from other patients, your local hospital, your community health center, your doctor or oncologist, your health food store, or ask for assistance from the cancer or AIDS council in your state or an equivalent organization which understands your needs. Many of my referrals come from oncologists/immunologists who know this approach is beneficial to their patients and that their patients won't be dissuaded from medical treatments.

As I'm always asked about the diet which I prescribe, the

following guidelines are included. These guidelines are such that every individual in the community would benefit from them, regardless of their state of health. They're based on sound common sense and sensible nutrition. They are general outlines only, and again, if you're seriously ill, then find a qualified person to help you use these recommendations to your best advantage. Dietitians within the hospital system are highly trained to understand the components of foods. However, they're not trained in the therapeutic effect of various foods. For those who have cancer of the stomach, liver, pancreas, gall bladder, bowel, or who have any digestive discomforts, please refer to chapter 8, Burps, Burning, and the Dreaded Bloats (see pages 181-251).

Foods to Avoid Totally

Avoid any foods containing:

- *Preservatives*
- *Artificial colorings*
- *MSG (monosodium glutamate—a flavor enhancer)*
- *Artificial flavorings*
- *Emulsifiers*
- *Stabilizers*
- *Added sugar*
- *Cow's milk and its products—with the exception of yogurt, butter, cream (see individual notes)*
- *White flour*
- *Any other chemical additive*

The following list takes each foodstuff and looks at whether it should be included in your diet or not. These are the foods which are asked about most commonly. If there isn't a list for a particular food then it means that it's probably not recommended. For instance, I have assumed you know foods like smoked meats are *not* good for you!

Alcohol

Most people who feel unwell will lose their desire for alcohol. For those undertaking chemotherapy, alcohol should be avoided altogether for several days before and after having their chemotherapy. For most people with a life-threatening disease I'd suggest limiting alcohol intake to one or two glasses of wine on special occasions. For those whose hemoglobin is low (see page 185), it might be beneficial to have a stout type beer as it is rich in iron and other blood-forming elements. If you have liver metastases, have a primary liver tumor, or are on a drug treatment such as chemotherapy or AZT, you will probably benefit from leaving out alcohol altogether. Some people find a glass of sherry before the evening meal will stimulate a jaded appetite (see in chapter 8, Loss of Appetite, page 224).

Avocados

Avocados are an excellent source of nutrition. If you're having chemotherapy or your liver is affected by disease, you might need to eliminate or reduce their intake because of their high fat content. Some people use avocado as a spread instead of butter. For the normal healthy person, half an avocado per day is fine. Avacados are rich in potassium, chlorine, sulphur, and Vitamin A.

Bread

Use only whole grain breads that have no artificial additives. Many breads are available now from organically grown wheat or rye. It might be preferable for you to use a yeast-free bread, depending on your particular health problem. For those who are allergic to wheat, rice crackers, rye crackers, or pumpernickel bread are fine. The aroma of freshly baking bread is second to none in stimulating jaded palates. If you've had a hankering to learn how to make bread, this might be the time. Whole-wheat bread contains protein, most minerals, and the B vitamins.

Butter or Margarine

My preference is for no-salt butter, but used very sparingly. Sparingly means one to two teaspoons per day of either butter or cold pressed oil. You might need to eliminate butter (and oil) altogether if you have a liver problem or any problem with nausea. Butter is a saturated fat and is high in Vitamin A and calcium.

Canned Fruits, Vegetables, or Fish

Canned fruits and vegetables are best avoided altogether as much of their valuable vitamin and enzyme content has been destroyed through the canning process. They've lost their freshness and vitality.

However, canned tuna, salmon, or sardines (preferably in brine, not oil) are good sources of protein, and especially trace elements and minerals. Drain them well and include in your diet if you enjoy them. You're principally eating fish for its minerals, trace elements, and protein content; these are not destroyed in the canning process.

Cheese

Goat and sheep cheeses are readily available in our cities now and these are fine for adding sparingly to your diet. For cow's milk cheeses, refer to the section on milk.

Crackers or Crispbreads

Choose whole-grain crackers or crispbreads which have no preservatives, colorings, cheese, sugar, or other chemical additives. Rice cakes and crackers, particularly pumpernickel or rye crackers, are fine as a substitute for bread if you're allergic to wheat.

Dried Fruits

Avoid sulfur-dried fruits. Even though sun-dried fruit doesn't look as appealing, it's far better for you. Dried fruits are extremely concentrated foods and are best consumed in small quantities. Many people soak dried fruit overnight and add it to their cereal as a sweetener. It's best avoided if you're on a low-sugar diet. Dried fruits are generally a good source of potassium and iron. Levels vary from fruit to fruit.

Eggs

Avoid eggs laid by miserable hens. Eggs from happy hens—that is, hens who get to scratch around in the dirt and who have healthy diets—are certainly preferable. Generally I wouldn't recommend more than four a week. The number of cooked eggs might have to be restricted or eliminated altogether by people who are experiencing digestive upsets (please refer to chapter 8, Burps, Burning, and the Dreaded Bloats). Avoid fried eggs altogether. Raw free-range eggs in banana smoothies (see page 176) can usually be tolerated very well by people who are feeling unwell. Eggs are an excellent complete protein and are high in iron and Vitamin A.

Fast Foods

There are many "fast foods" available today which are entirely free of chemical additives and which are nutritious. Most health food stores carry a range of tofu burgers, lentil burgers, tofu sausages, and other similar foodstuffs. In the interests of expediency, sanity, and taste, I believe they're a valuable addition to the diet. Again, they can be frozen so they're on hand for the times when you choose not to spend a long time in the kitchen. If you have a vegetarian restaurant in your area, you might have the staff prepare the occasional meal for you. This will depend on the diet you've adopted and your financial situation. Some good delicatessens have homemade soups and other products which could be entirely suitable for you—like, for example, humus, made from chickpeas, tahini, and garlic. Make life as simple as possible for yourself.

I'm not suggesting you live on take-out or frozen foods, but that you have your priorities right, remembering peace of mind as your one goal. Ask those friends and relatives who've offered to help if they'd make you some soup, or a (free-range) chicken casserole (see recipe on page 177), to have stored in the freezer for times when you come home frazzled and weary and want something on the table in ten minutes flat.

Fatty or Fried Foods

Avoid these altogether, as they're an unnecessary stress on the liver, are often high in cholesterol, and are of no benefit to your body. It's likely that you'll find the thought of these foods is enough to upset your tummy!

Ferments and Molds

These might be best eliminated from your diet depending on your particular health problem. They include foods like miso, tamari, and soy sauce. Be guided by your practitioner as to the necessity of eliminating them.

Fresh Fruits

An abundance of fresh fruit in your diet is to be encouraged unless you're on a sugar-free diet, in which case you might need to restrict the fruit to three pieces per day or less. Choose from a wide range of fruits in season to ensure you acquire all your vitamins and mineral needs. If you have any problem with nausea or squeamishness in your tummy, then it's very likely oranges will make it worse. Avoid them while undergoing chemotherapy. Grapefruit are generally tolerated well. See the section on nausea in chapter 8 (see pages 230-242). Make sure all fruit is ripe and wash it thoroughly before eating. If you can easily procure fresh and vital organically grown fruit and vegetables, so much the better. It is best not to cook fruit, unless you're following some of the therapeutic guidelines listed in chapter 8 (see pages

189-242). Fresh fruits are generally high in Vitamin C and potassium. Again, the levels vary from fruit to fruit.

Frozen Foods

Avoid frozen foods because they may have lost much of their freshness and vitality. The exception to this rule can be made in the interests of expediency, sanity, and harmony within the home. When you make soups, casseroles, or pies, make extra and freeze. I believe it's an excellent idea for people to have on hand nutritious, easy-to-prepare foods, for those times when you come home late, tired, or frazzled. There might be times when you aren't up to preparing fresh meals and a store of palatable, on-the-table-in-minutes food is a boon. This especially applies to people who live alone. As pointed out in the section Fast Foods (see page 165), most cities and large towns have vegetarian or health restaurants and you could purchase from them soups, casseroles, vegetarian pies, and so on, then freeze them for the occasions mentioned above. Check out the ingredients with the chef before buying. In this way you can streamline your culinary activities and leave more time for healing yourself.

Garlic

There's no reason why garlic cannot be utilized in your diet if you enjoy it. It can be used in dressings, with stir-fried veggies, or in any other way you enjoy. Garlic is high in potassium and sulphur.

Ginger

Ginger, for those who like its flavor, is a welcome addition to stir-fried or steamed vegetables and/or fish. It stimulates the production of gastric enzymes (which is very useful for those whose digestion or appetites are poor). For more information on poor appetites, please refer to chapter 8 (see page 224). Warm ginger tea is very settling to upset stomachs. Slice a quarter of a cup of raw ginger thinly and add to a liter of boiling water. Simmer for fifteen minutes. Let cool and add a little honey and perhaps lemon juice. Sip slowly. This is a very warming drink and, for those who feel cold from the bones out, it can be very soothing.

Honey

For those on a sugar-free diet, honey, even though it contains many nutrients, is best avoided. For others, it's important to remember that honey is a very concentrated food and thus must be used sparingly. Royal jelly, propolis, and pollen also contain many nutrients which are readily assimilated into your body and all of these can be utilized. Propolis is particularly beneficial for problems in the mouth and throat. For more information about mouth problems, see page 194. Pollen is particularly rich in zinc, which is of value to the immune system. Honey has potassium and other minerals present.

Meats

The addition of meat to your diet will depend very much on the state of your health. Some people, believing cancer thrives on meat protein, decide to adopt a very low protein diet. This is a little short-sighted, since all repair and rebuilding of cells in the body is dependent on protein. In the Western world we have tended to rely heavily on meat protein in our diet, though this has changed quite dramatically in the last few years as people have adopted healthier eating patterns. Whether you choose to include meat in your diet will depend on more factors than just your health. Those people who choose to adopt a totally vegetarian diet should move slowly in that direction rather than doing it "cold turkey"!

The problem with red meat is that when it's kept in a warm dark place for any length of time it putrefies. Animals which are accustomed to eating red meat have a very short alimentary tract in comparison with human beings. Lions and tigers have only a couple of meters of alimentary tract in comparison with ours, which is more than ten meters long. If red meat "sits" in our bowel for a long period of time, the toxins which result from the putrefaction will enter the bloodstream. Again, this is an unnecessary stress for the body. Ideally, food will take about eighteen hours to pass through your body. In this time it is broken down into small enough particles to be assimilated into the bloodstream and the remaining roughage is passed through until it reaches the rectum for elimination. You may want to check your own transit time for food. You can do this by eating some sesame seeds or corn and then keeping an eye on the toilet bowl. If transit time is less than fifteen hours, it will probably mean you're not holding the food long enough for all its nourishment to be assimilated. If your transit time is longer than twenty-four hours you probably have a problem with constipation: toxicity may be entering through the bowel wall into the bloodstream. Some drugs will lengthen or shorten this transit time as, of course, will surgery where some of the bowel has been removed.

White meats do not putrefy like red meats. I usually recommend the inclusion of deep-sea fish or free-range chicken several times a week to ensure adequate protein intake. Chicken and fish are best prepared by either grilling or steaming. If you're undergoing medical treatment such as chemotherapy, you must ensure you're having adequate protein. When you're on chemotherapy your body loses large amounts of protein through the destruction of some healthy cells as well as cancer cells. It's essential you provide your body with excellent complete proteins at least six times per week. Too often, people who undertake a low-protein diet become weary and lethargic. Incomplete proteins will also be provided in plentiful amounts by nuts, pulses, legumes, and grains. However, they're not complete proteins, that is, they don't contain the eight essential amino acids. Soy beans are the only source of complete vegetable protein (see tofu, this chapter). Complete vegetable proteins can be derived by the following combinations: legumes and seeds; grains and legumes; milk and grains; almond, cashew and brazil nuts. Be guided by your practitioner.

Most people will find their taste for red meat diminishes when they're unwell. It's the body's natural knowledge of what's appropriate for it that makes this so. If you have a really strong craving for red meat, choose lamb and eat a hearty green salad with it to provide the extra fiber needed to assist it through your digestive system.

Milk

The consumption of milk is every bit as controversial as the custom of meat eating. I think cow's milk is fantastic food—for baby calves! The enzymes involved in the digestion of milk are rennin and lactase. These enzymes are present in our bodies as babies, but are reduced in quantity by the time we reach the age of three. Human beings are the only mammals who continue to drink milk after weaning. As we often no longer have the necessary enzymes to digest milk properly or completely, I believe we're certainly much better off without it. Debilitating disease and some drugs, including chemotherapy, seem to decrease many people's ability to digest cow's milk. This applies equally to cheeses. The best of the hard cheeses is Parmesan and low-fat soft cheeses can be kept for "treats." If animal milk is an essential in your diet, replace cow's with goat's or sheep's milk. Otherwise use soy "milk," as it's called. You can buy light varieties of soy milk which are more palatable than the more grainy ones. Avoid soy milk with sugar added to it.

To argue about the necessity for cow's milk on the basis of its calcium content is also unfounded. All green leafy vegetables and soy products have good quality calcium in a form much easier to assimilate than cow's milk. The calcium in cow's milk is bound up with casein which forms curds in the tummy, making it difficult for our bodies to assimilate. Raw sesame seeds are also rich in calcium and can be added to soups, casseroles, or salads. Most fruits and vegetables contain good amounts of calcium, as do nuts.

Cream is not recommended for most people. However, for those who are severely underweight and who don't have any nausea or squeamishness in the tummy or diarrhea, the addition of cream might be beneficial. It can be added to banana smoothies (see page 176), soups, casseroles, and so on.

Yogurt has its own entry at the end of this section.

Milk is high in Vitamins A and D, and calcium.

Nuts

It's preferable to eat all nuts raw. They're an excellent form of protein and supply good quantities of calcium in an easy-to-assimilate form. They're more concentrated than fruits and vegetables and shouldn't be eaten excessively. They're best avoided by people with stomach, liver, or bowel complaints. Avoid eating roasted nuts as they're acid forming. Nuts are generally high in potassium, phosphorus, and iron. Cashews are high in Vitamin A as are pecans and pistachios.

Oils

Cold-pressed oils low in saturated fats are the only oils recommended, and should be used sparingly. Sparingly means no more than two teaspoons per day of either no-salt butter or cold-pressed oil. These might need to be restricted or eliminated altogether, depending on your health.

Packet and Processed Foods

Avoid these, as they're generally not fresh and have substances added to them to prolong shelf life. As always, there are exceptions: Prepared whole grain noodles, pasta, crackers, crispbreads, pumpernickel crackers or bread, some breakfast cereals, popcorn, noodles, seaweeds, miso, horseradish, and so on. *Make it a habit to read labels and understand what the numbers and abbreviations stand for.*

Pasta

It's a rare individual who enjoys whole meal pasta or who knows how to cook it properly! You might like to experiment with freshly made store-bought pastas (ask about ingredients), or use prepared whole grain noodles in place of pasta or to add to a casserole to thicken and add flavor. There are some delicious prepared whole grain noodles available with buckwheat, brown rice, whole wheat, carrot, and spinach. Ask about them at your local health food store.

Salt

Sodium chloride should not be included at all. Replace with either coarsely ground sea salt (use a salt grinder) or vegetable salt. The vegetable salts rely on sea salt with the addition of "salty" herbs, such as parsley, celery, and tomato. Don't cook with salt; add it at the table so you're aware of how much you're having.

Seeds

These include sunflower, sesame, pumpkin, poppy, and caraway seeds. Seeds, like nuts, are a very concentrated form of protein and are high in fat. They are best eaten sparingly. Eat them raw, as roasting renders them acid forming. Make sure your seeds are fresh. They can be sprinkled on casseroles and vegetable dishes for added flavor. Sesame seeds are high in calcium, B vitamins, potassium, and phosphorous. Sunflower seeds are high in protein, potassium, phosphorous, Vitamin D, and calcium. Pumpkin seeds are high in phosphorous, protein, Vitamin A and the B vitamins.

Tofu

Tofu is made from soy beans and can be bought in blocks. It's sometimes referred to as bean curd. It's a good source of complete protein and can be added to vegetable dishes, casseroles, soups, and even banana smoothies. It has very little flavor and certainly needs the addition of other flavors, like garlic, ginger, or miso, in order to make it palatable. Tofu is available from

health food stores and many supermarkets. Some health food
stores also sell tofu ice cream which is fine for the occasional
treat.

Tofu is high in lecithin, calcium, and potassium.

Vegetables

Use a wide range of vegetables in your diet to ensure you receive all your vitamins, enzymes, and minerals. Use both raw
and cooked vegetables. When cooking, they're best prepared by
either steaming or dry-baking. The occasional vegetable stir-fry
is fine for most people, so long as it is cooked in a wok. Use
only a teaspoon or two of cold-pressed oil in the wok to stop
the vegetables from sticking and then rely on the juices from the
vegetables to provide the moisture. Many people find difficulty
in digesting raw vegetables. If this is the case, try the vegetable
juices and when you *do* eat vegetables cook them well. If you
have digestive problems you might find that it's better to peel
the vegetables before they're cooked. Refer to chapter 8 for
more information.

Vinegar

Ordinary vinegar is best avoided, as it contains malic acid which
is damaging to the mucosa of the digestive tract. Use lemon
juice or apple cider vinegar (an alkaline product) instead.

Water

I would highly recommend you buy a water purifier. The water
tastes so much better, since the purifier removes the unwanted
chemicals. The variety I usually recommend is a reverse osmosis
unit; however, cheaper models are better than none at all.

Yogurt

Yogurt is made from milk and so all of what has already been

said about milk applies. Yogurt, however, does have some re-
deeming qualities in that it's predigested—to a certain extent
anyway. The varieties of yogurts I'd recommend are either goat's
milk yogurt (which is marginally better for you though seldom
enjoyed!) or cow's milk yogurt made with the lactobacillus acidophilus culture. Sheep's milk yogurt is very smooth and almost
sweet. It's becoming more commonly available. Many people eat
yogurt in vast quantities to "replace" gut bacteria which have
been destroyed through drug and radiation therapies. Antibiotics, chemotherapy, radiotherapy (if it is to the abdominal area)
and AZT all destroy beneficial (and indeed essential) gut
bacteria.

This kind of yogurt is also very beneficial for people who are
or have been suffering with diarrhea. Two tablespoons per day is
usually recommended. Most cow's milk acidophilus yogurts can
be bought with a reduced fat content.

Recipes

The following section contains simple suggestions for healthy
eating. Many people undergoing treatments have jaded appetites
and yet are in need of optimal nourishment. These recipes are
simple to prepare and easy to assimilate, even for people feeling
quite frail.

Juices

Freshly made vegetable juices are an excellent addition to the
diet. With vegetable juices you receive an excellent intake of
fresh and vital vitamins, enzymes, minerals, trace elements, and
other substances in a form which is easy for the body to assimilate. They're palatable, easily made, and will pick up people's
energy level more quickly than anything else. For those who are
recovering from surgery or who've been feeling unwell and have
become quite run down, the juices work like a charm. I can say,
with complete confidence, that if these people drink three
glasses of this juice a day, they won't know themselves within a

week. The juice has a remarkable capacity to kick-start the internal engines! There are very few contraindications for juices. These include some kinds of diarrhea (which are caused through infections which need to be treated, or postoperatively when much of the bowel has been removed); liver disease (in such situations people need to be carefully monitored in order not to overtax their livers); and when people can't learn to love them.

Juices should always be freshly prepared. The vegetables don't need to be peeled, though washing them is essential. Drink the juice slowly, mixing it well with saliva. I believe the following recipe is the best there is:

- *85 percent carrot juice (chop the top one-and-a-half centimeters off the carrot)*
- *10 percent beetroot juice (made from the fresh raw beet)*
- *5 percent green juice (made from celery, spinach, outside lettuce leaves, parsley, beet tops—but not if they're limp)*

Some people have difficulty with the beetroot and it's advisable not to go above 10 percent unless you really enjoy it. I've found this juice will help people to remain as healthy as possible while undergoing chemotherapy or AZT. It seems to minimize the side effects to a remarkable degree. I usually recommend three 250 ml glasses per day, but it depends a little on the individual's health and ability to prepare them. If you are about to undergo chemotherapy or surgery, three glasses per day in the preceding week will nourish you well in preparation. Always drink juices at least half an hour before a meal, or one and a half hours afterward. Some people might prefer to drink their juice with a straw. If you don't like the taste of the vegetable juice, leave out the beetroot and see how it tastes. If you still don't like it, then perhaps veggie juices aren't for you!

Vegetable juices are preferable to fruit juices, especially for those undergoing chemotherapy, other drug therapies, surgery, or radiotherapy. Fruit juices tend to cause headaches, dizziness, and weakness, whereas vegetable juices are far more gentle in their cleansing action in the body and these symptoms don't occur with them. For those who aren't feeling ill and who enjoy freshly made fruit juices, these can, of course, be included. Some people advocate emulsifying the vegetable juice with a little oil. I haven't seen any benefit in this practice.

Banana Smoothies

Banana smoothies are a delicious way to nourish someone who's feeling a little frail, who's underweight or who's having digestive problems (such as those covered in chapter 8, see pages 181-251). They're simple to prepare and can be stored in the refrigerator all day without loss of goodness. They're sometimes best drunk with a straw (if the mouth is sore, or the person is feeling a little squeamish), so that the fluid is delivered to the back of the throat. "A little and often" might be the best approach for most people. Very slightly warmed and taken before bed, it can help prepare a person for sleep as well as provide extra nourishment. The recipe is very flexible and many things can be added to the basic formula, which is:

- *1 large banana or 2 small ones (or other soft fruit)*
- *2 free-range eggs*
- *1 cup of soy milk*

Blend the ingredients together until smooth. Cinnamon or nutmeg can be sprinkled on top if desired. Banana smoothies are regarded as food, not fluid.

Optional Extras:

- *2 teaspoons of slippery elm powder (see page 189)*
- *1 heaped dessertspoon of yogurt (particularly if the person doesn't like eating yogurt)*
- *Other soft fruits like peaches, apricots, mangoes*
- *1 heaped dessertspoon of cream or tofu (particularly if the person is underweight)*

Chicken Casserole

I'm including this recipe because it's so simple and the casserole can be used in so many ways. This recipe is really easy for any person who's offered to cook something for you. You can either take it out of the freezer and leave it in the fridge to defrost during the day, or you can heat it very slowly so that it thaws at the same time.

For people who can't eat very much, the liquid of the casserole is very nourishing and delicious. For those who can tolerate a little more, then include the barley (or brown rice) and a few of the vegetables. For those with ravenous appetites you'll have to restrain them from eating the bones! This is what you do.

Take a free-range chicken, remove the fatty parts (including skin) and place in a casserole dish. Joint the chicken first if you prefer. Cover with water and add onions, garlic (if liked), 2 bay leaves, a heaping teaspoon of dried mixed herbs, and a cup and a half of pearl barley or brown rice (or half and half). Cook slowly. When almost ready, add any other vegetables, roughly cut. Cook until all is tender.

If you're cooking one, you might like to cook a second one to freeze for one of the frazzled days.

Pumpkin Soup

This might not be the richest pumpkin soup but it's certainly simple to make and will be tolerated more easily by frail tummies than some of the fancier varieties. For variety you can use other vegetables instead of pumpkin (potato, zucchini, carrot) and I suggest you make a large pot so you can freeze some for later.

Place into a pot cubed peeled pumpkin and diced onions (if tolerated). Cook in a little water until soft. Blend until smooth and gradually add soy milk. Add nutmeg to taste. Garlic can also be added if the person can tolerate it.

Sample Menus

Keeping the preceding guidelines in mind, here are some sample menus. These are for the person with cancer or HIV who appear to be in good health with no digestive disturbances. They are only suggestions and you don't *have* to include all the things mentioned. A typical daily dietary program might include:

Breakfast

- *Oatmeal (well cooked for those with upset tummies; made with soy milk for those underweight)*
- *Muesli (to be avoided by those with bowel disturbances)*
- *Puffed wheat, rice, millet, or corn served with soy milk (use sun-dried fruit, soaked overnight, for sweetener, or chopped banana)*
- *Lightly scrambled, poached, or boiled free-range eggs (if you're experiencing any indigestion do not combine with any cereal [as above] or bread, toast, or muffins)*
- *Whole meal bread, toast, or muffins*

Or...

- *Fresh fruit and yogurt*
- *Fresh fruit and nuts, pine nuts, sunflower seeds, etc.*

Remember These Points:

- *It's better to choose either grains, fresh fruit and nuts, or yogurt. Don't mix fruits and cereals (with the exception of banana, which is a complex carbohydrate).*
- *Use soy, goat's, or sheep's milk on cereal.*
- *Always chew slowly, mixing the food well with saliva.*
- *Enjoy your food, and eat with gratitude and joy.*
- *If you're concerned because you're losing weight, then use cereals for breakfast and keep fruits for snacks.*
- *If you're concerned because you're putting on weight, then use fruit and yogurt for breakfast instead of cereals.*
- *Don't drink with your meal. Drink at least half an hour before the meal or one and a half hours after.*

Mid-morning/Afternoon Snacks

- *Banana or other fruit smoothie (see recipe on page 176)*
- *Fresh fruit and nuts, sunflower seeds, pine nuts, etc.*
- *Crackers, pumpernickel, and avocado/salad veggies*
- *Small amount of dried fruit and fresh fruit*
- *Miso or vegetable soup*
- *Yogurt and fruit*
- *Fresh vegetable juice*

Lunch or Dinner

- *Always have some salad veggies, either as a salad sandwich, a side salad, or as the whole meal*
- *Jacket potatoes, sweet potato, or pumpkin, dry baked in the oven (use yogurt and chopped chives instead of sour cream)*
- *Vegetable soups (pumpkin, broccoli, cream of spinach—use soy, goat's, or sheep's milk)*
- *Stir-fried veggies (cooked in a wok to ensure that you start with only a teaspoon of oil)*
- *Grilled, steamed, or baked fish or free-range chicken*
- *Steamed vegetables (or microwaved if desired)*
- *Free-range chicken casserole (see recipe on page 177)*
- *Lentil, tofu, or tempeh burgers*
- *Pasta and vegetables*
- *Lentil, split pea, barley, lima bean, etc. dishes*
- *Whole wheat, buckwheat, or rice noodles*
- *Brown rice*

Remember These Points:

- *Use only cold-pressed oil and lemon juice plus garlic and dried or fresh herbs for salad dressings.*
- *Use a wide range of salad veggies so you meet your needs for vitamins,*

minerals, and enzymes. Include lettuce, tomato, cucumber, capsicum, broccoli, cauliflower, mung and alfalfa sprouts, zucchini, and so on (if you like them).

- *Chew food thoroughly.* The first stage of digestion takes place in the mouth when the food is mixed with an enzyme in your saliva.

- *If you're having baked chicken, eat the meat closest to the bone. Avoid the fatty areas and skin.*

- *Use the microwave sparingly and only for vegetables.* When feeling stressed, it's better to get food rapidly onto the table than to compound the chaos by fiddling around in the kitchen. Don't overcook the veggies.

- *Lentil, tofu, or tempeh burgers are usually available in the fridge of any good health food store.*

- *Whole meal pasta tastes pretty awful unless you're very creative.* Use ordinary pasta made from unbleached flour, or freshly made store-bought pasta—after having checked its ingredients with the chef. Many of the prepared sauces in good gourmet shops are fine, though do check the ingredients and avoid oily ones.

- *Prepared noodles are great to have as a stand-by in the pantry.* They're good on their own as a soup or can be added to vegetable, chicken, or fish dishes to flavor and thicken. They are available in health food stores and some supermarkets.

- *Many unwell people are weary by the evening.* If you're weary, so is your digestive system. You might find it best to make your main meals breakfast and lunch, and have just a light meal (like soup and muffins) for dinner at night.

- *Don't drink with your meal.* Drink at least half an hour before the meal or one and a half hours after.

Sometime in the near future the Quest for Life Foundation plans to produce a book that contains recipes for delicious and appetizing foods for those who are unwell. If you have a favorite recipe, or a solution to some dietary problem, you might like to send in your contribution to share with the world! Of course, you'll be acknowledged and our readers will be grateful for your creative ideas. Please write for information to the Quest for Life Center.

Chapter Eight

BURPS, BURNING
AND THE DREADED BLOATS
(AND MUCH MORE)

. . . .

Don

After my HIV+ diagnosis, I continued my work as a teacher as if nothing had really changed. It was not until I actually became ill that I was emotionally affected at all. The doctor said that the relentless diarrhea was HIV related. I was coping with extreme physical debilitation and finally had to give up work because of the weakness I experienced. Also, I began having "accidents" when I couldn't make it to the bathroom, and I found these episodes particularly undignified and humiliating.

My doctors tried everything to find and treat the cause of the diarrhea but were unsuccessful. Sometimes it would improve for a day or two and then come back even worse than before. Some of the drugs they experimented with made me horribly ill and the side effects were worse than the ever-present symptom they were trying to treat. My life became terribly restricted as I was afraid to leave my apartment. Having to visit the bathroom up to twenty-eight times in twenty-four hours made me feel that my quality of life was diminishing rapidly.

At times when the diarrhea was not too severe I used to attend support and meditation groups. At the time, these groups were my life-line as I was able to explore and express all the thoughts and feelings I was experiencing. It was also good to meet with other people who were coping with their own difficulties in a positive manner and it melted down a lot of the barriers which my isolation created.

I decided to consult Petrea as I knew she did a lot of work with people who experienced various symptoms associated with their disease. It was difficult to be motivated enough to even make an appointment when I held no hope that anything could make a difference. However, a friend insisted on taking me and I began on a new path to control the diarrhea. At this time I weighed just under 98 lbs. and the only way I could keep my pants up was with suspenders.

I made several changes to my diet and began taking the homeopathics and slippery elm that were suggested. Within twenty-four hours I could notice a difference. I had to experiment a little with the combination of homeopathics and slippery elm and found this latter substance to be of enormous benefit. I take slippery elm every hour and find that's the most effective dose for me. The slippery elm gave me a good feeling knowing that I could actively participate in my recovery and it gave me back a sense of control. This has been a really impor-tant factor because to feel out of control is to feel not at peace. Peace has become my main goal but I couldn't find peace within myself while my body was so unmanageable. Now I feel I'm back in control and that I can make a difference.

Now, two and a half years later my quality of life is much im-proved. I still have diarrhea, but it's not severe and has become quite manageable. I am able to lead a fulfilling life. My weight is not up to its normal level but I have plenty of energy and can do the things I choose to. I have found there is always beauty to enjoy and some ac-tivity to pursue. I am able to honestly say that I am perfectly happy, which is a rare and valuable gift that I cherish. I can't believe that heaven can be any nicer than where I am right now.

❧

This chapter covers many of the unpleasant symptoms of the disease and the side effects which might be experienced from your treatments. You're encouraged to read the whole chapter because you'll find there are a lot of overlapping suggestions among the alphabetically listed subjects.

Much of the information is based on simple common sense, the use of home remedies, and the addition of nutritional or herbal supplements. The ideas, suggestions, and recommendations in this chapter are a result of years of working with thousands of people who've suffered not only the symptoms of their disease but the many discomforts that their treatments sometimes cause. None of the information is intended as a prescription and you're encouraged to speak to your doctors before implementing these suggestions, and give them feedback as to the results. You could also benefit by consulting a naturopath or doctor trained to tailor a dietary program to your specific situation. The remedies and guidelines within this chapter are in no way designed to *treat disease*. The intent is to give you, the patient, some information about minimizing the *symptoms* of your disease or the side *effects* of your treatment.

Very often, your doctor is more interested in the treatment of your disease and is less interested in the symptoms you might experience. If you complain about a lack of appetite; a mouth full of ulcers; chronic squeamishness; restlessness at night; indigestion; lymphoedema; decreased libido; memory, weight or hair loss; watery eyes; night sweats; or any of the myriad discomforting things which may occur, he or she might well show little interest because he or she is more concerned about the treatment of your primary condition. This can be very disconcerting. In fact, I find most people will say, "I can cope with the disease but *my hair falling out really gets to me*" (or *losing weight*, or *lack of energy*, or *living with uncertainty*).

In the health food store, you might have difficulty replicating the exact formulas mentioned in this chapter. However, there'll be formulas which closely resemble the ones listed and I suggest you seek the assistance of the proprietor in deciding which is most appropriate for you. All of the substances, herbs, and homeopathics may be taken in addition to your medical treatment. They will not interfere with your treatment.

Where it's suggested that a remedy be taken at regular

intervals, it is with the understanding that you *don't* need to wake up at night to continue the process. For instance, when there's severe indigestion it's recommended that digestive enzymes be taken at two-hour intervals. It might be necessary to continue this right up until bedtime, but once sleep has been achieved, enjoy it!

Throughout this chapter you'll see that homeopathics are referred to frequently. Homeopathic healing is based on the principle that "like cures like." The medicinal substances used in homeopathic medicines can be of animal, vegetable, or mineral origin. A simple description of how homeopathy works is this: if you ingest the herb ipecac it will make you feel nauseous and can easily lead to vomiting. However, if you dilute the ipecac to the point where it is no longer evident, it can stimulate the body to "cure" itself of nausea. This is a little like the vaccination theory: A small amount of killed or ineffectual virus material introduced into the body can stimulate a positive healing response from the body.

Most of the formulas and homeopathics mentioned in this chapter are available from any good health food store or naturopath. You might like to inquire at your local AIDS council or cancer council for a naturopathic practitioner who has had extensive experience working with people with your illness. If you have difficulty in finding any of the remedies mentioned in this chapter you might like to contact: Healthcrafters, Best Avenue, Norwalk, California, 90651 (310) 926-5522.

You might be wondering about the difference between homeopaths, naturopaths, herbalists, and so on. First of all, holistic medicine means an overall approach to healing or well being. This involves looking at the mind, body, emotions, and spirit of a person rather than focusing on the symptom or disease. A homeopath, using the tenet of "like cures like" to heal physical and emotional symptoms, uses prepared homeopathic remedies. A naturopath uses nutrition, herbs, vitamins, minerals, juices, and other supplements to encourage the body to heal itself. Both homeopathy and naturopathy are holistic in that they treat the whole person not just the disease. All holistic practitioners include the "mind" of the patient in their therapy. This may be through counseling, educating, meditation or visualization techniques.

Anemia

With anemia, there are not enough red blood cells to carry oxygen around the body. You need oxygen for energy and many other cellular and metabolic functions. If you've lost more blood than your body can readily replace, you become anemic. Sometimes it develops because cancer impairs the bone marrow's ability to produce blood. Some of the drugs prescribed for various treatments can depress the bone marrow's ability to produce sufficient red blood cells. These drugs include AZT and many of the chemotherapeutic drugs. Some cancers can make the red blood cells very fragile. As you can see, there's not a great deal *you* can do about your hemoglobin (the oxygen-binding protein in the red cells in your bloodstream). The most likely symptoms of anemia are:

- *Low energy level or general weakness*
- *Exhaustion or breathlessness on exertion*
- *Giddiness or light-headedness on rising*
- *Headaches*
- *Increased pulse rate*
- *Pallor of skin*

Clearly your doctor will be the best person to prescribe the appropriate remedy. However, the following dietary suggestions have been found to be useful by many people. These are foods rich in iron and other essential nutrients which help to form red cells in the blood.

Remember These Points

- *A glass of a stout type beer before the evening meal or before bed*
- *The vegetable juice (see page 174) three times daily, particularly in the week leading up to chemotherapy*

- *A supplement which contains iron, zinc, folic acid, Vitamins B12, B6, C and E*
- *Meats which are rich in iron*
- *Leafy greens in your diet (or juice)*

The benefits of adding these foods or substances to your diet will depend very much on the cause of your anemia. If you're bleeding continuously from an area of your body, then drinking juices and not attending to the hemorrhage would be worse than useless. However, if nothing can be done to prevent the bleeding, or if anemia is a side effect of your treatment, then by all means use everything available, including blood transfusions, to ease the situation.

Blood in the Feces

Blood may not be easy to detect in feces, though if it's bright red, it's easy to see. This bright color usually only occurs if the bleeding has occurred in the last section of the bowel. If the stool is dark and looks somewhat like coffee grounds, it could well indicate bleeding from higher up in the bowel. It's essential you have it investigated immediately by your doctor to ascertain its cause.

Beetroot and/or beetroot juice will turn the stool and/or urine a beetroot color. It definitely looks like beetroot, not blood!

Bowel Blockages

Blockages in the bowel can cause extreme pain and discomfort. They can be partial, which means that only a small amount of fecal matter and gas can pass through the bowel, or they can be complete blockages in which case nothing can pass. Needless to say, if nothing passes through, then nausea and vomiting will result if the person continues to eat. Often nausea and vomiting are the first signs of a blockage. People suffering in this way often need hospitalization in order to monitor and assess their situation. Sometimes surgery is suggested so that the blockage can be removed and the bowel rejoined. Occasionally a colos-

tomy or ileostomy is the best solution. This is a surgical procedure where the bowel is brought out through an artificial opening in the abdomen so that its contents can empty into a bag. A
colostomy is an opening from the large bowel; an ileostomy
from the small bowel.

Sometimes, a wait-and-see approach is adopted. This approach usually entails removing any fluid from the stomach via a
naso-gastric tube while giving intravenous fluids. This allows the
bowel to rest so that any inflammation or pressure may subside
and, perhaps, resolve the blockage. Once this has happened,
clear fluids are permitted and gradually the person can return to
a fuller intake of foods. In the weeks following a bowel blockage, it's important that the person eats foods which are easy to
pass through the bowel and which won't cause constipation.

**If you would like to adopt the approach outlined in this
section, you must discuss it with your doctor first. He or she
will understand your particular situation clearly and will be
able to advise you accordingly. The guidelines are included
here because very few people seem to be given any assistance
in finding appropriate foods to eat after a bowel blockage. If
your doctor says it doesn't matter what you eat, then these
guidelines could prove invaluable.**

After a bowel blockage, or to avoid one, it's best to eat foods
which will remain soft as they pass through the bowel. Don't eat
constipating foods such as cheese, dairy products (with the exception of yogurt), white flour products, red meats, cooked eggs
and whatever else *you* find constipating. Nor should you eat
foods which are high in fiber such as bran, muesli, and fruit and
vegetable skins.

A young member of our support group, Jan, was hospitalized
with a bowel blockage as a secondary problem to her extensive
ovarian cancer. Her doctors adopted the wait-and-see approach
mentioned previously and within a few days she felt far more
comfortable. The naso-gastric tube was left in place for three
weeks in which time she received all her nutritional needs
through an intravenous drip in her arm.

She used her time wisely, meditating, relaxing, concentrating her calming thoughts upon her distressed interior. After the first week, her abdomen began to gurgle and bubble which meant gas was able to move about and be passed. Great celebrations took place, as this was a sign of improvement. (Once we have an illness we celebrate the most bizarre occasions!) Finally, Jan could eat small amounts of food, having gradually progressed from clear fluids, and she was, at last, released from the hospital.

On her departure, she was given no information about the foods which would probably help her to avoid a recurrence. Once she arrived home, Jan faced the dilemma of what to eat. She telephoned the hospital, spoke with the dietitian, and was told to eat low-fiber, nourishing foods. When Jan asked what sort of foods were nourishing, she was told to concentrate on milk puddings, cheese, pastries, meat, and eggs. When asked if she could eat pizza, the dietitian replied "Yes." Jan's physical problems compounded with the fact she also needed morphine which *causes* constipation left her with more than a potential problem.

When I asked the staff at the hospital why she'd been given such unhelpful advice, they replied they were expecting her back within a week or two with another blockage, and they didn't think what she ate would make much difference.

Fortunately, Jan decided to seek more information before she adopted their advice. I encouraged her to eat along the lines suggested in this section and she continued to improve, gaining in strength and energy. Until her peaceful death several months later, she never had another bowel blockage. Even though Jan was young when she died, it's the way we *live* until we die which is important. Anyone who's ever witnessed the extreme pain and distress a bowel blockage can inflict would go to any lengths to avoid its recurrence.

I have another client who had experienced two bowel blockages due to the spread of her uterine cancer. She was hospitalized on each occasion for surgical removal of the blockage. The first obstruction occurred more than five and a half years ago, and her doctor cannot understand why she's still alive. She adopted the program outlined here and for four years she re-mained free of problems, even though her abdomen felt almost "solid" with tumors. She then developed another blockage which resulted in a colostomy. The colostomy has been working well for the past twelve months and she's in good spirits, even though her abdomen feels much the same. Her doctors are still surprised (and delighted) that she's alive and her quality of life is excellent.

Slippery Elm Powder

After a blockage, or to avoid one, the use of Slippery Elm powder is invaluable. It's made from the bark of a tree and has been used for centuries by the American Indians as a gruel for their babies to soothe upset tummies and to nourish them. It puts a slimy or mucilaginous coating over the whole of the gastrointestinal tract. This substance is very soothing to the smooth muscle of the stomach and small intestine and promotes healing to damaged tis-sue. It tends to regulate the bowel and is useful for those who suf-fer with nausea, diarrhea, or constipation. Slippery Elm is readily available from any health food store and has no side effects.

It's best used in powdered form as it's the most readily uti-lized/assimilated. It's also available in capsule or tablet form and, for problems occurring lower down in the bowel, these can be used instead if powder is unavailable. Frankly, I always prefer to use it in powdered form. The powder itself can be mixed with water but the easiest way to ingest it is mashed into a little low-fat, acidophilus-based yogurt or soft, peeled, stewed fruit. For minimizing a recurrence of a bowel blockage, try mixing two heaping teaspoons of the powder in this way and have it three times daily, about twenty minutes before each meal. You can have it as frequently as seems necessary for you and, in fact, many people have virtually lived on Slippery Elm and yogurt for one or more weeks.

Digestive Enzymes

Digestive enzymes are normally produced in the juices of the mouth, stomach, small intestine, and pancreas. These enzymes are essential so that food can be broken down and assimilated into the body. Many people have a diminished ability to produce digestive enzymes. Sometimes this inability to produce sufficient digestive enzymes is evident in people who:

- *Are over the age of fifty*
- *Are having or have recently had chemotherapy*
- *Are unwell*
- *Have had major surgical procedures to the digestive tract*
- *Are recovering from any major surgery*
- *Are having or have had radiotherapy to the stomach/abdominal area*

Those wishing to avoid a bowel blockage might find the following recommendations of benefit. As stressed previously, check these guidelines with your doctor before following them. If the blockage has been very severe:

- *Abstain from all food and drink water, chamomile, or peppermint tea without honey. You may wish to make the herb teas into ice cubes to suck. They can be very refreshing when your mouth is feeling stale.*

Then, implement the following:

Take two digestive enzyme tablets every two hours. The formula should contain:

- Pancreatin 4NF   200 mg
- Bromelain   100 mg
- Pepsin   100 mg
- Trypsin   30 mg

After eight hours (or if very hungry):

- *Take two teaspoons of Slippery Elm powder mashed into two tablespoons of low-fat acidophilus-based yogurt.*

  This must be eaten very slowly and be well mixed with saliva. Do not have any fluids for at least thirty minutes before or at least ninety minutes after.

  Give two tablets of the digestive enzyme formula mentioned at the same time with the minimal amount of water to swallow. Repeat this every four hours (Slippery Elm and digestive enzymes).

- *Stay with this program until the bowel is passing something other than gas.*

- *Once the bowel is working, you might like to try some well-stewed (peeled) apple and yogurt.*

- *If all is still calm after 48 hours, try some very well-cooked peeled vegetable (avoid seeds) or pumpkin or other vegetable soup (see page 177) or a banana smoothie (see page 176). Use only very ripe, sugary bananas or other soft fruit.*

- *Gradually expand the diet, keeping to only two foods per meal. For example, steamed fish and well-cooked carrots; peeled and cooked zucchini and mashed potato (no additives except a little vegetable salt).*

- *Continue with the Slippery Elm at least three times daily.*

- *Listen to your body and heed its messages.*

These suggestions must be approved by your doctor before you implement them. They are additions to your medical management and are in no way a replacement for it. These suggestions will not eliminate the cause of the blockage but may reduce the likelihood of you developing one. You'll gain the greatest benefit from these suggestions by having them tailored to your individual needs.

Bowel Cancer

It's common knowledge in the medical community today that there's an increased incidence of bowel cancer in those who consume a high-protein, high-fat, low-fiber diet, and yet I'm still to hear of an oncologist encouraging patients to improve their diet after surgery. Even when patients ask if there's anything they can do to prevent a recurrence, they're told there's nothing that will make any difference. The medical argument for this is that, even though dietary factors may contribute to bowel cancer, there's no evidence that correcting the diet will make any difference to the final outcome. Common sense and experience certainly suggest that an holistic approach to health, which includes an appropriate diet, *will* make a difference.

If you've had a goodly portion of your digestive tract removed, then you'll need some assistance in finding a diet which helps you to feel comfortable until your body adjusts to this new situation. The recovery of your bowel function will depend very much on the amount of bowel removed and (perhaps) whether there are any lymph nodes affected in the adjacent area. You should allow six weeks for the bowel to heal and settle down after surgery. Only then will you be able to ascertain what is now "normal" for your bowel. All the factors I've mentioned in the text relating to bowel and digestive function will be of relevance to you. Particularly useful will be the Slippery Elm powder mashed into yogurt or banana. This tends to regulate or normalize bowel function as well as soothe and heal the traumatized lining. Experiment until you find what works for you.

Burps, Burning, and the Dreaded Bloats

The mucous lining of the mouth, esophagus, stomach, intestines, and other internal organs have a high proportion of rapidly dividing cells—for instance, the cells forming the lining of the mouth are replaced every twenty-four hours—and are therefore affected by chemotherapy. Most chemotherapy drugs interfere with this process and so the mouth can become raw or sensitive and can form ulcers. Likewise, the surface of the digestive tract will be damaged and will take several days to recover.

Many people develop symptoms of indigestion when having chemotherapy or other drug treatments, particularly those people over the age of fifty. This might take the form of burping repeatedly after eating, a burning sensation just below the sternum, or a feeling of bloatedness. From experience, I believe that some forms of chemotherapy and some other drug treatments interfere with the body's ability to secrete hydrochloric acid, and gastric and pancreatic enzymes. The addition of hydrochloric acid and digestive enzymes in tablet form in conjunction with an appropriate diet can often eliminate these distressing symptoms altogether. The formulas which I recommend contain:

Digestive Enzyme Formula

- *Betaine HCl*   400 mg
- *Pancreatin 4NF*   200 mg
- *Bromelain*   100 mg
- *Pepsin*   100 mg
- *Glutamic acid*   100 mg
- *Trypsin*   30 mg

One to two tablets with each meal should be sufficient to alleviate symptoms. Some people find they need to take digestive enzymes and hydrochloric acid any time they ingest any food or fluid, with the exception of water.

Do not drink any liquid for at least thirty minutes before a meal, or at least ninety minutes after eating (with the exception of minimal fluid in order to take the digestive enzymes).

As previously discussed, chemotherapy, antibiotics, and some other drug treatments destroy the "good" bacteria that normally reside in the intestines. These bacteria are essential because they help break down the food you eat so your body can assimilate the nutrients. I recommend you eat two tablespoons of an acidophilus-based low-fat yogurt per day during the time you're on a drug treatment program, so that you replenish the gut bacteria which the drugs destroy. For the first few days after chemotherapy your body won't be able to fully assimilate the foods you eat, no matter how nutritious they might be. Your main objective in the first few days is to replenish gut bacteria and maintain your physical comfort as much as possible. If you're having radiation treatment to the abdominal area this also applies. The yogurt must be based on the acidophilus lactobacillus. Several low-fat cow's milk varieties are available as well as goat's milk yogurt (which few seem to enjoy!) and sheep's milk yogurt (which can be difficult to obtain but which is delicious). These kinds of yogurt are generally the *only* dairy foods which I recommend for people with cancer, AIDS, or any other acute or chronic illness.

Bloating can be caused by a build up of fluid in the abdomen. This fluid generally collects in the peritoneal cavity. The peritoneum is a fine double membrane that lines the abdominal cavity. Fluid might collect between the membranes if cancer cells start growing on them, or because of liver disease. This fluid is called ascites and won't be improved by the digestive enzyme formula. Your doctor is the best person to diagnose and treat ascites. Often indigestion is experienced *because* of this bloating and this will certainly be eased through the addition of the digestive enzymes and yogurt. If the symptoms are very severe, see Gas (see page 212).

Chewing and Swallowing Problems, Mouth Ulcers, Dry Mouth, and Thrush

A dry mouth can be the result of various forms of treatment, or because of disease. Treatments might include some kinds of chemotherapy, or radiation which is to the mouth/salivary gland area. Some analgesics, like morphine, dry out the secretions in the mouth. The problem doesn't necessarily stop at the discomfort and inconvenience of having a dry mouth. The saliva serves a valuable function in maintaining hygiene within the mouth and gullet area and, with these secretions missing, infections, mouth ulcers, increased sensitivity, bleeding gums, and thrush can all become problems. Having a mouth which feels and tastes like the bottom of a bird cage is no fun either. With a sensitive mouth it becomes increasingly difficult to eat. If the dry mouth and its resultant problems are caused by radiation, then improvement will begin once the treatment has ceased. In some instances, some of the salivary glands don't resume their former functioning capacity; however, there are many salivary glands which will be able to take over adequately.

A dry mouth at night can be very distressing, as it interferes with your ability to sleep. To awaken gagging from the dryness can be frightening. Always keep some fluid nearby. Artificial saliva can be useful since it evaporates much more slowly than water. Your pharmacist can order artificial saliva if he or she doesn't have it in stock. Five to ten drops on the tongue is usually sufficient to give relief. You might need to use a little more at night to keep your mouth lubricated while you sleep. Your dentist or pharmacist can also supply you with a chewing gum which increases salivary production. There are some excellent ones available. If you have difficulty in chewing, then the artificial saliva will be preferable. Ice cubes of peppermint or lemon tea can be both soothing and refreshing to the mouth. Do not use lemon tea if the lining of the mouth is raw or sensitive. In severe cases where the mouth is very sensitive or raw, a liquid or gel local anesthetic will bring relief.

If thrush is present then your doctor will prescribe a liquid for the mouth or some lozenges for you to suck. Thrush can be very painful and can make swallowing difficult, particularly when it extends down the esophagus. Your doctor will prescribe some further medication if this is the case. Thrush sometimes develops after a course of chemotherapy or antibiotics.

Zinc lozenges containing Vitamin C and lysine are also very helpful for mouth ulcers or broken areas in the mouth.

Propolis is a bee product which contains many nutrients that are readily assimilated by your body. It's also a valuable antibiotic against the anaerobic germs which might live in our mouths and throats and which might extend right throughout the digestive tract. Propolis is very helpful for people who have recurring infections in the mouth and throat.

Depending on the severity of the dryness, rinsing the mouth several times a day with tea-tree oil diluted in water can be beneficial. The dosage is five drops of oil in a third of a glass of tepid or warm water. Rinse the mouth, gargle, and spit out. This might sting a little if there are any broken areas. You can reduce the tea-tree oil to one or two drops if that's more comfortable. It's very helpful for bleeding gums, mouth ulcers, thrush, cracked or sensitive mouth linings (in addition to, or as replacement of, any prescribed medications).

Those with chewing problems will find it easier to eat moist, soft foods and might even benefit from a liquid diet of nutritious foods drunk through a straw. Smoothies, soups, and vegetable juices can all be ingested in this way. This delivers the food to the back of the mouth and minimizes any mouth irritation. As mentioned above, the use of a topical anesthetic can also assist in "numbing" the pain in the mouth before eating. Techniques of relaxation can also be used for this purpose.

Tom had severe thrush which extended from his mouth down through the esophagus and into his stomach. His weight loss had accelerated considerably due to his inability to eat without experiencing the most severe pain. He used all the practical suggestions I've listed here and found that one of the most helpful was to use a visualization technique. With this technique he imagined a clear blue soothing gel spreading over the whole of the affected area. This gel would "anesthetize" everything it touched. He would practice this technique for several minutes before each meal, and found that if he ate only cool foods he was able to maintain the effectiveness of his visualization.

Remember These Points:

- *Artificial saliva is available from pharmacists, and chewing gums which increase salivary output are available from dentists and pharmacists.*
- *Eat soft, tender and bland foods such as pasta and noodles.*
- *Eat cool, moist foods such as stewed fruits, yogurt, cold soups.*
- *Make ice cubes of peppermint and/or chamomile or lemon tea and suck on the cubes.*
- *Drink non-acidic juices such as nectars, grape, or apple juice (you might need to dilute them with water).*
- *Rinse mouth frequently to keep mouth and gums clean, put a fresh taste in the mouth, and prevent infection.*
- *Avoid highly acidic, spicy, or salty foods such as citrus fruits or juices, tomatoes, strawberries, pineapples, pepper and chili powder.*
- *Very hot foods can be irritating; cool/cold foods can be soothing.*
- *Avoid chewy or hard-to-chew foods like fresh fruits and raw vegetables.*

- *The warm liquid from a nourishing chicken casserole might be tolerated quite well (see page 177).*
- *Tilting the head back to swallow might ease the discomfort.*
- *Use a blender to prepare soft, smooth foods.*
- *Drinking through a straw delivers food to the back of the mouth. Suitable foods to be consumed in this way are soups, smoothies (see page 176), vegetable juices, yogurt, and Slippery Elm.*
- *Relaxation or meditation techniques practiced before eating can allow swallowing to be more easily tolerated by those who experience pain in their esophagus.*

"Cold Bones"

Many people with cancer and AIDS find they experience a coldness that seems to come from right inside the bones. No matter what they put on in the way of extra clothes, or whether they sit right in front of a fire, they *still* feel cold. I used to feel as if my bones were made of ice! The only remedy which I have found to be helpful is ginger tea. This is made by thinly slicing a quarter of a cup of fresh ginger root and simmering it for fifteen minutes in a liter of water. Let it cool to body temperature, then strain. You might like to add a little honey to sweeten. Drink a small cupful every hour or two, or before bed.

Colostomies and Ileostomies

Much of what's written in this chapter applies to those who have a colostomy or ileostomy. After any bowel surgery, it takes six weeks for "normal" function to reestablish itself. Your hospital will have put you in touch with the nearest colostomy/ileostomy or stoma group, who'll be able to give you information regarding the first weeks and months of learning to live with this new situation. If it hasn't, *ask!*

Bowel upsets may occur as you're becoming used to your ostomy and even when you're quite familiar with the foods that agree with you. It's good to remember that these upsets can be caused by emotional stress, medication, tiredness, or travel and are not always related to diet. You might also find that foods that don't agree with you today will be tolerated very well if you go for a few days before trying them again.

It's important that you keep up a high fluid intake—at least two liters of fluid per day to prevent dehydration. The output from an ileostomy will always be of a liquid consistency, and restricting fluids will not make it any thicker.

You lose more salt from your ostomy than if your bowel functioned normally, so it's important that you maintain your salt intake. You do not need to increase it; just maintain your normal intake.

Some foods increase odor in some people. Avoid these foods *only* if they cause this problem repeatedly: onions, baked beans, peas, cabbage, fish, Brussels sprouts.

You will find that the information contained within the text relating to the digestive tract will be applicable to you, especially that on diarrhea. It is important to control diarrhea as you can easily become dehydrated due to excessive water and salt loss.

It's important to eat meals at regular hours. Snack in between times if you're having any problem with weight loss. It's important to eat slowly, chewing well and keeping your mouth closed when eating to minimize swallowing air with your food. It's best to swallow *before* taking the next mouthful of food. If you're eating nuts, corn, or cereals, it's important that you chew them *very* well because you can run the risk of blocking the passage to your stoma with improperly broken-down foods. It's better for you to avoid seeds and nuts altogether unless you have them made into a "milk." This is done by taking sunflower, sesame seeds, or nuts and grinding them finely (in a coffee grinder) and then blending them in a little warm water. You can add a little honey if you want.

It takes most people a while to adjust to the idea of an ostomy. Be gentle and compassionate toward yourself as you learn to manage it. It *will* take time to learn how best to cooperate with your ostomy, but you *can* make the adjustment. Each person will have a "different relationship" with his or her ostomy. You'll probably find it very helpful to speak to someone who's been through the same experience and who understands the implications of living well with an ostomy.

Constipation

Like gas, constipation has the power to create intense pain, particularly after surgery or if there are tumors or other causes for pain within the abdomen. You're constipated if your bowel movements are hard and you have difficulty passing them. All sorts of things can cause constipation and, as with any condition, it's essential to find the cause. We all know some of the factors which cause constipation—lack of exercise, insufficient fluid intake, most analgesics (painkillers), lack of fiber, not eating enough, and some foods like cheese, cooked eggs, and so on. The causes of constipation are too numerous to enumerate. Constipation is only the symptom of a problem. Once the problem has been pinpointed, appropriate treatment (if any) can be planned. If possible, don't wait until you're really badly constipated before doing something about it.

If the constipation is caused through the necessary intake of analgesics, then you'll need to take a laxative. Most analgesics, in addition to relieving you of pain, also cause constipation. They do this by slowing down the peristaltic movement of the bowel and by drying out its contents. These two things in combination cause you to develop constipation. Your nurse or doctor will know what's causing *your* constipation so ask his or her advice. Community and palliative-care nurses are also experts at managing constipation. They'll recommend to you an appropriate laxative which contains a softening agent. The addition of extra fluids, prunes, bran, and so on will need to be discussed with your medical advisers. They may perhaps prefer you to be on a low-fiber diet, depending on other factors relating to your health.

It's important to drink plenty of fluid and to exercise to the extent you're able. Sometimes a massage to the abdomen or the application of warmth will be sufficient to stimulate action of the bowel (in addition to your laxative). This warmth can be applied in the form of a hot-water bottle, an electric heating pad, or a towel soaked in hot water and wrung out, then placed gently over the abdomen. If massage is used, it should always be performed in a clockwise direction. Slow and gentle massage with a warmed and perfumed oil can be very soothing.

Your doctor or nurse might also suggest the use of suppositories or enemas. These days they're extremely easy to give (though some cause a burning sensation) and are very effective.

Coughs

Any cough should be checked by your doctor so that he can discover its cause and establish the appropriate treatment. There's one particular cough about which I want to say a few words. Some people develop metastases (secondary growths) in the lungs. Occasionally these small tumors interfere with the nerve receptors which can cause a constant and irritating "tickle" in the upper part of the chest. You might develop a cough which is exacerbated by talking, stress, trying not to cough, physical exertion, laughing, or lying down. Occasionally these tumors can be effectively treated by radiotherapy or chemotherapy, so it's essential you speak to your doctor. People who have, or are recovering from, Pneumocystis carinii often experience an irritating cough which might or might not be associated with excess mucus in the lungs. If there's no recommended treatment, you might like to try the following homeopathic remedy which has worked effectively in many cases. This formula isn't intended to treat the cause but to alleviate the effect of the nerve irritation, and can be taken in addition to any medical treatment.

Cough Drop Formula

Bryonia	2x
Drosera	3x
Spongia	5x

Coccus cacti   5x

Belladonna   5x

To alleviate cough: Take ten drops in a couple of teaspoons of water every half to one hour. Hold in the mouth for a few seconds before swallowing.

If the cough is particularly persistent: Seventy drops in half a glass of water. Sip every two minutes, holding each sip in the mouth for a few seconds before swallowing, until cough settles. Then reduce the frequency to every five, then ten, then fifteen, then thirty minutes. Resume frequency if the cough returns.

Though this remedy will alleviate the cough in many cases, it doesn't "do" anything to treat the cause of the cough. It doesn't work by reducing tumor size or by treating infection, but does seem to soothe the irritation to the nerve receptors. It is also a beneficial formula for those who develop an irritating cough when under stress.

Some forms of asthma can be helped by these drops also. My daughter Kate has a very mild form of asthma which doesn't cause her to wheeze but produces a dry, irritating cough. When she's having a bout, she can cough until she dry retches. It's always worse when she lies down, which means her sleep (and mine!) can be very disturbed. These drops in combination with an Italian licorice sweet have made an enormous difference to her ability to alleviate the debilitating coughing. Three or four of the small licorice pellets will stop her coughing in seconds. I've used these sweets with many other people plagued by coughing from various causes with almost miraculous results. The cause of the cough does not seem to make any difference to the effectiveness of the sweets.

Cramps

Is anything more harrowing than being woken from a deep sleep with a painful cramp in the leg? It has you leaping from the covers to hobble around the bedroom, yelping quietly so as not to wake the neighbors. Sometimes these cramps are related to medication, sometimes not. In all cases they're painful. Speak to your doctor about them.

If they're not related to your medication (and even if they are), try this simple remedy. I know you're all going to laugh at me and I'm about to put my credibility on the line. However, this "remedy" has worked hundreds of times so I'll repeat it anyway. Take ten wine bottle corks, put them in a piece of cotton, like a man's handkerchief, and place at your feet in the bed. That's it! It's best if the corks came from their bottles in the past three months, *and note that you don't have to drink the wine first.* Your local restaurant will probably oblige by giving you theirs. I've used this remedy on everyone from a high court judge through to children, with similar excellent effect. Its success seems to have little to do with gullibility!

If this remedy sounds too unscientific for you, try a supplement which contains Vitamins B1, B3, B6, E, biotin, calcium, magnesium, and potassium.

Diarrhea

Diarrhea involves passing loose bowel movements often and usually with urgency. In other words, "when you gotta go, you gotta go!"

One's self-esteem must be in great shape in order to withstand the undignified presence of diarrhea for a long period of time. Next to constipation, it's what we dread most. As one of the members of our support group said, "It's better to have good bowels than good brains!"

Fortunately there are many home remedies available for diarrhea. Since the advent of AIDS, diarrhea has been a feature of my professional life! My "diarrhea skills" have had to reach new heights. The majority of those with cancer who suffer from diarrhea are relatively easy to assist in comparison.

For people with cancer, there can be many causes of diarrhea including bowel cancers which have necessitated surgery, the presence of secondaries in or around the bowel, infections, nervous tension, and the effect of medication or treatments. Diarrhea can also be due to malabsorption—in which case the bowel can't absorb certain substances into the bloodstream. The stools in this case consist of large, pale, soft material which contain a lot of fat. Because they contain so much fat, they're difficult to flush away. You could become deficient in Vitamins A, D, and K if this continues, plus minerals (such as calcium). Your doctor will check for these levels in your blood. He might suggest you take additional supplements of these in oral or injection form. Again, the cause must be determined in order to find the appropriate form of treatment.

If your diarrhea is caused by an infection then it must be treated. If it's the result of radiotherapy, your treatment could be adjusted (speak to your doctor), or you could follow the guidelines I suggest here. Likewise, if your diarrhea is caused through your chemotherapy treatment, it could either be adjusted by your doctor or you could adopt the very successful plan outlined here.

If diarrhea is present after surgery to the colon for bowel cancer, it's considered to be entirely normal. As previously mentioned, it takes at least six weeks for the bowel to heal and settle down after major surgery. If you've had a major portion of your large bowel removed, you're bound to experience soft, loose, or very loose bowel movements, depending on the amount of bowel which was removed. You'll need to relax and give yourself time to heal before making any major adjustments. Then, after six weeks, if you still have more looseness in the bowel than you're willing to put up with, following the guidelines here might be beneficial.

Remember, diarrhea often occurs after a course of antibiotics. If this is the case, it means that in addition to the "bad" bacteria the antibiotics have also killed off some of the useful bacteria which live in your gut. They need to be replenished with either yogurt or lactobacillus acidophilus in capsule or powder form. This might in itself be sufficient to remedy the situation.

Sometimes, stool cultures are necessary as a way of determining the nature of the offending "bug." This particularly applies to people infected with HIV. When the immune system is depleted, you are more susceptible to infection with intestinal "bugs." It is essential that the cause of the diarrhea be diagnosed so that appropriate treatment can be instigated. For some kinds of infections there isn't any effective treatment and, in this case, the program outlined here will certainly be of benefit. With or without treatment, the guidelines suggested here can still be followed.

It's important you don't become dehydrated while you have diarrhea.

If your diarrhea is severe, you should report it to your doctor. If it's accompanied by nausea and vomiting, you might well need intravenous fluids until it's brought under control.

Occasionally what appears to be diarrhea may, in fact, be an overflow from a full bowel. There are several different reasons why the bowel can be full and yet you don't feel the urge to empty it. When this happens, an overflowing sometimes occurs where some fecal matter is passed without you being able to control it. By examining you, your doctor will be able to establish if this is the case . Many people feel ashamed or embarrassed by these symptoms and some even want to hide their symptoms instead of seeking help. Although these feelings are entirely understandable, they're also inappropriate. Seek help from your doctor.

There are some excellent medications available for diarrhea and you might wish to speak to your doctor about these. The problem with some of them is that they "stop up" the system only to have it let go with a vengeance at a later time. If this is the case, then the approach suggested here could save the day. Please discuss these guidelines with your doctor before following them. The information here will also be helpful to anyone suffering with erratic bowel function.

A Holistic Approach to Diarrhea

In order to soothe and comfort the lining of the bowel, you can't use a more efficient and calming substance than Slippery Elm powder (see page 189). It's very soothing to the bowel wall, calms irritated and raw tissue, and promotes healing to those surfaces traumatized through surgery, infection, or radiotherapy. The bowel wall needs to be soothed in order for you to assimilate the nutrition from your food; you can have the best diet in the world but if the food passes through your body too quickly, you'll be unable to absorb its goodness. The treatment of diarrhea, as set out here, involves the "slowing down" of the bowel function and the addition of substances which will ensure that you have the necessary enzymes and bacteria to assimilate the food you're eating.

For ANY irritation in the bowel, I suggest one or two heaped teaspoons of Slippery Elm powder mashed into a little low-fat yogurt, or very ripe banana, or soft or stewed fruit, four times daily before meals and before bed.

This simple remedy will be beneficial in conjunction with a common sense diet for *any* bowel disturbance including colitis, ulcerative colitis, constipation, and so on. It's important to use it in conjunction with the diet. Slippery Elm has a marvelous capacity to *normalize* bowel function.

Foods to Avoid

The following foods should be avoided completely if you have diarrhea:

- *Cheese, cow's milk, cream, butter, sour cream, or any other dairy product with the exception of yogurt. Replace with a light soy milk.*
- *High-fat substances such as fried foods, gravy, creamy soups, or sauces.*
- *Seeds, whole nuts, bran, muesli, grain husks, whole grains, most unprocessed foodstuffs, salads.*
- *Caffeine, Indian/China tea, carbonated beverages.*
- *Cabbage, broccoli, cauliflower, onions, beans, peas, corn.*
- *Sweets, chewing gum, sugar, honey, molasses, golden syrup, cookies, chocolate, cakes, or any other sweet substance with the exception of those listed below.*

It's important you replace lost body fluids with your liquid intake.

Suggested Liquids

- *Water, broth, clear soups*
- *Apple, pear, apricot, and peach nectars*
- *Herb teas (without honey), dandelion coffee*

It's also important to replace electrolytes with high potassium foods such as bananas, potatoes, and apricot and peach nectars.

The use of homeopathics is highly recommended also. These will need to be supplied by a homeopath/naturopath or health food store. The most beneficial homeopathic formula I've found is:

Diarrhea Drop Formula

- *Phosphoricum Acidum*   3x
- *Tincture Chamomilla*   4x
- *Tincture Colocynthis*   6x
- *Tincture Veratrum Album* 6x

To prevent diarrhea: Ten drops in a couple of teaspoons of water four times daily before meals and before bed. Hold in the mouth for a few seconds before swallowing.

Taking the drops this way *before* having any treatment which you know will give you diarrhea helps to minimize its effect. If you still develop diarrhea, then take the drops as follows:

To alleviate diarrhea: Seventy drops in half a glass of water. Sip every fifteen minutes until diarrhea begins to subside, holding each sip in the mouth for a few seconds before swallowing. Once the diarrhea has settled, then reduce frequency to every hour, then every two hours, then three and so on, until you're back to taking it four times daily. If another wave of diarrhea appears, resume the prescribed frequency. Homeopathics work best not by the strength of their dosage but by the frequency with which they're taken.

Occasionally, when diarrhea is really severe and usually of long-standing, the above drops are insufficient on their own. In this case there are some extra drops which can be taken once a day in addition to the others and which double the strength of any homeopathic. They consist of:

Potentizing Drop Formula

Phosphoricum Acidum	12x
Sulphur Iodatum	12x
Ferrum Iodatum	12x
Calcarea Iodatum	12x

They're taken in the same way as the Diarrhea Drops except they're taken only once a day, preferably in the morning.

Many people with cancer, HIV, chronic fatigue syndrome, and other illnesses develop an intolerance to cow's milk. If you *really* don't like soy, goat's, or sheep's milk, then use Lactaid with a low-fat cow's milk. Lactaid is a brand name of the enzyme *lactase*. You can find Lactaid, or its equivalent, through your pharmacist.

Remember These Points

- *Note the foods to avoid.*
- *Keep up your fluid intake.*
- *Make ice cubes of peppermint and/or chamomile tea and suck on them.*
- *Drink fluids through a straw if it makes it easier (be careful not to swallow air when sucking through a straw).*
- *Well-cooked oatmeal is often tolerated—you can add Slippery Elm powder.*
- *Try small meals, frequently, served at room temperature.*
- *Try low-fiber foods such as stewed apple (without the skin).*
- *Try pureed or grated fruits or cooked vegetables.*
- *Don't drink with your meals—drink thirty minutes before or at least ninety minutes after eating.*

- *So long as the carrot-based vegetable juice (see page 174) doesn't increase your diarrhea, it's an excellent form of nourishment.*

- *Have your food neither too hot nor too cold.*

- *The herbal relaxant (see page 219 under Insomnia) is often very helpful for a bowel in spasm.*

Sometimes the bowel forms the habit of emptying itself constantly; the herbal relaxant mentioned above is very good for breaking this cycle if it's used in conjunction with all the other suggestions.

Many people find the following recipe good for stopping diarrhea in its tracks.

- *1 cup of cooked white rice*

- *1 large mashed banana*

- *1 grated apple (left to go brown before adding to this mixture)*

- *1 heaped dessertspoon of Slippery Elm powder*

- *Cinnamon or nutmeg to taste*

- *Mix all the above ingredients with Pediayte or the equivalent (available from the pharmacist, it contains compound sodium chloride and glucose in a powdered form) to the desired consistency.*

This might not sound appetizing; however, it works like a charm for those brave enough to give it a try.

Iron

Many people with chronic or severe diarrhea have found relief by taking iron pills. This often will work when nothing else seems to help. Iron is toxic to the liver, so it's essential that you discuss your situation with your doctor. It may well be that the relief experienced from controlled bowel function far outweighs the threat of toxicity to your liver.

Chronic Diarrhea

If you've had a considerable amount of the large bowel removed, you might have a mild chronic diarrhea. In cases like this, you could benefit by using a bulking agent on a regular basis. Only resort to this if all avenues have been explored by your doctor and the cause of the diarrhea is understood. Metamucil (or any of its generic equivalents, it is made from psyllium husks) is quite helpful in this situation.

Intermittent Constipation and Diarrhea

Another very common problem is constipation which alternates with diarrhea. This can be caused in a number of ways. People often experience this problem after a course of antibiotics. Following the guidelines set out here will help in regulating the bowel function. They will not *cause* constipation.

Irritable Bowel

Irritable bowel can also be helped by following the guidelines suggested here for controlling diarrhea. Slippery Elm is particularly helpful, as are the homeopathic drops. Eliminating all sugars except fruit sugars is essential.

Experiment until you find *your* perfect solution. Techniques of relaxation, visualization, and meditation are very useful and should be incorporated on a daily basis.

The herbal remedy mentioned in the Nervous Tension, Fear, and Anxiety section (see page 219) is also invaluable.

Fatigue; Too Tired to Prepare Meals

Feeling exhausted can be very depressing, and once depression settles, it can become difficult to motivate yourself enough to prepare healthy and nutritious meals. It's important, as always, to find out the cause of your fatigue. It could be because your hemoglobin (the oxygen-binding protein in the red cells in your bloodstream) is low; it could be because your lung capacity is restricted for some reason and the red blood cells can't pick up sufficient oxygen; it could be because your body is undernourished; it could be the overall effect of debilitating illness or depression. Once the cause is understood and treated as effectively as possible, then you'll need to find practical and simple ways to nourish yourself with a minimal output of energy. Many people find difficulty in asking for assistance and, in some cases, there *is* no one to ask, anyway. If there are friends, neighbors, or family who have offered their assistance, now is certainly the time to reach out for help. They wouldn't have offered if they didn't genuinely mean for you to take them up on it. It gives them the opportunity to do something truly constructive to assist you.

A supplement from the health food store containing methionine, tyrosine, asparagine, iron, folic acid, biotin, Vitamin C, and manganese may prove helpful.

Co Enzyme Q10 can be beneficial in reducing fatigue, depending upon its cause. This substance, available through health food stores and many pharmacists, usually gives quick results. It has other benefits as well for the immune system. Most people need to take 40 mg. per day. It can take four weeks for the full effects to be felt.

Remember These Points:

- *Prepare meals ahead of time when you're feeling well, and freeze in individual servings.*

- *Keep easy-to-prepare foods on hand: frozen dinners, canned tuna, salmon or sardines, free-range eggs, noodles, frozen soups, muffins, muesli bars, healthy snack bars.*

- *Eat small meals frequently.*

- *Accept offers from family, friends, and neighbors to help prepare meals.*

- *Take advantage of healthy take-out foods.*

- *If someone offers to make vegetable juices and you find you can tolerate them, accept them with as much enthusiasm as you can muster. Vegetable juices will pick your energy level up more quickly than anything I know (depending on the cause of your exhaustion). If you can manage three freshly made glasses of carrot-based juice (see page 174) per day, you won't know yourself in a week.*

- *Take advantage of home delivery services.*

- *Use Sustagen, Ensure (soy-based nutritional formulas) or a similar nutrient supplement.*

- *Take vitamin/mineral formulations to meet your essential needs.*

Very occasionally, artificial feeding is suggested. This involves the passing of a very thin tube through the nose down the esophagus into the stomach, allowing a nutritious formula to be "fed" directly into the stomach. Once the naso-gastric tube is in place it causes no discomfort at all. All kinds of nourishing fluids can be passed directly into the stomach without distress to the person.

George was having enormous difficulty with weight loss because of chronic diarrhea, Cryptosporidium in the gall bladder, and his general inability to assimilate food. He was eating quite well, but was continuing to lose weight. He was given a choice between a gastrostomy (a "hole" into the stomach from outside the body, into which foods can be fed directly), night feeds via a naso-gastric tube so that he would receive extra nourishment while he slept, or doing nothing and continuing to lose weight. George felt that the surgical solution would be debilitating and the resulting gastrostomy would interfere too much with his quality of life, so he opted for naso-gastric feeds. It isn't in his nature to choose the last option of doing nothing; he's a great believer in "while there's life, there's hope!" At home he's become quite adept at passing the tube into his stomach and finds that the night feeds don't interfere with his sleep at all. He was able to return home from the hospital quite quickly and gradually began to put on weight. This led to greater energy levels and an improved quality of life.

Flushes

Many women experience early menopause either through surgical removal of, or radiation to, the ovaries, or through the use of drugs which interfere with the action of estrogen. The symptoms can be very mild or they can be quite annoying.

The following homeopathic remedy, Climacteric Drops, assists most women in bringing the flushes under control. It consists of:

Climacteric Drop Formula

- *Sepia*   4x
- *Sanguinaria*   4x
- *Lachesis*   12x
- *Sulphuric Acid*   4x

To take: Ten to fifteen drops in a couple of teaspoons of water four times daily before meals and before bed. Hold in the mouth for a few seconds before swallowing. Once the flushes have gone or are greatly decreased in frequency or intensity, reduce to three times daily, then two times daily, and stay on one daily until you reach the end of the bottle. Occasionally, when flushes are really severe and usually of long-standing, the above drops are insufficient on their own. In this case there are some extra drops, called Potentizing Drops. They can be taken once a day in addition to the others, and will double the strength of any homeopathic. The formula is given on page 207. They're taken in the same way as the Climacteric Drops except they're only taken once a day, preferably in the morning.

Tamoxifen (a non-steroidal anti-estrogen) causes flushing in some women while others experience no side effects at all from this treatment.

Gas

By whatever name you call it—flatulence, gas, or wind—this condition has the power to render its host incapacitated if it's severe enough. I shall settle for calling it gas. In small amounts which are easily passed, it isn't difficult to deal with. In large amounts that become trapped within the convolutions of the bowel, it can become a nightmare. Usually this amount of gas is associated with other disturbances within the bowel, liver, pancreas, or stomach. To many, gas might seem inconsequential. To the person who's suffering, the pain might well be excruciating, particularly if there's been recent surgery to the abdominal cavity.

Each and every person's situation will be different, but there are some general guidelines which can be followed in most cases. You are encouraged to discuss them with your doctor before proceeding.

For the first twelve hours:

- *Avoid all food and take water, or chamomile or peppermint tea without honey. You may wish to make ice cubes of the herb teas and suck on them.*

- *Take two digestive enzyme tablets every two hours. The formula should contain:*
  - *Pancreatin 4NF*   *200 mg*
  - *Bromelain*   *100 mg*
  - *Pepsin*   *100 mg*
  - *Trypsin*   *30 mg*

- *Take 2 tablets of the following formula every two hours:*
  - *Betaine HCl*   *400 mg*
  - *Glutamic Acid*   *100 mg*

After twelve hours:

- *Take two teaspoons of Slippery Elm powder mashed into two tablespoons of low-fat acidophilus-based yogurt.* **This must be eaten very slowly and be well mixed with saliva. Do not have any fluids for at least thirty minutes before or at least ninety minutes after.** *Take two tablets of each of the digestive enzyme formulas mentioned above at the same time, with a minimal amount of water. Repeat this every four hours. Continue to take digestive enzymes plus Betaine HCl and Glutamic acid every two hours.*

- *Stay with this program until the gas has subsided.*

- *You can add two charcoal tablets every two hours if the above has not worked adequately within twenty-four hours.*

- *Once the gas has subsided considerably, you might like to try some well-stewed apple and yogurt. Continue with the Slippery Elm and yogurt at least three times daily.*

- *Take two of the digestive enzyme tablets plus two Betaine HCl and Glutamic acid tablets every time any food is ingested.*
- *The addition of methionine (available from health food stores) can sometimes be helpful.*
- *If all is still calm after forty-eight hours, give very well-cooked oatmeal with soy milk, or pumpkin soup (see page 177), or a banana smoothie (see page 176).*
- *Gradually expand the diet, keeping to only two foods per meal. For example, steamed fish and well-cooked carrots; or peeled and cooked zucchini and mashed potato (no additives except a little vegetable salt).*
- *Listen to your body and heed its messages.*

Hair Loss

There are some kinds of chemotherapy where you'll be told you'll lose all your hair. There are other kinds which result in some hair loss. For the people in the former category, it's heartening to remember that not everybody loses all of his or her hair; in the latter category, many people who are on a good diet, drinking vegetable juices, and taking vitamins and other supplements lose only a minimal amount of hair. These people also tend to grow their hair back quickly. Everybody's hair grows back after chemotherapy, sometimes with a wave in it, sometimes even curly, thicker, and often of a slightly darker shade than before.

People often find that their fingernails thrive on chemotherapy and become (and stay) much stronger than before!

The essentials for strong hair regrowth are folic acid, silica, biotin, and cysteine. These can be taken in a formula and are available in tablet form from your local health food store, naturopath, or doctor who specializes in nutritional medicine.

The emotional impact of losing the hair will vary from one individual to another. For some it can be quite devastating and will feel like the worst part of having cancer. Reassurance is necessary, as the self-esteem often falls with the hair!

Hair lost through radiotherapy to the head usually grows

back unless the dosage has been very strong. For many, particularly young people, the challenge of learning to live with bald patches can be almost insurmountable. Our self-esteem is nearly always connected to our self-image. Special consideration and encouragement are needed to ensure safe passage through the traumas of such hair loss. The constant wearing of head scarves, wigs, turbans, and hats has its own tedium. Some wig companies will make a wig fringe attached to a light cotton scarf. This gives the impression of hair while letting the scalp "breathe" more easily than if it were confined under a full wig or turban. This is, of course, particularly relevant in summer when a wig can feel hot and foreign, especially as hair regrowth begins.

A young patient, Peter, was much comforted by his classmates who chose to wear hats for the whole duration of his hair loss (due to chemotherapy). And another child, Stephanie, was deeply touched by the action of her school class who went as far as shaving their heads so that she wouldn't feel so strange. Such gestures bring extraordinary comfort and nourish the spirit more deeply than volumes of words.

Herpes Simplex/Genitalis

Ulcers which form around the outside of the mouth in the lip area respond very well to diluted tea-tree oil. Most people who develop herpes simplex are aware of a sensation of numbness or tingling *before* anything actually shows up on the skin. If you apply tea-tree oil diluted 50/50 with almond, grape seed, or apricot kernel oil twice a day as soon as any numbness or tingling occurs, the herpes rarely appears, or is very minor when it does. This applies equally to genital herpes. Many people find they have an outbreak of herpes either during or immediately after their course of chemotherapy, antibiotics, or other drug therapy. It is important to replenish the gut bacteria through the use of a low-fat acidophilus yogurt after any course of antibiotics or chemotherapy. Use of tea-tree oil in the manner mentioned will also bring relief. Many people who have genital herpes find that the only way they can urinate without excruciating pain is in a warm bath. Sixty drops of tea-tree oil can also be added to the bath water. If you're prone to attacks of herpes (either genital or in the form of cold sores) you might like to try a supplement containing lysine, folic acid, zinc, Vitamin B12 and the B complex.

Herpes Supplement:

Vitamin B1	50 mg
Vitamin B2	10 mg
Vitamin B3	50 mg
Vitamin B5	50 mg
Vitamin B6	25 mg
Vitamin B12	25 mg

Insomnia

Anyone who's unwell has an increased need for sleep. And yet it's at this very time when sleep might be disturbed or elusive. We might need to implement correct sleeping patterns if they become disturbed through hospitalization, pain, worry, or some other factor. The worry of *not* sleeping can, in itself, keep sleep at bay. Lack of sleep is nothing to be overly concerned about. We *can* catch up. Remember, a good day's worry is far more debilitating than a good day with an ax. When we've had a good day with an ax we fall into bed and sleep like babies; when we've had a good day's worry, we twitch all night. This applies doubly if we're going to spend our nights tossing and turning with fruitless worry. I'm sure you've had the experience, as I have, of everything seeming far worse at 3:00 A.M.! I call them the 3:00 A.M. freakies! Healthy sleeping patterns can be established by implementing a sort of ritual around bedtime.

If it's pain which wakens you through the night, you might want to check with your doctor or nurse that your pain medication is adequate before you retire in the evenings. Also see chapter 9, Beyond Pain (pages 252-279). Many techniques which could prove useful for those with pain can be found there.

Some people who normally sleep well have difficulty for a few days around their chemotherapy time. This is often not due to the chemotherapy but is a side effect of an anti-nausea drug which is often prescribed at the same time. If you're susceptible to the side effect of this particular drug, you'll feel "jittery" and restless and settling into a comfortable position may be very difficult. If this is your problem, speak to your doctor about changing your anti-nausea medication, and see Nausea, pages 230-242. Other people sleep restlessly because they're *anticipating* the chemotherapy in three or four days' time! These people will particularly benefit from the regular daily practice of relaxation techniques and following the guidelines set down here.

Many people experience "loneliness in bed" after the death of a loved one. To have shared the same bed for many years and then to find yourself alone can be very hard.

Greg, age thirty-seven, had been married for fifteen years when his wife, Kate, died from cancer. They'd been close companions and he felt her absence keenly. He said the worst time for him was at night when he tried unsuccessfully to settle down to sleep. Kate's childhood teddy bear had always sat upon a wicker chair in the bedroom. Greg took to bidding the bear goodnight each evening, and on particularly lonesome nights was not above taking teddy to bed. It actually helped. Sometimes we just need a ritual in order for us to break the habit of not sleeping.

Some people have fears and anxieties which keep them from nodding off at night, while they have no difficulty in falling asleep during the day. These concerns are best talked about with someone you trust. This might be your partner or a family member, or you might prefer to speak to your nurse, doctor, or counselor.

Many people find that even though medically prescribed drugs make them sleep, they don't wake up feeling refreshed in the morning. The hypnotic family of drugs allows you to wake up feeling refreshed, but they're effective for only four hours. Instead of sleeping the night through, many people wake up the moment the drug has worn off. You might like to use the following program in addition to your medically prescribed drugs or in place of them. If you've been using medically prescribed drugs for sleeping for a long period, I suggest you don't just suddenly stop. Use this program in addition to your medication and then gradually reduce your medication when you no longer have a problem sleeping.

When you follow the guidelines listed below I'm sure you'll find deep and refreshing sleep. For those who have a chronic sleeping problem, be patient; it may take three to four days or even a week before you notice an improvement. Here's the program:

- *Affirm, throughout the day, that you'll have no difficulty at all in falling asleep easily when you go to bed. Every time you're assailed by thoughts of yet another sleepless night, gently put them aside.*

- *Take two tablets of a herbal sedative formula (there's one listed on page 219) with dinner, and two tablets one hour before bed. This formula has no side effects and won't make you sleepy—just very relaxed. It helps by relaxing the muscles of the body and tends to quieten down the activity of the mind.*

- *During the evening engage in quiet activities. No riveting television, no mystery or adventure stories. Perhaps do some tapestry or other craft work; listen to relaxing music; read some inspirational or encouraging books.*

- *In the hour before bed, have a warm bath or shower (if practical), drink a cup of warm chamomile or valerian herb tea (a good complement to the herbal sedative formula), then go to bed.*

- *Settle into a comfortable position, then play a relaxation tape.*

Sometimes a gentle massage from your partner or other caregiver will settle and soothe an aching body or an agitated mind. Use grape seed, almond, or apricot kernel oil mixed with a few drops of lavender or geranium oil. Even a gentle massage of hands, feet, or head can bring incredible relaxation.

If your difficulty isn't in falling asleep but in staying asleep, then have a relaxation tape ready for you when you awaken. Go to the bathroom (if that's your habit), go back to bed, and play the tape immediately before your mind becomes active. The use of a relaxation tape as you settle into bed can be helpful in getting the mind focused and the body relaxed, allowing sleep to come as it will. I've made a tape for people who have a sleep problem and the use of this tape can help to reestablish healthy sleep habits. It can also be used when you feel anxious or physically uncomfortable. It's available from Dawn Publications (see page 368). We say, with (almost complete) confidence, that no one's ever heard the end of this tape!

Try this herbal sedative formula (or a similar one, available from most health food stores):

Herbal Sedative Formula

- Magnesium Orotate   50 mg
- Valerian   50 mg
- Passionflower   50 mg
- Nicotinamide   50 mg
- Hops   25 mg
- Pyridoxine hydrochloride   5 mg
- Chamomile   5 mg
- Oats   5 mg

The sleep achieved through this formula is usually deep and refreshing and is a valuable ingredient in a program to reestablish better sleeping patterns. It isn't addictive or habit-forming and has no side effects. It can be used safely with children (half-dosage under the age of twelve). This formula is also particularly good for people who are anxious, fearful, and distressed. Two tablets can be taken as often as every three hours without any side effects.

Another excellent homeopathic formula, called Quieta, has also proved invaluable for many people, especially children. It consists of:

Quieta Formula

- Avena sativa   3x
- Valeriana   3x
- Humulus   3x

- *Coffea*   4x
- *Ignatia*   6x
- *Zincum valerianum*   6x

To take: Ten drops in a couple of teaspoons of water four times daily before meals and before bed. Hold in the mouth for a few seconds before swallowing. Once restful sleep has been established, decrease the frequency to three times daily, then two times daily, and stay on one daily until you reach the end of the bottle.

These drops are also very effective for helping those who feel stressed, agitated, or nervous. They can be added to a glass of water that sits by your bed, travels with you in the car, or accompanies you into an examination room. Many a student has felt the benefits of their calming quality!

To alleviate anxiety: Seventy drops in half a glass of water. Sip every five minutes until anxiety begins to subside, holding each sip in the mouth for a few seconds before swallowing. Once you feel settled, then reduce frequency to every half hour, then hourly, then every two hours, then three and so on until you're back to taking it four times daily. If you feel another wave of anxiety, resume the prescribed frequency.

I went to visit Miriam in the hospital quite late one night. She was a member of one of our support groups and was having great difficulty sleeping. We sat and talked for a while and it transpired that it wasn't actually the pain which was keeping her awake so much as the fear that she might not wake up in the morning. Miriam had recently been moved from an acute-care hospital to a nearby palliative-care unit. Going through her mind was the thought, "They only move you here when you're about to die." She needed to talk about the unresolved issues in her life which centered mainly around her son. Miriam had harbored anger toward him for many years because of some expensive family business decisions he'd made twenty years previously. She said she'd been punishing him ever since by never letting him feel close to her. When she said that, she fell silent for a moment and then looked at me with eyes that sparkled with tears of recognition. Miriam realized she'd been punishing herself every bit as much as she'd been punishing him. She healed that relationship then and there within herself, and was resolved to speak with her son first thing the next morning, after a good night's sleep.

Michael is a university medical student who loves his course of studies but who became very stressed in the weeks leading up to his exams. He manifested his stress physically through an irritable bowel. This gave him severe pain, diarrhea, and bleeding, and he tended not to eat very well and to sleep little (and even then restlessly). For the past two years he's been using relaxation techniques in addition to some dietary changes as part of his daily program and, overall, is generally feeling less stressed about life. He finds he's able to concentrate for longer periods and he doesn't become nearly so anxious in the pre-examination period. Initially he took the herbal sedative formula very frequently (two tablets every three hours) but now he uses it only occasionally.

Another gentleman, this one age eighty-two, had a mind as sharp as a pin. However, it used to cause him sleepless nights because it wouldn't quieten down. A combination of the herbal sedative formula and a relaxation tape restored his sleeping pattern to normal.

I've often used this program with people who are addicted to sedatives. Many people start taking sedatives because they are having difficulty sleeping. Perhaps this is because they have some emotional or psychological pain they need to address, but don't know how. Instead of being helped to deal with the real issues, they've been prescribed sedatives. Before long, sleep becomes impossible without them and the unresolved issues become buried more deeply within.

For those who are addicted to, or dependent on, sedatives, I highly recommend that you find a support group wherein you can deal with the painful issues in your life. **You use sedatives (or alcohol or other drugs) to dull the pain which exists within yourself. Deal with the pain and you deal with your addiction.**

I'm not saying it's easy, but it's certainly possible. Deal with the issues which stop you from fully living.

In the meantime, you could find it useful to take two tablets of the herbal sedative formula every three hours *in addition* to your drug of addiction. Then gradually reduce the amount of your drug. You might need to reduce it by half a tablet at a time until you're off them altogether, and it could take weeks or months depending on the strength of your addiction. This program will only work if:

- *You want it to.*
- *You're dealing with the painful issues which stop you from fully living.*

Libido

Many people experience a decrease in their sex drive during their illness. There are many possible explanations ranging from the effects of fear, depression, and worry through to side effects of treatments or surgery. Most people are reluctant to talk to their doctor or nurse about a decrease in their libido. In fact, most doctors and nurses are reluctant to raise the subject at all! This can leave the patient in a very isolated situation.

Sex is a very important part of most people's lives and to lose the sexual urge can be quite worrying. Your doctor will be able to ascertain what's caused your decreased libido. If it isn't caused through injury to the nerves in the genital area, then, in some cases, Chinese herbs can be very effective in restoring the sex drive. Talking things through with your partner can also help in dealing with fears, depression, or anxiety. Many people find that when they're dealing with their emotional issues (perhaps with a counselor or support group) their tension level is reduced and the problems with their libido also subside. A decrease in libido is very commonly experienced by those on chemotherapy. Rest assured: once your treatment program is complete and you've recovered from its debilitating effects, your sex drive will increase.

For many people, their sense of identity and self-esteem is strongly attached to their sexuality. It can be extremely traumatic for them to feel a loss of identity at a time when they're also feeling unwell and perhaps facing other issues around the purpose and meaning in their lives. A safe, supportive environment in which these fears can be aired and explored is invaluable.

Some women who have gynecological cancers could well find they need to adopt a more creative approach to lovemaking. You might find intercourse painful or less pleasurable. Some surgical procedures and treatments can lead to a dryness in the vagina and the use of a lubricant will become essential to enjoyable sex. The most important things are to be gentle with yourself, decrease your expectations, and talk about the issues involved with your partner or a sympathetic health professional.

Liver Disease

Primary cancers of the liver or metastatic disease in the liver may or may not cause pain and discomfort. Many people believe that liver cancer in particular is extremely painful. It can be, but I've also known many people who've experienced no pain at all. Sometimes pain is experienced in the right shoulder area rather than around the liver itself. This can be "referred" liver pain.

Colin was operated on for extensive bowel cancer almost four years ago. The surgeon removed a large amount of his colon and examined his liver, where he found some smaller inoperable tumors. Colin's prognosis was very poor and he was given a matter of months to live. In the past three and a half years Colin has changed his life dramatically. He's a keen meditator, watches his dietary intake, plays tennis several times a week, travels extensively, and generally loves life. He and his wife, Joan, facilitate support groups for other cancer patients and bring a lot of comfort, hope, and encouragement to them. He says he's too busy to be sick! Colin has never experienced any discomfort or pain from his liver, and though the tumors have remained they cause him no distress. He eats and enjoys oranges, butter, the odd glass of wine, and complex combinations of food without any problem.

Unlike Colin, many people *do* experience digestive problems at some stage: nausea or squeamishness, burping, and so on. It's

important that these people adopt a "liver-friendly" diet. This
means avoiding:

- *Oranges and orange juice*
- *Fats, oils, butter, margarine (fried fatty foods)*
- *Alcohol*
- *Cooked eggs*
- *Cheese and all dairy products with the exception of yogurt*
- *Complex combinations of foods*

There are some people with metastatic liver disease who love
orange juice and who seem to suffer no side effects from it. If this
is true in your case, keep on enjoying it. It seems to depend very
much on the location of the tumors in the liver. For others who
love orange juice, but have a chronic squeamish feeling in the
tummy, it's definitely worth leaving it out altogether for a couple
of days to see if it's the juice that is the culprit. If anything will
make you feel squeamish, it'll be oranges or their juice. Some
people find they can tolerate grapefruit, lemons, and limes without
any discomfort while others would be better off leaving out all
acidic foods—including strawberries, pineapples, and tomatoes.

Digestive enzymes are also beneficial for many of these
people, particularly if there's burping and discomfort in the upper
part of the digestive tract. The digestive enzyme formulas listed
under Gas (see page 212) will very likely bring relief. One to two
of each of these tablets can be taken any time food is ingested. If
there's discomfort further down the intestinal tract, then following the other guidelines listed under Gas will be helpful.

Remember, if *you're* tired by the end of the day, so is your
digestive tract. Make your main meals breakfast and lunch and
have only a light dinner: for example, soup and muffins or
stewed fruit and yogurt.

Loss of Appetite

Loss of appetite has been referred to here and there in the
preceding pages. It can be quite depressing to lose one's appe-

tite, particularly for those of us for whom food has played a major role in life. Now we look upon it with disinterested eye and jaded palate. We wonder if life's worth living if we cannot enjoy the tasty morsels of the past. Loss of appetite can stem from many causes. It can be the side effect of a treatment we're on, a result of our disease, or the product of depression or anxiety.

Many people find that chemotherapy destroys their taste for food and subsequently lose interest in what used to be enjoyed. Some complain that all foods have a metallic taste after chemotherapy. This diminishes as you recover from the treatments. Some find they crave salt, while others can't stand anything salty—and so on.

Whatever its cause, the results can be a worry, unless we started off particularly well covered in the first place. As with all symptoms, it's important to seek out and, if possible, eliminate the cause. If anxiety, depression, or fear are causing loss of appetite, then it's essential these feelings be dealt with. This can be done with a friend, support group, caring nurse, doctor, or counselor.

Subsequently it's possible to stimulate the appetite in a number of ways. Again, homeopathics can be helpful. Ask your homeopath for a formula which contains homeopathic dosages of the following ingredients, contained here in the Appetite Drop Formula:

Appetite Drop Formula

- *Lycopodium*   30x
- *Ceanothus*   8x
- *Cinchona officinalis*   6x
- *Ferrum muriaticum*   6x

Ten to fifteen drops can be taken as often as every hour or two in a couple of teaspoons of water. Hold each sip in the mouth for a few seconds before swallowing.

Some people find that a glass of sherry stimulates the appetite if taken half an hour to an hour before eating. Two to three pieces of ginger in its crystallized form is excellent for calming a squeamish tummy and stimulating the appetite.

Remember These Points:

- *Eat small, frequent meals five times throughout the day.*
- *Schedule eating times every two hours and stick to them.*
- *Keep high-calorie snacks available for nibbling between meals; for example, nuts, seeds, yogurt, dried fruit, soups, and crackers.*
- *Make eating a pleasant experience by eating with friends.*
- *Make your food and surroundings attractive.*
- *Choose your favorite foods to stimulate your appetite.*
- *Prepare foods that give off a pleasant aroma, such as simmering soup and casseroles, baking bread.*
- *Give all food a chance; what's unappealing one day might be appealing the next.*
- *Prepare foods at times when you're feeling "up."*
- *Always have in the fridge foods like banana smoothies (see page 176).*
- *Use dried or fresh herbs, garlic, and spices to enhance flavors.*
- *Avoid low- or no-calorie foods such as coffee, tea, and clear soups.*
- *Don't skip eating times; treat them as you do medications or other therapies.*

Corticosteroids, in small doses, are sometimes used to stimulate the appetite. You could discuss the use of corticosteroids with your doctor.

Lymphoedema

Lymphoedema is caused by lack of circulation of lymphatic fluids. It principally occurs where the lymphatic glands have been removed, irradiated, or are blocked by tumors or pressure. It's most commonly seen in the arms or legs and can cause discomfort and immobility. It occurs frequently after a mastectomy where many of the glands in the armpit have been removed and/

or the area has also been treated with radiotherapy.

It's important after you've had a mastectomy that you avoid trauma to the arm on the same side. For instance, don't have injections, especially chemotherapy, in that arm. Have the nurse or doctor take your blood pressure on the other arm. Avoid anything which causes an unnatural or increased pressure or workload on the vessels in the affected arm. It is better to avoid lymphoedema than to treat it.

When lymphoedema is present in the leg, it's because the lymph nodes in the thigh/groin have been removed, damaged by radiotherapy, or are blocked from functioning by the presence of tumors or pressure in that area.

Lymphoedema can occur in other parts of the body, but these are the most common sites.

Most doctors will tell you the only measures which can alleviate lymphoedema are taking diuretics (fluid tablets), wearing a support stocking or bandage to the limb, and keeping it elevated. These measures are certainly of some benefit but don't do a great deal for the people who've a really major problem with lymphoedema.

Proper lymphatic drainage can make an enormous difference to these people. The kind of lymphatic drainage I'm referring to here is a very specialized one, and proper training must be undertaken in order to practice it effectively. *This is not the kind of lymphatic drainage which is available through beauticians or massage therapists.* It must be done by someone who understands cancer, its treatments, has a good understanding of the lymphatic drainage system throughout the body and who's been trained in the technique. This training isn't widely available yet in many countries, but I urge you to find out from your oncologist the name of the nearest clinic which can teach your caregiver how to do it. At Royal Prince Alfred Hospital in Sydney, there's a clinic that will take referrals and will teach nurses, physiotherapists, and occupational therapists how to train caregivers in the technique. Very often it isn't until the patient asks for something to be done about a particularly annoying symptom that it gets addressed. Too often doctors are preoccupied with your medical treatment; a symptom like lymphoedema is of no importance to your overall medical management (in their view).

My experience of people is very different. People say, "I can deal with having cancer! It's the fact I've got this heavy leg which really slows me down that depresses me."

Memory Loss and Lack of Concentration

Many people complain of memory loss and/or lack of concentration after they've been diagnosed with a life-threatening illness. Most often this is due to the effects of shock, stress, and a change in priorities and will certainly improve with time. One woman, Carmel, described her experience very well when she was commenting on the adjustments forced upon her after a diagnosis of cancer. She said her life had taken on "a changed kind of reality."

It's important not to have high expectations of yourself after you've been through the trauma of a life-threatening diagnosis. You'll undoubtedly find your priorities change. This might show itself in simple and yet aggravating ways. For instance, you might find that right after being introduced to people, you've completely forgotten their names; you've forgotten where you left your keys; you forget phone numbers and where you put your glasses (even when you're wearing them!) and so on. This can extend to forgetting what your doctor told you and, in some cases, forgetting to take your medication. It can be very frustrating, and sometimes worrying, to find you no longer are functioning at your usual level of competence. Remember you're under considerable stress and you need to be gentle with yourself.

A formula containing Vitamins B1, B6, B12, choline, tyrosine, serine, iron, and glutamine could be of benefit.

You might need to make lists which will help you remember things and establish a place where you *always* leave your keys/ glasses and so on. A tablet dispenser which has compartments for each day might be helpful. Some people record their consultation with their doctor on a small tape recorder. Others write down their questions and seek their doctor's cooperation in writing down the answers. This is then a reference for the future. If at all possible, enlist the support and assistance of your loved ones. For instance, most people benefit by having someone close to them accompany them when they visit their doctor. Remember, four ears are always better than two.

Some people find a herb called gingko biloba, available at health food stores, very helpful. It's been used for centuries by the Chinese as a remedy for memory loss and poor concentration. It increases the blood flow to the brain. Start off with one tablet or capsule a day and gradually increase to between three and six per day.

Monilia

Many women who are having chemotherapy or taking antibiotics or AZT experience almost constant monilia or vaginal yeast thrush. This aggravating complaint can be quite difficult to treat. There are some medications which work well against monilia and, in fact, for women who must constantly take AZT or antibiotics there's almost no alternative to regular anti-yeast thrush medication. Most women will find an improvement if they follow these guidelines:

- *Totally avoid all sugars in your diet; this means no cakes, cookies, honey, chocolate, maple, or golden syrup.*
- *Add sixty drops of tea-tree oil to the bath water.*
- *Soak a tampon in a solution of 90 percent almond, grape seed, or apricot kernel oil and 10 percent tea-tree oil, and then insert. Change tampons every three hours until improvement. Do not use these treated tampons for more than three consecutive days.*
- *Take six drops of sandalwood oil each day. Use a small piece of bread to soak up the sandalwood or have it in water.*
- *Add four drops of lavender oil to two each of rose and bergamot oil and add to a liter of warm water for a douche.*

- *A tampon soaked in an acidophilus-based yogurt and inserted into the vagina can bring relief. Change the tampon every four hours.*

Muscle Pain and Weakness

Many people experience muscle pain during their illness. This can stem from inactivity, tension in the muscles due to anxiety or pain in the region, or to the drug treatment. When muscles are held in a state of tension they produce lactic acid which is very irritating to the tissues. This irritation leads to greater tension and the cycle is perpetuated. Massage can be very helpful in easing the pain and can often increase the mobility of the area. I've seen many people who fear they have a secondary growth from a cancer because they're experiencing pain in their back, neck, or shoulder area when, in fact, it's only muscular tension. A supplement containing biotin, inositol, selenium, and the Vitamins B5, B1 and E could also benefit in this situation.

Many people who are taking AZT experience a wasting and weakness in their muscles. Regular, strenuous physical exercise will certainly assist in minimizing this symptom. Obviously, if you're feeling unwell, then physical exercise might be out of the question. In this case you might find that massage will be of great benefit.

There's a great deal more information about muscular pain in chapter 9, Beyond Pain (see pages 252-279).

Nausea

Food plays such an important role for most of us that to have its intake or enjoyment diminished can be frightening or, at the very least, unsettling. Many people encounter nausea or an unsettled feeling in the tummy at some stage during their illness. This nausea could be induced by chemotherapy, radiotherapy, or some other treatment, or it could be part of the disease process itself. The important thing to find out, as with all symptoms, is what's causing the nausea. It can be directly related to the illness itself if, for instance, there's a tumor in the stomach area or liver. It can be caused through a bowel or kidney obstruction or through pressure on the brain. Sometimes cancer can cause nausea indirectly through the release of too much calcium into the bloodstream. Anxiety, fear, or depression can be responsible for or increase this condition. It could be the result of an infection, overindulgence in food/alcohol, a stomach ulcer, gastritis, or something eaten that doesn't agree with you.

Don't forget you probably experienced nausea occasionally before you had this illness! Once we're diagnosed, we tend to think *everything* is related to the disease or its treatment.

There are numerous myths surrounding chemotherapy, most of them fear-inducing! There's a vast array of chemotherapeutic drugs. Some of these are extremely mild and create no side effects while others produce nausea, squeamishness, or vomiting. Radiotherapy to the abdomen or surrounding areas can also produce nausea.

People will respond individually to their treatments so comparing yourself and your reactions with someone else's could be totally inappropriate. If your treatment involves the kind of chemotherapy that creates nausea, your doctor will also prescribe an anti-nausea drug. Some people find they can control their nausea without requiring this medication. Others prefer to take their anti-nausea medication as soon as they begin their chemotherapy, while some prefer to wait and see if they actually become nauseated before taking theirs. Often these anti-nausea medications are given automatically at the same time through the intravenous drip that delivers the chemotherapy.

If your anti-nausea medication is to be taken by mouth, the sooner you start taking it the better will be its effect. Halting mild nausea is easier than when it's really giving you a hard time. Some people find the side effects of the anti-nausea drug more difficult to deal with than the nausea itself. If so, speak to your doctor who will review your treatment program and perhaps suggest another drug in its place. Others find they feel very jittery or restless after chemotherapy and this interferes with their sleep and emotional well-being. If this is the case for you, speak to your doctor. It's very likely a side effect of the anti-nausea drug, which can easily be changed, rather than the chemotherapy.

Sometimes, after a long period of treatment, or after a strong reaction to chemotherapy, *anticipatory* nausea can be a problem. People might experience this in the days leading up to their chemotherapy, some even at the sight, thought, or smell of the hospital or clinic in which they receive their treatment. Some people think they're being weak or have gone a little crazy when they experience this. Not so! The mind and body are interconnected and your body has acquired a conditioned physical response to a mental process. Some people feel squeamish or even reach the stage of vomiting just by driving on the same road which leads to their place of treatment.

Chemotherapy and AZT are broken down in the body by the liver, and so it's a good idea to adopt a liver-friendly diet during this time. If the cause of the nausea cannot be removed then you'll need to implement a program or treatment plan to minimize its effect on your life. Many people experience nausea in the first few days/weeks of beginning AZT and the guidelines here should help to minimize this. Nausea is nausea, no matter what its cause, and there *are* some helpful guidelines which are worth following to try and alleviate this problem.

Many people find their taste for food is disturbed during chemotherapy treatment and their food has a metallic taste to it. This will gradually disappear once the treatment has stopped. Some find they cannot tolerate salty or sweet foods, while others crave them. Taste changes can occur regardless of the treatment schedule. Don't force yourself to eat foods which you no longer enjoy simply because you think they're good for you. Find suitable alternatives. Some people thrive on chemotherapy and continue working or maintaining their usual lifestyle without interruption.

Some find the side effects of the chemotherapy/radiotherapy increase (or decrease) as the treatment program progresses. Some grow weary of the side effects and might wish to discuss with their doctor the possibility of a "break" from treatment or a change to a less intense treatment program. Hand in hand with nausea goes a lack of appetite, which is often distressing when weight or energy loss is also a factor (see Loss of Appetite, page 224). Some people find eating dispels nausea. All of these responses are normal and individual. Remember, avoid comparing yourself with others.

People sometimes feel they'll never return to their usual healthy selves again. It's an understandable fear, and yet many people who've been *very* sick with their treatment feel on top of the world within weeks of its completion. Those who are eating a nutritious diet, taking appropriate supplementations of vitamins, drinking vegetable juices, meditating, and maintaining a positive outlook seem to suffer only minimal side effects from their treatments. There are naturopaths who suggest a low-protein diet if you have cancer. I've found people who adopt this kind of diet often suffer debilitating weariness. Remember, while you're having chemotherapy or radiotherapy treatment, which destroy both cancer and some healthy cells in your body, you'll have a higher demand for protein. Proteins are the building blocks of the body. You might prefer to get your proteins from beans, nuts, seeds, and soy products (see chapter 7, Recipe for Life, pages 152-180).

The following information is based on practical experience of having worked with several thousands of people with cancer, AIDS, and other diseases both inside and outside hospitals. It isn't designed in any way to be a treatment program. Most of it is common sense, often a rare commodity in time of crisis.

Foods to Avoid

There are some foods to avoid when you're feeling squeamish in the tummy, or are about to have chemotherapy or start AZT. They are:

- *Oranges, orange juice*
- *Fats, oils, butter, margarine*
- *Fried fatty foods*
- *Alcohol*

- *Cooked eggs*
- *Cheese and all other dairy products with the exception of low-fat acidophilus-based yogurt*
- *Complex combinations of foods*

There might be other foodstuffs which make *you* squeamish while another person could tolerate them easily. Listen to your own body. If anything will make you feel nauseous, it will be oranges or orange juice. Remember, sometimes we think we're doing the very best thing for ourselves by having freshly squeezed juice, when in fact it could be *causing* the nausea. If your liver is upset (as it will be with most chemotherapy), avoid oranges or orange juice. It's a mystery to me why orange juice is served in hospitals to cancer patients while they're *having* their chemotherapy. The liver seems to tolerate grapefruit, lemons, and limes, but dislikes oranges. However, some people find that grapefruit, strawberries, tomatoes, pineapples, lemons, or any other acid foods will increase their nausea. Listen to your own body and heed its messages.

If you're feeling nauseous, probably the last thing you feel like eating are foods containing fats or oils. Likewise, most people will want to avoid red meat entirely. There are exceptions; some people crave red meat at this time. Similarly, most people lose their interest in alcohol when feeling nauseated. Cooked eggs are best avoided during treatment, though raw eggs in banana smoothies (see page 176) are often tolerated very well. Some people tolerate soft boiled, poached, or lightly scrambled eggs.

Cheese isn't recommended as it's too high in fat to be tolerated easily. Even low-fat cheeses aren't recommended. Most people who suffer from nausea don't tolerate foods containing lactose. Use soy milk instead, remembering that there are some very good light brands of soy milk available. Goat's and sheep's cheeses are often tolerated well and can be included.

Keep your diet very simple when suffering with nausea; perhaps as simple as having only two or three foods (without additives) at one meal.

Chemotherapy

If you're having the kind of chemotherapy which makes you nauseous, try the following plan. Practice your techniques of relaxation/visualization and meditation on a daily basis. Many people actually use a relaxation cassette tape (see page 379) while having their chemotherapy in the hospital or clinic. Often a familiar voice helps us to remain calm and positive. These techniques can be harnessed to help you maintain a positive attitude toward your treatment. You can view your treatment as a highly toxic poison which is bound to make you sick *or* as liquid sunshine, light or healing which is designed solely for your benefit. It's up to you.

Sometimes, talking your feelings through with a friend, support group, nurse, or doctor can help to alleviate your fears or anxieties. Well-run support groups (see chapter 4, Friends for Life) are invaluable because you meet others who've been through similar treatment programs and who can encourage you. Your attitude will change the way you experience the side effects. People who feel positive about their treatment program and trust in its ability to help them fare better with side effects than those who view their treatment in a negative way.

It is possible to change your attitude, and there's much more on this subject in chapter 2, Techniques for Living.

In the week leading up to your chemotherapy treatment, try to maintain an optimal diet which includes vegetable juices (see page 174) and appropriate vitamin supplementation. You might wish to consult a naturopath to ascertain your individual need for vitamins. The following ones are those I most commonly suggest for any person with cancer, AIDS, or other serious disease affecting the immune system.

- *Vitamin C—use a formula which combines sodium ascorbate, calcium ascorbate, ascorbic acid, and the bioflavinoids. The powdered form is easy to take, can be added to juice or water, and is certainly the most economical way to take Vitamin C.*
- *Vitamin B Complex Formula*

- *Selenium*
- *A mineral formula containing zinc*
- *An herbal formula which benefits the immune system*

The dosage of these vitamins/supplements will depend upon your individual state of health, weight, and so on. It's essential therefore to have them tailored to your individual needs by seeing a naturopath or doctor who specializes in vitamin therapy. Ask other patients, your doctor, clinic, cancer or AIDS council, or friends to recommend such a person. Then make sure that person has had a lot of experience with people with your illness.

Please inform your oncologist/doctor before taking vitamins/supplements. Don't expect enthusiastic encouragement, as most doctors are fairly uninformed about the benefits of this approach. It's important that they be made aware of your intention to take vitamins as, very occasionally, there are contraindications for them. Let them know if you feel you've benefited from this approach; it's only when enough people return to their oncologist/doctor with encouraging reports that all this information will be offered within the hospital system.

Slippery Elm powder is also a wonderful aid to counteracting nausea (see page 189).

Radiation Treatment

It's unusual to experience nausea with radiation treatment unless it's to the abdominal area or to parts of the brain. If this is so, all that has been said about nausea applies equally. You might need to use a system of trial and error in order to find what works best for you. If you've had radiation to the abdominal area, it's almost inevitable that you'll experience diarrhea or, at least, looseness of the bowel movements. For diarrhea, please see page 202.

Nervous Tension, Fear, and Anxiety

Stress affects the body in many ways. One of its favorites is to make us feel nauseous. If you feel that stress plays a part in your feelings of nausea, then don't just worry about it! Find some constructive ways of dealing with your stress so you can channel your energy into more useful directions. For instance, talk about your fears or anxieties with a friend, support group, nurse, or caring professional counselor. They'll help you deal with the situation and assist you in finding constructive ways of minimizing your stress. Learn the techniques of relaxation, visualization, and meditation and practice them at least twice daily. These techniques will change the way you view life and your illness. Find the things which bring you joy and make sure every day you have those things present. This may be solitude; the company of goods friends; inspiring books; the company of your pet; music; nature; exercise; a walk along the beach; your favorite craft or pastime. Whatever it is that brings you peace, include it in each day.

With clients who are particularly stressed, I often use an herbal formula which helps calm them. This formula induces relaxation, which allows sleep to come and tends to quieten down the chaos in the mind. Ask at your health food store for a formula as close to this one as possible.

Herbal Sedative Formula

- *Magnesium orotate*   50 mg
- *Valerian*   50 mg
- *Passionflower*   50 mg
- *Nicotinamide*   50 mg
- *Hops*   25 mg
- *Pyrodoxine hydrochloride*   5 mg
- *Chamomile*   5 mg
- *Oats*   5 mg

For people who are very frightened and distressed, two tablets can be taken as often as every three hours. For others who are less distressed, one tablet every four hours are sufficient.

For those who wish to ensure a night's sleep by using this

formula, I suggest they take two with dinner, and then two tablets one hour before bed (see also Insomnia, page 216).

Slippery Elm Powder

Slippery Elm powder is a wonderful substance to counteract nausea (see pages 230-242). Try mixing two heaping teaspoons of the powder with yogurt, banana, or stewed apple and have it three times daily, about twenty minutes before each meal. You can have it as frequently as seems necessary for you.

If you're having chemotherapy, you might like to take it an hour or two before your treatment is administered, and again a couple of hours after. Slippery Elm mashed into whichever medium feels right for you might be the only food which "sits" happily in your tummy for a day or so around chemotherapy time. This will vary enormously from person to person and will depend also on the side effects of the chemotherapy. Some people find very well-cooked oatmeal with soy milk serves them well for their first "meal" after chemotherapy. Oatmeal for dinner might not sound appetizing; however, it can be soothing for a nauseous tummy. If the Slippery Elm doesn't control or alleviate the nausea by itself, the addition of homeopathics is nearly always effective. You'll need to get these from a homeopath, naturopath, or health food store. They're entirely harmless and are remarkably effective in the control of nausea. There are also homeopathics which stimulate the appetite and which restore taste buds to their former efficiency (see Loss of Appetite, page 224). The homeopathic formula that I use for nausea is:

Vomisan Formula

- *Aesthusa*   8x
- *Colchicum*   12x
- *Cocculus*   12x
- *Ipecacuanha*   12x
- *Petroleum*   12x
- *Nux vomica*   12x

This formula is in liquid form and can be taken in two ways.

To prevent nausea: Ten drops in a couple of teaspoons of water four times daily, before meals and before bed. Hold each sip in the mouth for a few seconds before swallowing.

To alleviate nausea: Seventy drops in half a glass of water. Sip every three minutes until nausea begins to subside, holding each sip in the mouth for a few seconds before swallowing. Once nausea has settled, then reduce frequency to every five minutes, then every ten, then fifteen, then thirty and so on, until you're back to four times daily. If another wave of nausea appears, resume the frequency as mentioned above.

Homeopathics can also be in pilule form; these are like sugar pills the size of a pinhead. Because they dissolve easily under the tongue they're suitable for use by children as well as adults.

Note: Those who've been using Slippery Elm powder for a while to counteract nausea may find that even the *thought* of taking Slippery Elm could make them feel worse! You need to be flexible and perhaps alternate the powder with the homeopathics or find creative ways of disguising its taste. Because you're often nauseous when you take Slippery Elm powder you can easily create an aversion to its taste. Some people blend it into their carrot juice or banana or other soft fruit smoothie. Canned fruit can also be used in a smoothie. Just because Slippery Elm works wonderfully for nausea doesn't mean you have to make yourself sick by eating it!

Ginger Tea

Ginger tea is very helpful in settling upset tummies. Thinly slice about a quarter of a cup of fresh ginger and add to one liter of boiling water. Simmer for fifteen minutes, then allow to stand until lukewarm or cool. Strain. You can add a little lemon juice or honey to sweeten if desired. Sip very slowly.

Many people with cancer experience a coldness which seems to come from the inside out. Ginger tea warms you and seems to almost create a glow from the inside (see Cold Bones, page 197).

A Dietary Approach to Nausea

As well as avoiding certain foods (see page 233), there are other factors which need to be taken into account when one is trying to minimize or eliminate nausea. Experiment with the following suggestions so that you find what works for you.

Remember These Points:

- *Take a moment to calm yourself before eating by practicing some deep breathing.*
- *Remember to be grateful for the food you're about to eat.*
- *Eat slowly!*
- *Two to three pieces of crystallized ginger eaten half an hour before a meal will often settle the tummy and stimulate the appetite.*
- *Eat more food during the times you feel better.*
- *Salty foods are often tolerated well; try soup and crackers.*
- *Avoid foods that produce a strong odor when cooked.*
- *Make sure your cooking area has good ventilation.*
- *Have only two or three foods at one meal. For instance, oatmeal and soy milk, soup and muffins, yogurt and slippery elm, yogurt and stewed apple.*
- *Avoid foods that may produce gas, for example, onion, cabbage, broccoli, cauliflower, cucumber, beans, or green pepper.*
- *Chew food thoroughly so it's mixed with saliva; the first stage of digestion begins in the mouth.*
- *Avoid your favorite foods during the times when you experience nausea in order to avoid developing an aversion to the foods you enjoy.*
- *Don't drink with your meals—your tummy knows it's done a good job of digesting its contents by the amount of liquid there is in there. If you drink with your meal, the little sphincter at the far end of your tummy interprets that as a sign that your stomach has done its job and relaxes to let the food pass into the small intestine for further digestion. If you've had a cup of tea, water, or juice, the tummy's interpretation will be that the food is digested, when really it's only been mixed with the fluid you*

drank. For most people this won't be a problem but for anyone with a fragile digestive system, it is. Drink thirty minutes before or at least one hour and a half after a meal.

- *It's better not to eat fruit with meals unless the whole meal consists of fruit. The exception to this is banana used as sweetener on cereal in the morning. Bananas, like cereal, are complex carbohydrates and will be digested similarly.*

- *Peeled and well-cooked vegetables are preferable to raw or fibrous ones for those with nausea.*

- *Small frequent meals tend to be tolerated better than three larger meals each day.*

- *Presentation is important; make the meal look attractive.*

- *Use Slippery Elm powder in yogurt or banana, plus homeopathics before eating.*

- *Drinking soups, flat lemonade, smoothies (see page 176) through a straw might be better. A straw can deliver the food straight to the back of the mouth.*

- *Have food neither too hot nor too cold; warm or tepid is best.*

- *Moist foods are often better than dry foods for those who suffer with a dry mouth in addition to nausea.*

- *Dry foods, such as toast or crackers, might be better for those who don't suffer with a dry mouth.*

- *Don't lie down after eating unless you've found it to be helpful in the past; recline with your head elevated.*

- *Don't become overly preoccupied with nourishing yourself in the first days after chemotherapy.*

To Sum Up

The suggestions contained in this section aren't in any way intended to be a "prescription." They're suggested only as effective, natural means of controlling nausea or squeamishness. They're totally without side effects and, in this way, can be very useful. Remember, some people have quite a marked reaction to the medically prescribed anti-nausea drugs. You might find a combination of both prescribed and natural substances works best for you.

Night Sweats

Many people experience the unpleasant effects of night sweats at some time during their illness. These sweats aren't associated with a fever and their cause is unclear. (For sweats which *are* associated with fevers, see next page). Sweats can be frustrating and depressing because they interfere with sleeping. They can be very mild, where people barely wake with them, or severe, where the pajamas and bed linen might need to be changed several times during the night. They can often be set off by the taking of antibiotics or analgesics (painkillers).

The following homeopathics work wonderfully in stopping these sweats. They're also effective for those who perspire excessively during the day. Many people with HIV and cancer are troubled with night sweats and these drops have been amazingly successful in stopping them. The formula consists of:

Antihydrosin Drop Formula

- *Tincture veratrum album*   12x
- *Belladonna*   12x
- *Sepia*   12x
- *Lachesis mutus*   30x
- *Kali carbonicum*   6x
- *Tincture sanguinaria*   6x
- *Tincture jaborandi*   4x
- *Tincture sambucus nigra*   4x

For night sweats: Take ten drops in a couple of teaspoons of water four times daily, before meals and before bed. *Hold in the mouth for a few seconds before swallowing.*

When sweats have greatly diminished (or disappeared) reduce to three times daily, before lunch, dinner, and bed. If there are no more sweats for three nights, reduce to two times daily, before dinner and before bed. It there are no sweats for another three nights, reduce to once daily, just before bed.

You might find the sweats will return if you begin a course of antibiotics or start taking some new analgesic medication, in which case you might need to repeat the above procedure with the drops.

Occasionally, when sweats are really severe and usually of long-standing, the above drops are insufficient on their own. In this case there are some extra drops which can be taken once a day in addition to the others which double the strength of any homeo-pathic. The formula for the Potentizing Drop Formula is given on page 207. They're taken in the same way as the drops above except they're only taken once a day, preferably in the morning.

Sweats and Fevers

The following remedies work very effectively when there are sweats *with* fevers which don't respond to any medical treatment. It's not uncommon among people with AIDS to have sweats with fevers without any obvious cause being present. The following combination of homeopathics has been used many times both inside and outside hospitals with excellent results. The Antihydrosin Drops Formula mentioned previously is used with the addition of the following homeopathics:

Inflammation Drop Formula

- *Belladonna*   4x
- *Apis mellifica*   4x
- *Lachesis mutus*   30x
- *Mercurius corrosivus*   5x
- *Baryta muriatica*   6x

Take the Antihydrosin and the Inflammation Drop Formula in the following manner (do not mix together in the same glass):

1. *Ten to fifteen drops of each remedy in a couple of teaspoons of water four times daily before meals and before bed. Hold each sip in the mouth for a few seconds before swallowing.*

2. *When sweats and fevers have subsided, reduce to three times daily (before lunch, before dinner, and before bed).*

3. *If, after three days, there are still no sweats/fevers, reduce to two times daily (before dinner and before bed).*

4. *If after three days, there are still no sweats/fevers, reduce to once daily (before bed). Continue taking the remedies once a day until the end of the bottles.*

5. *If sweats/fevers return, increase the frequency of the doses as in (1).*

Overeating

For all those who have a problem with eating too little, spare a thought for those whose problem is eating too much. Some treatments containing corticosteroids (for example, prednisolone) stimulate the appetite. For these people, the novelty of having an appetite soon wears off as they begin to put on extra kilos they'd prefer not to have. However, they're the easiest to feed, as they'll eat just about anything that doesn't eat them first. Most of this extra weight is retained fluid and so, fortunately, with the completion of treatment, the appetite and size returns to normal.

For some women this excess weight can be very difficult to shift. It's almost as if the experience or treatment of cancer has altered their metabolism irrevocably. They need to readjust their eating patterns to consume far less calories in addition to employing a regular and fairly strenuous exercise program.

Oxygen at Home

One of the most frightening feelings for people is not being able to catch their breath. Those who become very breathless on exertion might benefit by having access to oxygen at home. For some, getting up and showering can be an exhausting process. Any small exertion can result in complete collapse. The value of having oxygen nearby is that you can spend ten minutes receiving oxygen *before* you attempt your shower or other activity. You'll need to discuss your particular situation with a visiting nurse or doctor who'll be able to advise whether the use of oxygen would be beneficial. Your doctor can arrange for a cylinder of oxygen to be delivered to your home. I've had many clients who've been able to maintain their independence by having oxygen available. One lady, Sophie, had a very small portable cylinder which enabled her to continue coming to groups. The oxygen gave her a sense of security whenever she had to exert herself.

Pancreatic Cancers

Some of the most discomforting digestive problems stem from cancers of the pancreas, though not all people experience these problems. However, these cancers tend to create a great deal of gas which results in lots of burping, discomfort in the stomach and small intestine, and gas passed through the bowel. Rarely, on leaving the hospital, are they given any guidance as to the foods most suited to them in this situation and I advise you to adopt the same procedures described for controlling gas (see page 212).

It's quite likely that digestive enzymes will need to be taken with each food ingested if indigestion is a problem. It's possible to get a composite of digestive enzymes in one tablet, so that swallowing tablets is kept to a minimum. The formula *must* contain pancreatic enzymes in order to be effective. Slippery Elm powder mashed into yogurt or banana or mixed into a banana smoothie (see page 176) and taken with digestive enzymes often settles things down. It's important not to drink fluids within the thirty-minute period before a meal or for at least ninety minutes afterward. Remember, banana smoothies are considered food, not fluid.

Peripheral Neuropathy

Peripheral neuropathy can be one of the most distressing symptoms to experience. Some people feel this as a tingling, a numbness or pins and needles in their hands and feet following multiple doses of a particular chemotherapy called Vincristine. It's rarely severe and generally improves once the treatment program is complete.

People with HIV can experience peripheral neuropathy as a result of the activity of the virus on the nerves in their hands and/or feet, or as a side effect of their treatment program. Some describe it as feeling as if broken glass is lodged in their tissues. It can make walking extremely painful and in some cases can totally incapacitate. It can be severe enough to require strong analgesics. A dear friend of mine, George, suffered terribly with peripheral neuropathy as a result of HIV, particularly in his hands and forearms. He found that a combination of meditation and morphine gave him the relief he sought. He needed to readjust his whole life to accommodate his incapacity.

The following homeopathics have proved useful in minimizing the pain associated with peripheral neuropathy.

Neuralgia Drop Formula

- *Aconitum*   4x
- *Cedron*   4x
- *Colocynthis*   6x
- *Kalmia*   3x
- *Verbascum*   2x

For severe pain: Take ten drops in a couple of teaspoons of water every quarter to half an hour. *Hold in the mouth for a few seconds before swallowing.* Gradually reduce the frequency once the neuropathy has eased. Take once an hour, then every two hours, and so on. If neuropathy returns, increase frequency.

Occasionally, when the peripheral neuropathy is really severe and usually of long-standing, the above drops are insufficient on their own. In this case there is the Potentizing Drop Formula (see page 207) which doubles the strength of any homeopathic. The drops are taken in addition to, and in the same way as, the Neuralgia Drop Formula except that they're only taken once a day, preferably in the morning.

Massage can also be very helpful in controlling or alleviating the discomfort of neuropathy. You might find that the hands/feet are too painful even to be touched initially, but if the therapist/caregiver begins to massage from the top of the limb (that is, beginning at the thigh or upper arm), they can gradually work their way down to the hands/feet. The massage should probably be very gentle to begin with, but the deeper and more firmly the therapist can work the more effective it will be.

By the time the therapist gets to the painful hand or foot he or she may need to "lighten" his or her touch considerably. The therapist will probably need to return to very gentle (feather-touch) massage on the hands or feet but again, after about twenty minutes or so, can begin to work more and more deeply. This will often give twenty-four hours of pain relief. I recently massaged someone with AIDS in this way and his joy at being able to walk unassisted to the bathroom to have his first *private pee* in ages was incredibly gratifying. Quality of life is improved immeasurably by such treasured victories.

Pressure Areas

People who are confined to bed for more than a few days must be careful of the areas on which their body rests. These areas are principally the heels, hips, buttocks, sacrum, shoulder blades, ears, and elbows. It's especially necessary for those who are fairly inactive in bed, since the constant pressure can lead to the skin becoming very thin and perhaps breaking. This frequently happens with the elderly or with those who've retained a lot of fluid in their tissues because of their medication. A daily intake of one gram of Vitamin C has been shown to increase healing of bed sores; however, they're best avoided altogether if possible.

Regular gentle massaging of the areas at least every two hours and changing the position of the person so that other areas take the load on an alternating basis will help in alleviating this problem. Sheepskin rugs also help to distribute the pressure of the body, as do "ripple mattresses." These are mattresses which have compressed air forced through alternating channels.

One of the most effective ways to toughen the skin is to rub in methylated spirits. The most important part is simply to stimulate the circulation to the area. One doesn't have to be particularly sick for these areas to become a problem; it happens whenever a person is in any one position for too long.

Radiotherapy Side Effects

The side effects of radiotherapy will depend very much on the amount of radiation administered and the area of the body to which it's given. People are often told that there are no side effects from radiotherapy. However, this claim is inaccurate unless we're talking about palliative radiotherapy which usually involves only a small amount of radiation given to a fairly limited area.

I've touched upon the effects of radiotherapy when it's given to the abdominal area (see Diarrhea and Nausea, pages 202 and 230, respectively). Here, I want to talk about radiotherapy which is given to other parts of the body, and its effects.

A course of radiotherapy which runs over a number of weeks nearly always makes the individual feel somewhere between tired and completely exhausted. Some people find they can continue working during their course of radiotherapy while others find it very taxing and they need to rest for many more hours in the day. Some people find they become despondent, depressed, and/or tearful during radiotherapy, or they experience unusual mood swings. *These symptoms are associated with the treatment.*

Many doctors don't explain that radiotherapy continues to be active for a while after the last treatment. For instance, if you've been prescribed a course of five weeks of radiotherapy five days a week, the treatment will continue to work *as strongly for the first couple of weeks as if you were still going to the hospital daily, and will continue to work at a lesser level for as long as you* had *the treatment.*

This means that the side effects of the treatment will last for that period of time also, and you won't begin to recover your energies and emotional equilibrium until several weeks after you've finished your treatment. For example, where radiotherapy is prescribed for five weeks, it will be ten weeks from commencement of treatment before you begin to recover your full energy and emotional equilibrium.

If your support person knows this, he or she can reassure you that you *will* pass through this time and what you're experiencing is an effect of the treatment. You won't *always* feel that way.

It can be very difficult to keep your spirits up when you're feeling exhausted and depressed as a result of treatment. It's easy to forget you're not your usual self. The support person's role is very important because her or she can reassure and comfort you with the knowledge that it will pass.

I often see people who say, "I can't understand what's wrong with me. I finished my radiotherapy three weeks ago and I still feel exhausted and emotional. Am I ever going to feel better than this?" If they'd been properly informed, they'd understand they're *still* "having" therapy even though they're not going to the hospital for treatment; it's continuing to work in their bodies.

I believe the vitamins mentioned previously in connection with Nausea (see pages 230-242) are valuable for all people who have cancer, AIDS, or any other disease which affects the immune system. People who are having radiotherapy will benefit from the addition of vitamins and minerals which are particularly in demand for tissue repair work. These are Vitamins A, C, E, and the B complex, plus selenium, magnesium, methionine, histidine, copper salicylate, and zinc. Seek guidance from a doctor trained in nutritional medicine, a naturopath, or your local health food store.

Scarring After Radiation

Many people benefit from the application of aloe vera gel alternating with a Vitamin E cream after radiation treatment has ceased. Your radiotherapist will have instructed you about the care of your skin while you're having treatment. Once you're allowed to apply creams and so on to the skin, you may find they assist the healing process and minimize any permanent scarring in the area. Some radiotherapists will allow aloe vera gel or a non-metal-based cream to be applied during therapy. *Ask your radiotherapist.* Aloe vera gel is the juice from the aloe vera plant and is widely available from health food and department stores. Vitamin E cream is also readily available. Some people add Vitamin A oil as well.

Others claim they've benefited by drinking one cup of aloe vera juice per day both during and after their treatment.

Shingles

To be treated effectively, shingles needs to be diagnosed as early as possible. It's often a very painful and debilitating condition that can develop when the immune system is not functioning very effectively. If you are immune-suppressed, it's essential that you avoid children who might have the chicken pox virus (which also causes shingles). Your doctor will prescribe appropriate treatment for you. If you have any residual nerve pain after shingles, or simply want to hurry up the healing process, you might find the following homeopathics helpful.

Shingles Drop Formula

- *Croton tiglium*   6x
- *Mezereum*   3x
- *Natrum chloratum*   6x
- *Rhus toxicodendron*   4x

For shingles: Take ten drops in a couple of teaspoons of water every quarter to half an hour. *Hold in the mouth for a few seconds before swallowing.* Gradually reduce the frequency as improvement becomes evident. Take once an hour, then once every other hour, and so on. If pain returns, increase frequency.

These drops are also very effective for those who suffer with post-shingles neuralgia. Sometimes the pain or sensitivity can continue for months in the previously blistered area, and the Shingles Drop Formula is effective in alleviating this sensitivity. The drops are taken in the same dosage and manner; however, they only need to be taken four times daily, gradually reducing the frequency as improvement is evident.

Occasionally, when shingles are really severe, the Shingles drops are insufficient on their own. In this case there is the Potentizing Drop Formula (see page 207) which can be taken in addition to the others. The drops are taken in the same way as the Shingles drops except they're taken only once a day, preferably in the morning.

Skin Irritations

Most people who have cancer find that their skin is drier than usual. This doesn't cause any problem in itself and a good moisturizer will probably help. Many people with HIV find they experience this same dryness. In fact, people with the virus are prone to many difficult and irritating skin conditions. These problems need to be diagnosed by your doctor so that appropriate treatment (if any) can be employed. Many people experience "itchy" skin without any particular cause. If it's severe, antihistamines are sometimes prescribed to relieve it. Often it's confined to one area of the body; for instance, the scalp, face, or neck area. Some people find the use of an anti-dandruff shampoo on their skin will alleviate the itchiness. Others find an anti-bacterial wash works well for them. Your pharmacist will be able to recommend one. Tea-tree antiseptic cream can be very helpful for this itchiness also.

Watery Eyes

Occasionally people undergoing chemotherapy will experience a constant overproduction of tears. It's a side effect which is only experienced by some people. Often, however, the medical team will assure you that the tears have nothing to do with the treatment. This leaves you feeling uncertain about an annoying and unexplained symptom. I've seen enough people with this symptom to assure them that it *is* a side effect of the treatment and that it *will* settle down when they finish their chemotherapy. In the meantime, keep a tissue handy!

Chapter Nine

BEYOND PAIN

. . . .

Marianne

The most blessed childhood imaginable followed by seven years of carefree wandering in Europe and the Americas during my twenties, two marriages and three children plus a good stint of single parenting, and a healthy mid-life career change had mapped out my existence fairly substantially. My late forties found me settled, happy, and starting to gain a new level of awareness which I'd always imagined would replace the rather erratic excitement of youth. Then, about two years ago, I experienced a period of total lethargy, sudden and unexplained. I canceled my massage work and yoga classes, went to bed for a couple of days, and expected the symptoms of the flu, sore throat, streaming nose, and a clearing cough. The symptoms didn't materialize and I dragged myself back to my routine, still feeling totally drained of energy. Then I found a tiny lump in each breast and made a mental note to "watch it"; perhaps I needed to slow down a little.

The lump on the right side disappeared but the lump in my left breast grew slowly. Sometimes I thought about it, and at other times I chose to ignore it. My grandmother and my yoga teacher had both had breast cancer, mastectomies, and radiotherapy with no recurrence, and I realized the chances of malignancy were fairly high. Then the "universe" sent me three rapid fire messages: within a period of ten days, I had three clients recount their stories of discovering a breast lump, and my eldest daughter told me about nursing a terminally ill cancer patient who'd chosen to ignore medical advice upon having a diagnosis of breast cancer made. It seemed the time had come to seek advice.

I chose a young and capable GP, made an appointment and confided in a friend, asking her to make me promise I'd keep it! I had opted out of the system four years earlier, abandoning a "safe" paramedical job for a New Age career as a yoga teacher and masseur and I loathed the prospect of re-entering my former world as a patient, but somehow I managed to center myself and neutralize most of my negative feelings. The mammogram and cell pathology proved positive and within a very short time, I was faced with the prospect of surgery. "Whoa, what about a good cleansing fast, lots of meditation and a trial period to monitor the lump?" My belief system demanded a really good think before surgery! So I set a date ten days away to make my decision, told my daughters of the diagnosis, and after some discussion, we all agreed that probably the wise course of action was to follow the Western medical model: accept without fear the treatment available.

My courage deserted me briefly when I presented at the small community hospital on a Monday afternoon to be admitted. But I spent a reasonable night and was able to do an hour's yoga on the lawn and meditate intensely before I was wheeled into operating room exactly on time at 2:00 P.M. the following day. The anesthetist had agreed to forgo the preoperative medication and I felt the initial injection of pentethal flow up my arm, reach my chest, and there ended my awareness of procedures.

When I emerged from the "Mists of Avalon," I began to focus on my breathing once more and sent white beams of healing light to my left chest wall, now sprouting two lymphatic drain tubes. The surgeon had left the nipple and surrounds jauntily peeking out of the swathes of white gauze and I even managed a faint smile at his quirky sense of humor! The drip running in my arm meant my meditation was interrupted every hour or so as I levered myself onto the pan. Blissfully it was plastic, not shiny cold stainless steel! By morning I was determined to get out of bed and empty my bladder fully perched on the pan on a chair and after an afternoon visit to the bathroom and a gentle tepid shower, I could definitely feel my strength returning.

Three days later I went home. The nursing staff were wonderful, fully supportive of my chosen regime of meditation, and never insistent for me to take medication for pain. I resolved to make them a big Christmas cake. At home, I rubbed aloe vera sap from my plants on to the wound, gingerly explored some simple yoga stretches to ease the numbness and restricted movement of my left arm, kept doing lots of deep white light breathing and meditation and began to think about the next suggested step, radiotherapy.

"One lymph gland (armpit) and one central lymph node are affected. Suggest twenty radiotherapy treatments." Oops, where's my calmness? The idea of forgoing a month of precious summer and R and R at home, swimming and riding my horses, healing myself in familiar surroundings, the idea of radiotherapy proved to be more of a stumbling block than surgery! I began gathering available statistics to discover that four weeks of radiotherapy would, at best, merely slightly minimize my chances of a localized recurrence but would have no effect on my long-term prognosis. I balked.

With radiotherapy to commence on January 2, I still had almost two weeks at home and I was starting to feel really good again. Each afternoon I launched into the cold, swift currents of the Murray River and swam around the bend in midstream, breaststroke gently stretching the tightness in my left arm. I felt myself absorbing the pure energy of the water and allowed my thoughts to soar to the heavens as I floated on my back, borne by the currents. I was my own canoe as I nosed into the bank beneath the trailing green fronds of willows. I recalled my journey down the Amazon in the heady days of the traveling 1960's and then shivered as another of the "cosmic connections" hit home. After the South American journey was over, I'd read and researched the history of the continent and had been fascinated by Darwin's account of a voyage along the Amazon. He reported seeing the legendary Amazon women who had cut one breast off to improve, he assumed, their performance with a bow and arrow! So my daily applications of aloe vera sap and Vitamin E cream to my neatly healing scar became filled with love and reverence. On Christmas Eve I managed a creditable handstand on the back lawn! I gave thanks for the full use of my arm.

On New Year's Eve I traveled to Melbourne and chose to spend the last few hours of 1990 at the Siddha Yoga Ashram. The program of chanting and meditation seemed to give me strength and inspiration. I wrote in my diary on New Year's Day: "I think I understand momentarily a little more about vibrational levels. Living alone is perhaps a chance to fine-tune yourself; you don't have to expend energy using words in an attempt to harmonize your thinking with another person. We all like to feel comfortable and the constant (and very worthy) concessions which a relationship demands perhaps detract from the purifying process. We may all be a sound in the hearing of God, hence the chanting to tune the instrument. God is within us all; the purer we become, the closer we move to our God-like qualities—compassion, lightness, sensitivity, selflessness." So I determined to spend as much of the month of January as I could in a state of alpha waves.

By the start of the fourth week of treatment, my chest and back were a mass of itchy bumps and I was waking through the night scratching wildly. I was only about two-thirds of the way through the recommended twenty treatments and felt myself sliding into a trough of despondency. My skin looked like that of an aging reptile with a bad case of hives and I felt as though I was on fire. Heat, heat, too much heat. My sleeps were restless and sweaty; I awoke feeling washed out and listless. I plodded through the week until Friday's 4:00 P.M. appointment to be met by an overflowing waiting room and a chalked notice on the blackboard which read: "Due to a further breakdown, we're running two hours late. If you cannot wait, please reschedule for next week." I heard my inner voice yodel loudly, "Overload! That's enough! Listen to your body!" cried the yoga teacher within. My footsteps fairly flew down the stairs and out of the air-conditioned building; I ran out into the slanting golden sunlight of the summer afternoon, tears of joy welling up and spilling over on to my cheeks. I knew I wouldn't make another appointment.

February began gently at home in Albury. I advertised my classes and eased my way back into a light program of work. Still swimming each afternoon, meditating for an hour each day, and continuing with vitamin supplements, my irradiated skin slathered alternately with aloe vera sap and Vitamin E, I felt light and thankful and very positive. After a month my skin was totally renewed, I keep touching it to marvel at the body's ability to heal itself. I even sometimes wonder if the *breast tissue will regenerate if I were to really align my forces, but then I'd lose my perfect aim as I draw my bow and let the arrow fly!*

Who hasn't experienced pain? The important thing with pain, as with all symptoms, is to find and understand the *cause.* Even when we're free of it, pain is the symptom we probably worry about most. We might not be talking about physical pain only. There are many different pains from which human beings suffer. At its simplest level, we experience pain as something that "hurts." It might have many different causes, depending on what kind of pain is being experienced.

The pain which concerns us most is the physical pain we believe our illness will produce. It's important to realize that diseases like cancer and AIDS are *not* always painful, not even if they lead to death. In ninety percent of the cases where people *do* experience pain, it can be controlled and in many cases eliminated.

Most of us have heard stories about the pain of cancer or AIDS and it's understandable that anxiety and fear are experienced. You could even be feeling, right now, pain which isn't being adequately controlled. Very often oncologists, immunologists, general practitioners, and nurses aren't knowledgeable about appropriate pain management. When you've looked to them for guidance in the past they've probably had suitable answers or solutions to your medical problems. However, to treat pain adequately is a specialized field and *you* must become educated about your *own* pain and its relief.

In some ways, physical pain can be easier to deal with than the emotional pains which are more subtle. Physical pain is generally regarded as an enemy to be avoided at all costs and in Western cultures we go to great lengths to avoid it.

Perhaps we feel the pain of deprivation. It can be some kind of obvious deprivation, as in the loss of a limb or breast, or physical disfigurement. Or it can be more subtle, as in the loss of an organ or the ability to have children. Many people say they can come to terms with having their illness but are deeply affected by the loss of their hair, brought about through treatment. It could be loss of weight which preys upon the mind or loss of energy. For some, it will be the sacrifice of having to stop work.

We might not be feeling the pain of a physical loss and yet our pain can be intense. We might have suffered the loss of those we love, either through death or divorce, or we might simply have physically moved away from our loved ones. The pain felt by these separations can be deep and unacknowledged—our private pain. This pain is often more intense and makes us feel dispirited because no one quite understands our personal loss. Yet emotional pain is something to which we can all relate: unfulfilled dreams, loss of face, disappointing relationships, lack of success in our chosen careers, shattered expectations, and so on. We deal with these "pains" according to our past experiences. For one person, bankruptcy will be a devastating conclusion to all creative endeavors while to another it will be just another "educational" step along the way. Likewise, a childhood where there has been little with which to build self-esteem could leave scars which take a lifetime to heal. They could be scars which will *never* heal and which will influence the way a person makes all future choices.

There's the pain of separation: children leaving home to start life on their own; friends or family moving to another town or country; a child going to boarding school; leaving childhood and entering adolescence.

One pain often overlooked is the pain of clinging to life. For some, their ultimate pain will be the final separation by death— the leaving of everything familiar, the leaving of loved ones. The pain of not seeing children grow to maturity and beyond. Letting go and trusting all is well. Leaving a body which has completed its task. Leaving a body when we believe we *haven't* completed our task.

However, in retrospect, it's plain to me that many of the greatest traumas and "pains" in my life were fertile soil for growth and understanding. These "pains" included months in the hospital with extensive reconstructive surgery to my legs as a teenager, the death of my much-loved brother, a divorce, and leukemia—to name just a few of the more potent ones! The understanding and growth these experiences allowed was probably unavailable in any other way.

It's difficult for people to witness a loved one's pain. We can empathize, but beyond that we might feel helpless in our inability to give relief. The pain of our helplessness can be most acute. There are many misunderstandings about pain and its relief.

It's true we can learn much about ourselves through the experience of pain. However, we also need to temper our pursuit of understanding with gentleness and compassion. Unrelenting pain is both exhausting and dispiriting. Even the most positive attitude or resolve weakens when pain is persistent.

Pain is only a symptom of some distress which the body or mind is experiencing, and is a cry for help. And help is needed. Pain shouldn't be ignored. It is essential to investigate thoroughly and deal with its cause. This applies regardless of whether the pain is a physical or emotional one.

Unless emotional pain is dealt with, it will erode our peace of mind and ultimately cause stress to the body. Suppressed resentments, angers, jealousies, and hurts prevent us from living happy and fulfilled lives and inevitably damage our health. It has become apparent that many patients have suffered some major pain or loss in the six months to two years before the onset of their cancer. This observation is not a new one. For centuries both doctors and lay people knew that after a major stress, people were much more prone to disease. In the eighteen months prior to my diagnosis, my brother had died, I'd moved to a new country to undertake further studies, and had separated from my husband!

In chapter 2, Techniques for Living, we discuss many ways of dealing with these stressors, and you can refer to that chapter for further practical assistance. The techniques for forgiveness are particularly useful to apply to past situations which still cause us stress. Their use implies a willingness to let go of the pain of the past and an openness to seeing the situation differently. Why hang on to the pain of unforgivingness? As has been said before, physical pain requires investigation so we can learn what its cause actually is. It's a common trap, once we've been diagnosed with a serious disease, to believe every ache and pain is associated with "the disease." We forget we could be suffering from muscular tension, arthritis, indigestion, or a tension headache. Immediately we think we might have tumors in the brain, bones, or tummy! Rather than worry unnecessarily it's better to find out what the cause of the pain is, and find an appropriate treatment.

The mind will conjure up all kinds of frightening explanations for our pain and it can be far more worrying than knowing exactly with what we're dealing. When we know what is causing the pain, we can marshal our resources to work within that situation. The unknown is always more intimidating than the known. It's good to remember also that everything seems much worse at 3:00 A.M. What's quite tolerable in the clear light of day is sometimes overwhelming in the still watches of the night. The feeling of isolation in the middle of the night can be very acute. Sometimes I used to feel everyone was sleeping contentedly in their beds while I was quietly dying in my room. I was fortunate to have a very understanding mother to whom I could express my fears. Often just being able to talk to a sympathetic friend is sufficient to alleviate the stress associated with our fears and anxieties. Likewise with past resentments, hurts, jealousies, and so on. Once aired with an understanding person, they diminish in their intensity. If we don't have such a person in our lives, then we might need to enlist the aid of a trained counselor who can help us to resolve our difficulties. Often the emotional or psychological pain we "hold in" directly contributes to the physical pain we experience in our bodies. Barbara's story, which appears in chapter 10, What About the Children?, illustrates very well this connection between mental and physical anguish (see page 298).

Some avenues worth exploring for the relief of pain are listed here. It's a matter of trying out different suggestions and finding which ones are most appropriate for you. They're suggestions which have proven useful for others and require no prescription.

You may wish to discuss the following techniques with your physician before employing them. It is assumed that you will be under appropriate "pain-management supervision" from either your doctor or a palliative care team. However, here are some additional thoughts that might prove useful to you.

The Pain Scale

Using a scale to talk about your pain can be a very useful tool. This means you "measure" your pain on a scale of zero to ten. A zero means you're pain free; a ten means that something really needs to be done about your pain right *now*. To "scale" pain in this way seems somehow to objectify it. It puts it "out there" for discussion with your caregiver. After a time you'll also learn which number on the scale corresponds with the technique most useful in alleviating it. For instance, a rating of "three" could mean some diversional activity will take care of it. Perhaps a walk in the garden or a game of cards. A "five" could mean it's necessary to practice a particular relaxation technique for its relief, while a "seven" might mean you need to look for assistance in the form of appropriate or additional analgesics. It will be a very individual scale and it will take a little time to become familiar with exactly what will help most. People's pain tolerance can vary enormously. Some people have a very high pain threshold, while others will experience fear immediately and that will almost "lock in" their pain and make it all-consuming. Sometimes, when a disease progresses, our tolerance to pain becomes diminished and we require more effective techniques for its control. Factors such as the weather, weariness, boredom, fear, or the anticipation of some unpleasant procedure can influence how we will experience our pain.

Pain often restricts our activities, both mental and physical, and when boredom is added to pain it becomes much worse. If boredom is a facet of pain, it's helpful to have recourse to activities which stimulate the mind. These could include everything from a walk in the garden to doing a crossword to playing Scrabble or listening to a "talking book." These "books," com-

monly referred to as books on tape, are usually available from
your local library. Other activities such as needle-point, knitting, tapestry, painting, drawing, and other crafts can also be
beneficial in this way.

Beverley gains tremendously from doing tapestries. She finds
this relieves her pain by providing a distraction. She is determined to create and complete a tapestry for each member of her
family before she dies. I've met at least twelve members of her
family and I know how determined she is, so I have every confidence she will be here for a long time to come!

Massage

Often, gentle massage will relieve the symptoms of discomfort
and immediately increase ease and mobility. No one with a serious disease is free of muscular tension. Massage is a wonderful
means by which we can release tension and the vast majority of
people find it extremely relaxing and helpful. Often when we
experience pain, we "hold" that area in an unnatural position to
"protect" it from being bumped. For instance, if you have a pain
in your shoulder blade, it's very likely you'll tense the surrounding muscles in order to protect the painful area. This might well
lead to tension in neck and other muscles which will then cause
more pain. Massage can relieve all the surrounding tension. *Then*
you can deal effectively with the residual (and original) pain.

It can be useful to immobilize a painful part of the body.
This can be done through the use of a splint, a sling or by creating support through the use of pillows or cushions. If an area of
the body is immobilized, it might also be beneficial to use
gentle massage to the surrounding areas in order to minimize
tension held there. Elevating a limb on pillows or, again, in a
sling might also be advisable if there is any swelling. Massage
can be used to reduce swelling in arms or legs (see
Lymphoedema, page 226). If you're seeking professional massage, find a therapist who's had experience with people with
cancer or serious illness and who's familiar with some of the particular problems associated with these illnesses. You might wish

to check out the advisability of massage with your doctor. In some cases where there are metastases or "hot spots" in the bones, massage could be contraindicated. However, any therapist who's had experience working with such people would provide very gentle massage to those areas and pose no problem at all to the patient. The benefits are so valuable I would encourage anyone to give it a try. The principal benefits of massage are:

- *It induces deep relaxation.*
- *It provides nurturing.*
- *It improves the overall circulation.*
- *It relieves muscular spasms which could be causing pain, discomfort, or limited mobility.*

If you choose to have a professional massage don't be afraid to tell the therapist exactly what it is you want. Many therapists also visit the home and this might prove to be more convenient for you. In this latter case, they usually bring a portable massage table to your home. If they don't bring a table, they'll be quite happy for you to remain in your bed. If you're particularly weak or bed bound, then explain to the therapist over the telephone that you'll need to remain in bed.

Massage Induces Deep Relaxation

I recommend to people that they look on the time of massage as being their time to let go and deeply relax. It's preferable to do this in silence since chatting to the therapist both distracts you and prevents you from receiving the full benefits. It's an ideal time to practice relaxation techniques. In doing that, you can become acutely aware of the areas in your body which you habitually tense in sympathy with those in which you experience pain. If you can let your muscles "dissolve" before the therapist's fingers, you'll experience the most benefit.

Massage Provides Nurturing

Having a massage can also be a valuable time to learn to let go and actually receive some tender loving care from someone else. It's a time when you're ministered to. Let yourself luxuriate in the feeling of being tenderly looked after by someone who knows how! It's often difficult for us to let ourselves be nurtured. So many of us are only comfortable when "in control," letting someone take over for a while can be quite a new experience. We can feel rather vulnerable when being massaged, especially if we're in pain, and for this reason it's essential we have trust in the therapist.

Massage Improves the Overall Circulation

Massage increases the blood flow to the immediate and surrounding areas. With a restored and adequate blood flow, the area then receives both the nutrients and oxygen which the tissues require. It also means toxins from muscular activity or spasm can be effectively eliminated. Parts of the body which are cold and lifeless can be restored to warmth and mobility. As relaxation becomes deeper, the overall blood flow throughout the body is increased.

Massage Relieves Muscular Spasm

Hospital beds were never designed for physical relaxation! They're designed almost entirely for the ease of the nurses. Modern technology is gradually improving the situation for both nurse and patient. Of course, it's not just a matter of the bed. If we're hospitalized, there are all the added tensions of diagnostic tests, disrupted routines, endless people, noise, hustle and bustle, and frequently unfamiliar (and, perhaps, unpalatable) food. Add to this the stress of impending surgery or the anticipation of test results and it's no wonder our muscles are all of a-twitter.

Most people will say, after a massage in the hospital, that it's the best thing that's happened to them since they were admitted. Some massage therapists will visit people in the hospital, but it's essential you receive permission from your doctor first. To check with the doctor is a simple matter of courtesy. And don't forget a massage for the support person or caregiver! Everyone needs nurturing and support, and massage is a great way of having it.

Reflexology, Acupressure, and Acupuncture

These modalities work by stimulating the circulation and the energy flow to an area. They can be very helpful in alleviating pain. A trained therapist is usually needed; certainly for acupuncture. However, a therapist may be willing to show the support person the appropriate points to massage so the caregiver can bring relief to the patient. Some acupuncturists will leave small needles in place between visits. These needles will continue to stimulate the nerve endings in the area leading to pain relief. There's evidence to show that people who suffer with peripheral neuropathy (see page 245) often benefit from acupuncture.

Warmth

Don't forget the value of warmth. A simple hot water bottle can be very comforting for many pains. For safety's sake, regular checks on the integrity of the rubber and a cover for the hot water bottle is recommended. You can also find small electrical heating pads, like mini-electric blankets, which can be placed over areas of pain. (Conair, 1-800-726-6247, is one such manufacturer.)

A pain-relieving product called Warmease consists of underpants which have a "pocket" into which a heated gel pack is inserted. The gel pack gives sustained and comforting warmth to either the abdomen or lower back (depending on which "pocket" in the underpants you choose to utilize). The pants are very well made and the gel pack sits "flat" against the abdomen or lower back and thus is unobtrusive—jeans, dresses can still be worn without any evidence of the gel pack. They're safe, convenient, and provide excellent, comforting warmth to the area. For your nearest Warmease dealer, call 1-800-526-9464.

Exercise

A pleasant distraction involving exercise can be helpful in dealing with pain. This could involve a favorite sport or a gentle stroll in the garden. Sometimes all that can be managed is a slow shuffle up and down the hallway. Even quiet exercises done while in bed can relieve stiffness and poor circulation. Ankle rotation, and the tensing and releasing of muscles throughout the body are helpful for those confined to bed. The support person or caregiver can assist the patient by gently moving the various parts of the body.

For other people, quite vigorous exercise will bring pain relief. One of the effects of vigorous exercise is that the body secretes endorphins into the bloodstream. These endorphins are the body's own natural pain relievers. They're also released into the bloodstream when we laugh heartily or when we weep. You may well have experienced deep relaxation throughout your body after a really good cry or laugh.

Many people have adequately controlled their pain through their sporting activities. They generally find that it *increases* their pain initially; then they find they receive very valuable pain relief which lasts for a considerable period of time after their exercise.

Jody found her exercise bike was invaluable to her in this way. She had the bike moved into her bedroom and used it several times throughout the day. She would start off gently, as it was quite painful to begin; then gradually she was able to increase the length and strength of her cycling until she could sustain fairly vigorous movement for about ten minutes. She said this would give her pain relief for about one and a half to two hours.

In his book, *Anatomy of an Illness,* Norman Cousins gives an excellent account of dealing with his painful and crippling disease by the conscious use of laughter. He found ten minutes of good belly laughter gave him two hours of pain relief. Used in this way, laughter is a form of exercise and one of the most pleasant ones at that! Internal jogging! It's a very inclusive form of exercise and is quite infectious. We don't even need to leave our bed. Funny friends, videos, or books can be a godsend. Laughter makes everything much more tolerable and helps us to keep our perspective. It's one form of exercise in which everyone can participate. Learn to escalate a smile into a chuckle, a chuckle into a laugh, a laugh into a real belly laugh. Our own laughter is a very reassuring sound to our ears!

Poetry

Some people find release from their pain by listening to poetry. Its beauty and imagery can provide a very special oasis for the mind, taking the concentration away from the difficulties of the present. Having someone read to us when we're unwell can be very comforting. Cassette tapes of poetry or novels are becoming more widely available and can bring another world into our home. Don't overlook the possibility of writing poetry yourself either. This can be a useful means of expression for those whose activities are curtailed.

Will, a philosopher from way back, was now much slowed down by his cancer. He put many of his thoughts and feelings on paper, sharing his perspective on the world, his loved ones, how we spend our time upon this planet, and the meaning of life. In this way he was able to work through many of the issues to find his own path to peace. He also left a legacy of kindly words for his loved ones to remember him by.

Music

Like poetry, music can soothe, comfort, and uplift us. We can go beyond our pain to a space of calm and peace. Listening to music which is bright, cheerful, or inspiring can certainly lift our spirits.

Sometimes it takes an effort even to reach out for the things which we know will bring us comfort. It's almost as if we'd rather stay in a depressed or painful "space" than make the effort to shift our perception of things. Feel the pain, feel the inertia, then make the effort anyway.

Music has a tremendous capacity to lift us out of depression or pain. Experiment with the various kinds of music and be flexible in your choice. Music can also be used to put us in touch with our anger or frustration. By allowing it to "flow" over us we, like the music, find the resolution of these feelings. Some music is full of passion and torment and yet, having given full reign to these feelings, finds its way to rest and peace once more.

Touch

As with massage, the simple loving touch of someone can bring great comfort. A hand held, a brow softly stroked, a foot gently massaged. These small gestures sometimes convey all that's necessary. To be in pain is stressful in itself. To be in pain and to feel isolated from love is much worse. A gentle hug or caress is one of love's most natural means of expression.

By our response to the care and love shown to us, we can bring comfort to our caregivers. It's important for the caregivers to feel appreciated and that their "loving" of us is acknowledged. A simple smile or returned gesture often speaks more eloquently than words.

Prayer and Affirmations

The repetition of a positive statement or the "offering up" of our pain to a higher source can bring comfort and a changed perception of our situation. When we're in pain, at least we know with certainty that we are alive. To practice a technique of relaxation at this time can be challenging. It helps if we've been practicing on the "little pains" before we tackle the more intrusive ones. Once we're in a deeply relaxed state it can be very helpful to quietly repeat a word or phrase which we find comforting. To work with the inward and outward breath adds power to our practice. Some affirmations which have been found useful are:

Let go and let God.
All is well.
Healing Peace.

Peace and Calm.
Healing into Light.
Peace and Joy.
Om Shanti.
Ham Sah.

These words, repeated silently and slowly in the mind, can be rhythmically attached to the breath. For instance, on the inward breath, we can repeat silently "Let go and ... " and on the outward breath, "let God," and so on.

These techniques become powerful with practice and perseverance. With a strong faith all things are possible. It even becomes achievable to transmute pain into warmth and joy. It's often resistance to pain which makes it unbearable, not the pain itself. It is its limiting character which we resist. Some people have the determination and faith to go beyond their pain, to find a way of living at peace with their pain.

Early last year, I met a remarkable young woman by the name of Lois. She had had a melanoma removed from her leg some months previously and was seeking ways in which she could assist herself to increase and maintain her health, physically, emotionally, and spiritually. Together we explored the way she'd lived her life and, to her amazement, she found she was always trying to live up to *other* people's expectations. Her commitment became to *Lois;* to find out who she was, to learn to love herself without feeling a need to change a thing. The changes that *did* take place during that time were simply the falling away of everything she wasn't.

Lois learned to meditate, improved her diet, and became very interested in spiritual matters. Her meditations moved more and more into Christian prayer and she positively glowed with peace and serenity—and health. For many months I didn't see her, then she made another appointment. She limped unsteadily into my office using a walking stick and settled herself gently into a large comfortable chair. She looked quite different from last time. Her face was very puffy with fluid from her medication and her leg was at least three times its normal size. She sat un-comfortably in the chair at a slightly abnormal angle. In the in-tervening months since her last visit, she'd been very active and happy. Happier, she said, than at any other time in her twenty-one years.

However, three months before, she had experienced a severe pain in her back which wouldn't go away and responded only minimally to painkillers. It transpired that the melanoma had spread into her spine. This resulted in her having one and a half vertebrae removed and a rod and plate inserted to stabilize her spine. She now wore a brace as well. Further tumors had blocked off the return of the lymph fluid from her leg, hence the tremen-dous swelling. One would expect to see a disgruntled, angry, or depressed person, but not so. Here she was, telling this tragic story as if it belonged to another person. Her face had a serenity and softness which was unmistakably the face of peace.

The reason she'd come to see me was to ask a simple ques-tion. *How might she maintain her peace while enduring great and constant pain?* In the very asking, she was practicing the answer: her simple willingness just to be here now with whatever is unfolding.

We discussed living with pain at length. Lois talked about her need to curtail activities outside of home and her desire to spend time in more "inward" activities. Her greatest asset was her unshakable faith. I also put her in touch with a local hospital which teaches a lymphatic drainage technique which I knew would be helpful and which is discussed in chapter 8, Burps, Burning, and the Dreaded Bloats. (see page 227).

As she left my office, I mentioned to her that once a month we gather together people like herself to dress up as clowns to go to the Children's Hospital at Camperdown in Sydney. These clowns (**C**ompassion and **L**ove **O**ffered **W**hen **N**eeded) are very special because they have life-threatening diseases themselves. There's more about the clowns later (see page 366). I invited her to join us. No one was more surprised than I to see Lois on our doorstep on the designated day. She looked wonderful as a clown with hearts painted on her cheeks and a star on her brow,

and she was free of her walking stick. She said her clowning day
had been the most special day of her life and she's looking forward to subsequent visits. Her courage and faith are an inspiration to all who know her. She's totally at peace with dying,
because she's totally at peace with living. Lois has learned to live
moment by moment. She doesn't demand the future to be a certain way and she doesn't resist what today brings. She's found
that it doesn't take much to make a happy life.

Lois, like many of our clowns, had also discovered a great
truth. When in pain, whether emotional, spiritual, or physical,
one of the best ways of dealing with it is to go out and make
someone else happy. It's a mystery and a miracle but it works!
To forget one's own problem and give to others keeps our perspective large and our horizons unlimited.

Breathing Patterns

There are times when we need to "will" our way through pain. It
can be a real effort sometimes to go for a walk, or have a swim,
or finish "that job" when we're in pain. There are other times
when we need to stop what we're doing and consciously practice
some technique to help alleviate it. Sometimes one approach is
just right, other times a different one is needed.

Technique 1

A technique which is enormously valuable is simply breathing!
Often when we're in pain it's reflected in the manner in which
we breathe. Our breathing can become restricted or labored.
Sometimes we develop the habit of breathing in, holding the
breath, and taking an age to let it out again. Once we detect
this pattern we're in a position to establish a healthier rhythm.
More often than not, with this sort of breathing there are some
emotional factors at play, emotions such as fear or uncertainty.
To establish a better rhythm helps to calm those emotions. It
can be helpful to adopt a counting method with the breathing.
For instance, we can breathe in to the count of four, hold for
four, and breathe out to the count of four. We can gradually

lengthen the breath so we breathe in to the count of, say, ten or
even twelve, hold for that long—or a shorter period—and
breathe out for the same count. Experiment until you find what
works best for you. There's no right or optimum way to do it.
The right or optimum way is the one which works for you.

Technique 2

Another very restful technique is to breathe in and then focus on
the little pause at the end of the inward breath. Then breathe out,
and again focus on the little pause at the end of the outward
breath—each inward and outward breath leading to that comfortable pause. As the mind quietens, the pause naturally lengthens.
No effort is required to lengthen it. While breathing some people
like to hold in the mind the image of a crescent moon; one point
of the moon ten centimeters in front of the nostrils, the other
point of the crescent at the space between the eyebrows.

Technique 3

Some may find the techniques of "breathing in love, breathing
out fear" helpful. With each inward breath, focus on love; with
each outward breath, let all fear drain out of the body. Some
might wish to give "love" and "fear" different colors, perhaps
breathing in a soft pink, breathing out brown or gray.

One of these techniques, available on cassette, works to alleviate pain through the use of the breath (see page 379).

Breathing With the Person in Pain

A technique which is very useful when working with people in
pain is to simply breathe with them. This can be done in many
ways, according to the relationship which you have with the
patient. Choose a technique which is appropriate to your relationship. To look into each other's eyes and begin to breathe at
the patient's rhythm is all that's needed. After a short time, a
general sense of peace and calm is experienced and the breathing will naturally become slower and deeper. This produces a
very close feeling between the caregiver and the patient and this

might not be appropriate in all situations. Looking into the eyes of another for any length of time inevitably brings intimacy not experienced in any other way. Many people find such intimacy makes them feel too vulnerable and, of course, this must be respected.

Even just sitting by the bedsides of people in pain, and breathing according to their own patterns, somehow engenders a feeling of calmness. Very often the patients' own breathing deepens and becomes less labored as their pain and fear decrease. Perhaps the reassurance this practice brings is transferred to the patient and their anxieties or fears are somewhat allayed. It isn't necessary for the patient to understand, or even to know, what the caregiver is doing for the benefits to be felt. I've practiced this with people who are unconscious and whose breathing has conveyed distress. If I remain in a calm and peaceful state while breathing with the person in this way, it can have a surprisingly beneficial effect which is reflected in their breathing. I always "talk" to the person from my heart when involved in this practice. Unspoken words of reassurance have a powerful effect.

Breathing with a patient also helps us to enter into his or her "time zone." It's the most effective way I know of doing so. When we're unwell or in pain, our perspective on the world is entirely altered and we might well be in a different time zone from everybody else. To have someone who's on *his* or *her* "world time zone" rush into our room, when we're in a very different one, can be extremely jarring and certainly won't be felt as comforting. I make it a practice when visiting people in the hospital or in their homes to stop before entering their rooms and take some long, slow, deep breaths to calm and center *myself*. In this way I leave my world outside.

Our breathing is our most intimate connection with life. Without breath there is no life. It's the breath which ultimately connects us to our physical existence. If we're in pain and someone takes the time to breathe at *our* rhythm and at *our* depth, it provides reassurance, comfort, and confidence that all is well. When there's reassurance, fear diminishes and pain is more easily tolerated.

The techniques of breathing in harmony with someone in pain, more than any others, require great sensitivity to what's appropriate for the patient. To join with someone in their most intimate connection with life can be very valuable *and* it can be very intimidating. We're not *doing* something *to* the patient. We're not manipulating the person's experience. We're not even trying to change the person's situation. It's simply that, out of love or care for the patient, we wish to join with him or her in the experience, to share that person's reality, to feel as he or she feels. This co-joining of two people expands reality. It embodies a sharing attitude and the creation of emotional support. In order to use any of these techniques effectively it's necessary to put aside our own emotions. One cannot enter wholeheartedly into the experience of another while being preoccupied with one's own situation. We can be *aware* of our reality but not preoccupied by it. When we experience a deep sense of calm and peace within ourselves, we're more able to share in another's reality. If we're panicky and uncertain, it's these feelings which we'll bring to the patient. These feelings are likely to create more agitation and an *increase* in pain.

A technique I've often used with young people is to breathe through pain much as you would through a labor contraction. There's no reason why this technique wouldn't work for an older person; it's just I've only used it with under twenty-year-olds. This technique works for those whose pain arrives in fairly sudden "waves." We clasp hands if appropriate, look into each other's eyes and breathe together in harmony. We use a kind of panting breath which can become quicker and more intense if the pain does. It might sound surprising but we often find it quite an exhilarating feeling. It gives a great sense of "power over pain." *It* doesn't get us, we get *it*. It gives a sense we can work with this pain rather than live in fear of it.

Perhaps as we get older, we're less likely to try means that are innovative or unfamiliar and this must, of course, be respected. Something we've commonly noticed with these methods is that the pain begins to diminish in intensity and frequency as soon as patients feel they have a measure of control over it.

Developing techniques to assist us through the difficulties inherent in illness gives us a sense of being in control of our experience. These skills are the very antithesis of chaos and helplessness. From the practice of these skills we learn that even though life has its difficulties, its problems *are* surmountable.

The Role of Analgesics

It's a common yet erroneous belief that taking medical analgesics will somehow interfere with the process of healing. I've often seen people who haven't slept for days, who are dispirited and depressed through continuous pain because they refuse to take any prescribed medication. This is a really sad and short-sighted view. While the body is in pain, very little healing can take place, as all one's energy goes into dealing with it. Constant pain is very debilitating and it's difficult to keep one's spirits up when it's relentless. Often, all that's needed is forty-eight hours of good pain relief in which the patient gets some sound sleep. After this time the medication can often cease. Once we're rested and our spirits are restored, everything becomes easier. This pain-relief program needs to be administered by someone who's entirely qualified and competent to do so.

Some people are concerned that if they go on to strong analgesics, like morphine, they'll become addicted. Some fear that if they're taking morphine then their "end" must be close. Often these fears are held more by the surrounding family than by the patient. They're all understandable anxieties. With proper explanation from your prescribing physician these anxieties are easily eliminated. The technique described above, whereby strong analgesics are given for a short period of time, *does not* result in addiction. On the contrary, it results in a contented person who's gained some valuable rest and whose spirits are restored. Morphine, appropriately prescribed, never becomes addictive. People who have had drug addiction problems or are in recovery are often apprehensive about taking morphine. If this is your situation, speak to your doctor. It is important to have your fears allayed *and* to be as free of pain as possible. Your doctor will advise you as to which drug will be most effective.

It's a good idea to make arrangements in advance for after-hours medical care. You might never need to call on it, but it will comfort you to know that help *is* at hand should you require it. If your local doctor can't see you after-hours, make sure you have a summary of your medical history available with you for the doctor on call. This will save time and concern on your part.

If you are taking prescribed oral analgesics, it's essential that you keep a chart which clearly outlines the times when your medication is due. This is particularly important if you live alone and are the sole supervisor of your medication schedule. If you do not live alone, this chart should be kept by a friend or relative who resides there. Draw columns on a sheet of paper with these headings at the tops of the columns so that it looks like this:

Date	Time	Pain?	Drowsiness?	Other Remarks	Amount Given

Radiotherapy given to a specific area can often be of tremendous benefit in relieving localized pain. It's often used when a tumor is in the bone; you'll only know if it will help you when you discuss the possibility with your doctor.

Likewise, for those who have pain in the abdominal and lower back area, pain-killing suppositories can sometimes be more helpful than drugs taken orally. Many doctors overlook these drugs. In fact, many doctors don't seem to know about them at all. They can be particularly helpful at night as their action is spread over several hours and the drug releases slowly.

If pain is chronic and is being managed routinely by analgesics, then, again, they must be competently prescribed and administered. There are often "pain clinics" attached to hospitals. These clinics specialize in appropriate pain management. Often the analgesics prescribed are correct but the administration technique is at fault; these clinics can certainly assist with relevant information.

Many of the more powerful analgesics are given on a routine basis rather than on the basis of "pain demand." If they're given every four hours, for instance, the patient might well not experience *any* strong pain. If you wait for the pain to come before administration of analgesics, it takes *much* longer for them to be effective, by which time you're probably experiencing very strong pain.

Frankly, most oncologists and general practitioners seem to have limited knowledge of appropriate application of analgesics. They're fantastic at other things but pain is usually not one of their areas of specialty. In my experience, I've found there are three places to get expert advice on pain management. They are:

- *Pain clinics, that is, clinics with doctors who specialize in nothing but pain management. Some of these clinics use many of the techniques mentioned here, while others rely solely on drug analgesia.*

- *Local palliative-care/hospice units whose doctors and staff are all trained and well experienced in pain control.*

- *Your palliative-care nurse, who's part of the community nursing team. You can ask to be referred to your community nursing service by your oncologist or general practitioner.*

It's your right to have access to the best pain management skills available. It's your right to be pain free or as close to it as is possible. Don't be fobbed off with anything less than a great reduction in, and possibly complete alleviation of, pain. Keep asking until you get the assistance you need.

Constipation

Most of the medically prescribed, or even "over the counter," varieties of analgesics will cause constipation. This happens because analgesics cause the peristaltic (or wavelike contractions) movement of the bowel to decrease. They also dry out the contents of the bowel. These two factors are the cause of (analgesia-induced) constipation. This is one of the most common problems people experience. The person prescribing appropriate pain management should understand this and make sure adequate precautions are taken to prevent this unnecessary complication. Constipation can cause more distress than the pain! It's likely you'll have been prescribed something to assist with constipation. Dietary factors, appropriate to the person's needs, can also be useful. Please refer to Constipation in chapter 8, Burps, Burning, and the Dreaded Bloats (see page 199).

Surgical Intervention

In some instances your physician might suggest a more radical treatment for adequate pain management. This may involve direct intervention at the nerve supply to the painful area. If this is necessary, your doctor will discuss the procedure extensively with you so you understand exactly what it entails. I certainly wouldn't recommend it unless this advice came from a pain specialist who had tried all other alternatives first.

Pets

Don't underestimate the value of a pet in helping us deal with the stress of pain (see chapter 2, Techniques for Living, page 56). Many a pet has known exactly what's going on with its owner and has been able to bring about some magic by its presence.

Vitamin C and Coffee Enemas

These two forms of pain control are controversial so far as their effectiveness is concerned. The controversy largely exists between patients who've found them to be extremely effective in controlling their pain, and doctors who say there's no foundation for their use!

There are many people who claim to have had pain relief through the frequent administration of high dosages of Vitamin C. These dosages can be taken orally or intravenously. Obviously the administration of Vitamin C directly into the bloodstream can only be performed by a willing doctor. There are many such doctors in the community today who believe in and advocate the use of intravenous Vitamin C. Oral dosages of Vitamin C need to be administered on a very individual basis, since everyone's demand for it varies. It's essential you work with an experienced doctor or naturopath to establish the best dosage for you. When Vitamin C is given this way orally, it must be composed of sodium ascorbate, calcium ascorbate, ascorbic acid, and the bioflavinoids in order to give a balanced formula. Ascorbic acid on its own in high doses is very irritating to the stomach.

Coffee enemas have also been found very useful by many people to assist in their pain control, though for some people the very idea of a coffee enema is just not their cup of tea!

It's essential to have your doctor's permission for the use of coffee enemas. Your doctor may not be enthusiastic, but if he or she can establish that it won't do any harm, then you might wish to proceed. If there were any doubt about perforation of your bowel, he or she would be very much against it (and with good cause!)

The benefits of the enema are usually experienced within twenty minutes of administration. If you decide to try these enemas I suggest you be under the supervision of someone who's experienced in their use.

The following "recipe" is the one found to be most useful:

Place two to three heaped tablespoons of freshly ground coffee into a saucepan with 600 ml of boiling water. Simmer for ten minutes. Let cool to body temperature. Strain into an enema bag. This is then gravity-fed into the bowel. It's best to lie on your left-hand side while the enema is being introduced. You can lie on your back for the next twenty minutes to half an hour and then evacuate the bowel.

Enema bags can be ordered through your pharmacist if he or she doesn't have them in stock. Use petroleum jelly to lubricate the tip of the enema tube before insertion into the rectum.

Many patients with liver cancer have successfully controlled their pain solely through the use of coffee enemas. For some people these enemas are effective if given two times daily, while others will benefit by having them more frequently, up to six per day. Coffee enemas first became popular as part of the Gerson program (a strict dietary regime developed by Max Gerson) for cancer patients. Max Gerson was a German physician who lived in America and wrote a book called *A Cancer Therapy: Results of Fifty Cases*. Dr. Albert Schweitzer said that Dr. Gerson was "a medical genius who walked among us."

Note: Coffee enemas have also proved very useful to people who experience very itchy skin, often due to bile salts being present in the bloodstream. A noticeable "fading" of jaundice is usually evidenced in a matter of minutes of having a coffee enema. This is, of course, only a temporary solution and the bile salts do return. The enemas do nothing for the cause of the jaundice. However, the relief from itchiness can last several hours, which can be a boon when you are trying to get to sleep at night.

Techniques of Relaxation for Pain Relief

Techniques of relaxation are extremely valuable in relation to pain relief. While ever we're feeling uptight and anxious, it will compound our pain and make even the smallest twinge a cause for fear. It's important communicate with someone about *your* pain so you address the emotional or psychological components involved. Having done that, the regular practice of techniques which help to minimize or eliminate stress is invaluable.

Any of the techniques mentioned in this book will be helpful. There are two particularly which are most commonly used for pain management and I've put both these techniques on one cassette tape, Working with Pain (see Cassette Tapes, page 379).

Chapter Ten

WHAT ABOUT THE CHILDREN?

. . . .

Kay

When I was a little girl I remember thinking that forty would be a good age to die. I suppose when you're only five, forty seems a long way off. Thirty-five years later, shortly after my fortieth birthday, I was diagnosed as having breast cancer. It was an advanced cancer that had already metastasized. My chances of living more than two to three years were reported to be slight. When I visited my doctor after the surgeon had sent her the reports, she told me that it couldn't be worse and she cried with me as I talked about my children growing up without me.

Six years later and a long way from where I began, I'm still here. My life has been different from what it might have been and my priorities have altered. As a very special person called Carmel said once in telling her own story for a video we were both involved in making, "It's a changed kind of reality."

It has taken me quite some time to write my story, and writing this has been another learning experience for me. I didn't find it easy. I'm again reminded that no matter how far away in time I move from the pain of those first few dreadful months after diagnosis, with the busyness of surgery and follow-up treatment and the tearful times with family and friends, the reality that my life has been changed forever remains.

I've not been able to take myself back to those early months and write about them now as I might have done then. Instead, I'm writing somewhat from a distance. The painfulness is too much to go back to and I've needed to move on. It's easier now to analyze my experiences and to synthesize my learnings than it was then. For me, the journey these past six years has involved confusion, an inner struggle with feelings of self-worth, withdrawal, strong negative feelings and a search for personal meaning in my life. It's involved a confrontation with my fundamental attitude to living and an affirmation in faith that there is meaning in human experience. I'm far from having any answers but I've reached a point where I feel at home with a degree of mystery in my life. I've discovered that dealing with a life-threatening illness can provide an opportunity for personal transformation and the potential for growth. Strangely, cancer can be a very positive and life-giving experience.

At first I thought I didn't feel anger, but I probably did. I thought that I wouldn't be able to cope, but I probably have. In the early weeks and months, some days were definitely better than others. It's good to acknowledge this and, as well, not to assume responsibility for coping with everyone else's feelings. I needed to give myself space for coping with my own. When I first came home from the hospital, we closed the doors to friends for a while. Several weeks after surgery, when the doctors asked me if I was aware of the gravity of my situation, I was, but it wasn't easy to cope with. For a long time I couldn't talk about it to anyone except my closest friend. It was hard telling my three children, harder telling my mother, and almost impossible to tell my grandmother. I didn't tell them right away; there was a lot of sorting through I felt I needed to do first.

When I was ready I told my two sons, David and Benjamin, and my daughter, Elisa (thirteen, fifteen, and seventeen at the time). I felt then, as I do now, that the children had a right to know and also that I needed their help. It's difficult to make big changes in your life without the support of people you live with on a daily basis. Honesty in relationships is very important and the children wanted to know. They had sensed things anyway and, in general, children are capable of dealing with much more than adults give them credit for. My children were wonderful. It was important to give them an opportunity to accept some changes in their daily lives, because it gave them a sense that they were each making a personal contribution to helping me, as indeed they were. We spent some special times talking and crying together and I did my best to answer their questions. This wasn't easy. On the lighter side, they endured my less successful ventures into vegetarian cooking with patience and good humor. "Please God, don't make it lentils again," became the silent, secret prayer of my eldest son! We had a lot of laughs as well as tears along the way, and sharing what I was able to with them brought us all closer together.

I also needed and had someone who listened with gentle acceptance to my deepest feelings and fears, and who came with me as a partner to support groups where we both learned so much about the resourcefulness of the human spirit. People who are living with a life-threatening illness can learn a lot from each other, and hearing about other people's experiences helped me to get mine into perspective. It was important to know that, when I slipped into those tunnels of black despair, someone was there to help me through and to be with me in the long and difficult struggle to remain hopeful. Many friends and loved ones aren't able to cope with what they perceive as negativity and despair, but talking about death and what would happen to my children when I died, for instance, was necessary. I needed my feelings about it to be heard and acknowledged. Thank you, Wendie.

Thinking about your own death can be scary. I remember one afternoon when I was resting being startled by a very powerful awareness of what it is to die, to no longer exist, to leave. It was like death was in a drawer that suddenly flew open and I was very afraid. I went cold all over, and for days was terrified to be alone or to be the last one to fall asleep at night. It was such an overwhelming experience that I couldn't talk to anyone about it.

Over time, I was able to go back to the experience and each time I could open the drawer a little more until eventually I could pull it wide open and look right inside. Six years later I still do from time to time.

I am liberated by the belief that God made me and that, whatever happens in the future, my life has not been without purpose. I've learned that there is no such thing as a dying person. There are only living people and my plan is to live my life as fully as I can. I have learned that hope is a powerful healer.

❧

To have a member of one's family diagnosed with a life-threatening disease is a bewildering experience for children. Obviously their responses will depend very much on their age and maturity. A three-year-old's response to mother or father's absence due to hospitalization will be very different from an eight-year-old's, which will differ again from a teenager's. In this chapter, there are some overall guidelines which you'll need to adapt to the age and development of your child. These are guidelines only and you, as parent of your child, will know what's best in *your* situation, if you listen to the voice within your heart.

Helping Children Understand

Some parents wonder if it's really necessary to tell the children of their diagnosis.

Children invariably know something is wrong and, if not properly informed, they may conjure up fears far greater than the real situation warrants. A child has a right to know about anything that affects the whole family. The occurrence of a life-threatening illness in a parent will certainly have its effect on each member, and the child should therefore be included in the knowledge of this fact. The child might feel that to be excluded from this information is a breach of trust.

Children have an amazing capacity to deal with the truth and will come to terms with the diagnosis and what it means to them in their own time and in their own way. This might mean they retreat into their own world to adjust, or that they "act out" their feelings in some way. Even very sad truths will relieve the anxiety of too much uncertainty. You'll see from observing your children's behavior how they're dealing with the information.

If you exclude your children from the truth, they could very well interpret this to mean they're not important enough to be included in a family matter. If they hear about it from somebody else, they could be ill-informed and may believe that something too terrible to be talked about is happening. It's not healthy for children to grow up with an abnormal fear of illness. Children

are adept at overhearing conversations but they're very poor in-
terpreters of the information heard. Many children blame themselves for their parent's illness. For example, "I was mad at Dad
for making me tidy my room. Now he's sick. Maybe I made him
sick." Or, "Grandma died in the hospital. Now Mommy has to
go into hospital. She's going to die, too."

Many parents have been amazed at the support and comfort
their children were able to give them once they were informed.
To withhold your diagnosis and what it means to you is to withhold a great deal of yourself from your child. Nothing is more
painful for children than to feel excluded from those they love.
The experience of a life-threatening illness isn't a totally negative one. It's also an opportunity for the human spirit to gather
its resources and marshal its strengths. Your children will learn
much from you in this and it will provide them with the opportunity to grow in understanding and strength.

*Once you've decided to tell your children, then the next question you'll
have to think about is, "Who should tell my children?"*

You'll know if you're the best person to tell your children. If
you think you can explain simply to them what has happened,
while maintaining fairly good emotional control, then you're
probably the best person to tell them. Emotional control doesn't
mean without a tear. If you shed tears it gives your children the
permission and opportunity to cry, too. However, you won't
want to unnecessarily upset them. You might prefer to tell your
children in the company of a close relative or friend.

If you feel you're not the best person to tell your children,
then perhaps this relative or friend could speak to them. Make
sure the close friend is considered close by the children also.

Another possibility is to have the children told by your doctor or a member of the professional staff of the hospital. Who
should tell your children will also depend very much upon their
ages.

"At what point should my children be told?"

The answer to this question will depend on the age of the child. If your children are aware you're unwell and are having tests, then they might need or wish to know what the problem is just as soon as you do. If this diagnosis has come without warning, then you might prefer to take a little time to adjust to the situation yourself before including your children. This might mean several hours to a few days, depending on your initial reaction.

So, firstly you'll need to explain what is wrong. Then, once they understand what's wrong, you can explain to them how the doctor wants to treat you. They'll want to know if this means you're going into the hospital for treatment or will be remaining at home. Are there likely to be any changes at home or will things stay the same? If your treatment is on an out-patient basis, you could explain to them the likely side effects of the drugs, or radiotherapy. Tell them you'll let them know if there are any changes to the treatment and how you're feeling as you go along. Give the children time to assimilate your information and to formulate any questions.

Once your treatment has been completed you can explain to your children that you'll keep them informed about your health and will let them know about any changes. If a child continues to ask questions or seems overly concerned about your health, allow time to explain or reassure as necessary.

"How should I tell them?"

Initially, you might find it easier to speak to your children on an individual basis. This will give you the opportunity to gear what you're going to say to each child according to age and development. After this initial talk, you might find you can speak to them together. When speaking to them together always remember to use a language that each will understand, particularly if there are young children. To answer the questions of teenagers in front of seven-year-olds might be confusing unless it's put into a framework they understand.

You might want to rehearse in your mind what you'll say to each of the children and anticipate the questions which could arise in each mind.

"When telling my children, how much is too much?"

1. Children need to be told information which is clear and which they can easily understand. You'll want to tell them:

    *   *what has happened*
    *   *what will happen next*

    You'll want to reassure them you're having the best care available and you're very hopeful. In this way you'll encourage them to be hopeful with you, even though right now you and they might be upset. It will give them a sense of better times ahead. Sometimes the whole house seems to feel the effects of our fears and it's always wise to end these discussions with the reassurance that your child is loved and will always be cared for.

2. Let the children know how you feel as well as all the medical facts. This gives the children permission to have and express their feelings.

3. After you've told the children any new information, give them time to assimilate it so they can formulate questions of their own. Their questions and responses will let you know how much information they can handle. Answer their questions simply. If they wish to have further, or more in-depth information, they'll ask if you give them the opportunity. You can ask them what they think cancer or AIDS (or whatever) is. In this way you can ascertain how much they've actually taken in and correct any misinformation they might have. It's O.K. to say to children, "I don't know." It's much better to say, "I don't know," than to make up something which could prove to be inaccurate. There are some don'ts worth listing:

    *   *Don't lie.*
    *   *Don't frighten them with all the unnecessary medical details, or financial worries (unless they'll be affected by them).*
    *   *Don't trouble them with things which haven't happened yet; for example, test results which haven't arrived, operations or treatments which might not be needed.*

- *Don't make promises you might not be able to keep. Keep your options open by saying things like, "I'd love to watch you play baseball and I think I'll be up to it by Saturday," or "I'll be doing my best to...."*
- *Don't push children to talk. They will in their own time.*

Here are some ways of explaining things to children which will furnish them with information they can grasp. Obviously you will need to gear whatever you say to their ages and understanding.

1. *"You might have noticed that sometimes I feel sick and don't have enough energy to play with you as before. I have an illness which is called cancer. The doctor's giving me medicine to help me get well. Some days I'll feel tired or sick and other days I'll feel fine. Daddy (or Aunty Jane or whoever) will help me take care of you until I feel better."*

2. *"Sometimes our bodies don't behave as we would like. A part of my body became sick and the doctor had to remove it through an operation. I'll have treatment now so it won't come back. Sometimes people say scary things about cancer, so if you want to know anything about it, ask me."*

3. *"Because I have this sickness, sometimes I'm sad and angry. You might feel like that too when you see me feeling sick. It's O.K. to be angry; it's O.K. to be sad. Some feelings will change but the love we have together won't ever change. Having you around, your hugs, drawings, and rainbows are helping me."*

4. *"I have to have another operation because the cancer in my body has started to grow again. The doctor thinks this will get rid of it. After the operation he'll give me more treatment to see that it doesn't come back again. We believe this will work. I feel angry and sad this has happened. We all hoped I was finished with treatment."*

5. *"Because I have this sickness, I've decided to make some changes so that I can help myself get well. I'm going to eat foods which will give my body what it needs to fight this disease, and I'm going to spend time each day just being quiet and still so my body can help itself to get well. You can help me by doing activities which aren't noisy during my quiet time. You might like to come and sit with me so we can share some quiet time together."*

Wrapping Children in Rainbows

When I was diagnosed with leukemia my children were ages four and seven. Kate, the eldest, understood something was wrong, but Simon, at just four, was only aware that I wasn't my usual energetic self. He wasn't worried because he was at an age where he could easily adjust to a more sedentary mom. His father and I had recently separated and so, for much of the time, Simon and Kate were living away from me. When the children came to visit at the weekends, it was my mother who took care of their (and my!) practical needs. I found it very depressing not to be able to do all the things which I had formerly taken for granted. I wasn't only depressed, I was angry. I almost preferred them *not* to come than to see me as I was. The energy level of little children is very high and extremely difficult to tolerate for any long period of time when one is feeling so debilitated. I'm sure other unwell mothers of young children will be nodding in agreement. My children had difficulty in understanding why I was depressed and angry and this in turn made them more distant. They gradually preferred to run to my mother with their woes, and achievements, and for their peanut butter sandwiches. On the one hand I was very grateful for the assistance I had, but resentful that I couldn't do all those little things a mother usually does.

For the first two months I refused to say the word leukemia. I was afraid if everyone thought I had leukemia they'd start relating to me as a dying person. I wasn't ready for anyone to put me in a coffin, not even in their imaginations! However, this made it difficult to talk about my situation with both my parents and my children. Kate was surprisingly supportive for her years. She used to tell me if meditation was going to help me then I *must* meditate. Support is a gift or a gesture that lets us know we're loved. Kate would bring me a flower, or a drawing–some small token of her love–and it often changed my day. Even Simon was able convey his concern and love with a gentle pat, a wet kiss or a mini bear-hug.

They were difficult times. One of the gifts of that time was the discovery of wrapping the children in rainbows. What child doesn't love a rainbow—its beauty and magic?

Once Simon was tucked up in bed, I'd ask him to close his eyes and imagine I was wrapping him up in a cloud of red. As I talked quietly to him about this beautiful soft cloud of red light, I'd pass my hand very slowly and lightly over the whole of his body several times. Talking quietly about this beautiful, soft light, like a cocoon, I would be gently and slowly stroking him all the while. Then we would visualize the lovely clear color of orange: the color of nasturtiums (among his favorite flowers) in the sunshine. Wrapped in a cloud of clear color ... still moving my hand gently and softly over his body ... and so on through all the colors of the rainbow.

The yellow of early morning sunshine—or whatever is appropriate to your child's understanding or preference. The green of lush grass. Blue, like the sky. Indigo, the color of the heavens at night. And violet, the color of the flower. This ritual can take as long a time as seems appropriate to the age of the child. At the end, I would place my hand over Simon's heart and together we would visualize a strong rainbow beginning in his heart and then stretching out through the air to my heart. In this way we'd stay connected to each other all through the night. I'd also repeat a little poem which we made up, that went something like this:

> *I wrap you in a rainbow of light*
> *To care for you all through the night.*
> *Your guardian angel watches from above*
> *And showers you with her great love.*

It isn't just the child who benefits; parents enjoy it, too. During my illness I was separated from my children for weeks at a time and every night I'd send them a rainbow, as they did to me. Some of this time I was in Europe and America while the children were in Australia with their father, and yet we knew these rainbows were always being sent and delivered. Even after my recovery, sending rainbows was a regular feature of our going-to-bed ritual. Love can bridge all distances. Surely the substance of rainbows is love.

I've shared this technique with dozens of parents and children since, and I know many children to whom sending rainbows continues to be very important. These children became accustomed to sending them to a parent when the parent had cancer or AIDS. It was the child's way of sending love and healing. Even after the parent died, the ritual continued, the child knowing the rainbow was being received wherever the loved one was. For the child it's a sacred time of joining with someone they love who's no longer with them.

This technique gives us comfort and a tangible way of expressing our emotions. With a protracted illness often it's not solutions we're needing. Sometimes it's just the strength to continue, day after day with seemingly no end in sight, and still the uncertainty of what the future will bring....

Some people mistakenly believe that to be positive is to look only for the outcome which they'd like to see. So, to be positive is to have things 100 percent the way we'd like them to be. This presupposes that we know precisely what is the best outcome. One of my great realizations when I was sick was that not only did I not know what was best for everyone else in the world (!) but I didn't have a clue what was best for me either. Previously I genuinely believed if things weren't the way I thought they were meant to be, then they had to be wrong. Such was my attitude at that time. This attitude precluded any self-acceptance. At this stage I'd never heard of the concept of self-love or self-acceptance.

Talking About Death and Dying

Many people regard thoughts or conversations about death and dying as being thoughts of negativity, failure, or being morbid. If you're feeling concerned about discussing death with your children, you're not alone! Most of us hesitate to talk of death to children; however, it is an inescapable part of life. We must find ways of dealing with death and so must our children. One of the ways to help them (and reassure ourselves at the same time!) is to let them know that it is all right to talk about it. When we talk to them about the thoughts and feelings they have, we can discover what they know or don't know. They might have fears, misconceptions, or concerns which we can help allay through information, understanding, and reassurance. Talking through our feelings might not change the situation but it will certainly change the way we *feel* about the situation. It's important to show interest in and respect for what a child has to say. In this way we can better *hear* what their perceptions are rather than giving further information which might only confuse.

Your children are probably far more aware of death than you realize. Even very young children have seen dead lizards, birds, or insects. If they watch TV they probably see at least one death a day on the screen, and their games will often play out their fantasies about death and dying. However, a child can feel quite confused and frightened when the possibility of death and loss come close through the advent of an illness in a loved one.

Remember, *what* you will say to your child and *how* and *when* you will say it will depend very much upon their ages and understanding. For instance, preschool children often have the notion that death is completely reversible or temporary, while five-to-nine year-olds will realize that death is final and that all things which are alive must die. In this age group, though, the children often have the notion that it happens to other people and that it couldn't happen to them or their loved ones. They often feel they can control death through their own cleverness, bargaining, or efforts. From about the age of nine children begin to fully comprehend that death is irreversible, that all living things die, and that they too will someday die. The precise age at which children will comprehend death and its implications will vary according to a whole host of factors.

Death isn't the opposite to life. We live through the process of dying. Each and every one of us is going to pass through the experience of death, and not to talk about it can isolate us in our experience. Death is one of the most mysterious and awesome adventures upon which we're all obliged to embark, and to share openly with our loved ones the concepts, uncertainties, and apprehensions we hold can bring us to a much greater depth of intimacy and understanding.

Young children cannot fully comprehend death. Can any of us? Sometimes we can use symbols to help children understand the concept. A walk in the garden is full of possibilities for discussions on death and dying. Leaves that turn from green to yellow to brown; that let go the tree of life only when they're ready; to fly free through the air and land softly; to become mulch and soil to give new life to the tree. Or a cicada shell; a thing of beauty in itself which was left behind as an even more beautiful creature emerged from its shell. The seasons constantly demonstrate the ebb and flow of life.

One mother, Susan, explained about life and spirit and bodies in a tangible way to her three small children whose father was very ill. She took a balloon and blew it up. She explained to the children that the balloon was only made beautiful and special by the air which was inside of it. The balloon was like a body; a shell in which they each lived. When she let the air out of the balloon, she explained how the life and spirit leaving the body becomes part of everything else.

Communication Needs: Verbal and Non-Verbal

Remember, how much you include your children in your thoughts and discussions will depend entirely upon their age and development. Trust in what you know of your children and listen to your own heart. You'll then know how much of yourself to share with them.

What makes living with a life-threatening illness especially difficult are the many unknowns. Living with such an illness means living with uncertainty. There are some questions you won't be able to answer. We as adults need to accept that fact, and we need to assist our children to accept it also. It's fine to answer a child's query by answering, "I don't know." If it's the kind of issue to which someone (perhaps your doctor) knows the answer, reassure the children you'll find out and let them know.

You'll find you go through many stages in coming to terms with your illness. Perhaps disbelief, anger, depression, hope, and acceptance. Like you, your children are endeavoring to understand this in their own way and their behavior might well reflect their inner struggles.

Very young children fear separation, being left alone, strange people, and surroundings. If possible, when you're hospitalized, have a familiar person take care of them in their own home. Talk to them and, when you do, reassure them you're coming home soon and you're thinking of them (and sending them rainbows)! One of the most challenging aspects of talking to children is getting the timing right. When you're all ready to have a deep and meaningful talk they disappear to a neighbor's house to play. Or they ask you the most profound questions just as their baby brother is screaming for his dinner. It isn't always easy to get the timing right and we certainly need to hang on to our sense of humor. Maintaining a sense of humor when you're feeling frazzled or debilitated is a challenge in itself!

Hospitals aren't always geared for very young children so, when they come to visit you, be sure they bring some activities with them or a favorite toy. Perhaps you could keep some things at the hospital which will amuse them and differ from their toys at home.

Young children often feel they can control what happens to them and that they have magical powers. They often believe what they wish for will come true. It's not uncommon for children to feel guilty about their "bad" thoughts; they might feel guilty their parent is ill. *Reassure them from time to time that nothing they've thought, wished, said, or done has in any way caused your illness.*

Some children become overly concerned about a parent's health. It's important not to overload the children with too much information so they become worried about details. It's important to let your child's teacher know about your illness early on so he or she can support the child at school and can let you know of any unusual behavior.

Disturbances in eating, sleeping, schoolwork, and friendships are not unusual. This applies to children of all ages. Teenagers as well as younger children sometimes regress in behavior.

Teenagers have an especially hard time because their own emotional balance is often still precarious. At a time when they're just beginning to explore the idea of emotional and social independence from family, they're thrust into a situation where the parent might need to depend upon *them*. Some react by rebelling and becoming difficult to deal with, while others will want to take on responsibilities which are really beyond their years. Some will retreat into their own world and seem not to care, while others will not seem to overreact in any way and will remain their usual selves. All these reactions fall within the normal range. However, if you find your children's behavior becomes a real problem, seek assistance from your church (if you have one), your child's school counselor, your hospital, or the children's hospital in your area. Seeking professional help isn't a sign of failure on your part. Your hospital will be able to put you in touch with some books, videos or groups which could assist your teenager in understanding what he or she is experiencing.

In some families, communication wasn't particularly good *before* the diagnosis of an illness. Just because someone has a physical problem doesn't mean everyone's now able to be loving and supportive. There are often strained relationships within families and these won't automatically dissolve. There are professional counselors who'll see a family together, to help iron out the difficulties and to assist in reestablishing healthy communication. This can be a tremendously enriching experience for the family who is committed to improving relationships. Even if all family members choose not to participate in this kind of counseling, it can still be valuable for those who do.

Helping Children Deal with Change

Many changes will take place in your home because of your illness. These might range from emotional upheavals to the fact that you have no hair and are drinking carrot juice instead of coffee. Children are very observant of all these changes and will require explanations to ease their concerns. Don't take for granted your child will understand why suddenly you have to rest every afternoon. Explain to them in a language they can understand why you're doing these things. Children love routine and habit, and when you start breaking routines they need to adjust. This is much easier if they know why. For instance, it's preferable to tell your children about the side effects of chemotherapy when your hair first begins to fall out rather than when you're almost bald. Some mothers are happy to show their mastectomy scar to their children while others prefer not to. Children are intensely curious and, having had their curiosity assuaged, are usually content—until their *next* question arises.

You'll need to explain you're not able to do all the things you did before; that rest is essential; that their aunt (or whoever) will pick them up from school today; that you can't make their chocolate brownies this week; and that your love for them is always there.

As much as is possible endeavor to maintain a daily routine. Make sure all the essential things are attended to. Perhaps one family member can take over much of your role. Perhaps your twelve-year-old can take over mowing the lawn. It might not be done perfectly, but does it really matter? One of my favorite sayings is, "Would you rather be right, or happy?" Sometimes we need to let go the way we've always done things and let others make their own contribution it their own way. That's how we learn.

If you can afford it, you can employ someone to help you at the times which are most stressful in your day. There might even be a teenager in your area who'd be willing to do a couple of hours work for you after school. If friends or relatives offer to help, accept it. Let one of them organize the others so you don't have to supervise. Again, they won't do things the way *you* do them, but at least they'll be done. If you allow other people to support you, it enables you to spend time with those who are really important. If possible, make space each day to spend some quiet time with each of your children. If not daily, then weekly. If you've very young children who are in need of consistent care, try to have the same person helping.

One of our young moms, Tessa, decided her two-year-old should go into day care. The toddler loved the company of the other children and it enabled Tessa to rest and do the things she needed to, and be relatively fresh for his return in the afternoon. She would've preferred to be a full-time mom to her son, but that was impractical. He doesn't seem to have suffered any ill effects from this experience. Remember, many single parents who are working require day care facilities. You're not being a "failure" in placing your children somewhere where they'll get the consistent care they need.

Children are usually more accepting of physical changes and disabilities than adults. If you look or feel different from your usual self, give your child a brief explanation. Don't go into all the unnecessary details unless you're asked for more information. If you're not upset, it's very likely your child won't be and he or she will accept the changes easily. You may find your children's friends discussing your illness and you can let your children know you or your partner are happy to talk with them if they've any questions. Sometimes children will go to extraordinary lengths *not* to let their friends know things have changed at home. Just continue to be reassuring and leave the door wide open for discussions or questions.

Discipline

A breakdown in discipline can be very distressing for a child and can convince him or her something has definitely "gone wrong" at home. It may be more difficult to maintain law and order, as the children themselves are under stress and are likely to act up more than usual to get attention. Remember it wasn't always perfect *before*. It's important to set firm limits and find suitable ways of enforcing them. If you let your children know you especially appreciate their cooperation now, you can reward their good behavior while enforcing the discipline necessary to halt their misbehavior. You're doing this for your own sake and for theirs.

"I've Never Felt This Way Before!"

If you're the kind of person who never shows how you feel, it's very likely your child won't either. Your child might be experiencing all kinds of feelings which are quite new and unfamiliar. When you allow yourself expression of your feelings it will give your child the permission and opportunity to do the same. To suppress strong emotions is like sitting on a volcano. You might be used to living that way but it can be very scary for your children to feel strongly and not be able to express their feelings. By expressing your feelings you help your children to feel O.K. about the feelings they have.

It's natural for you to feel sad about what has happened. Have the courage to express your feelings. If you can let the sadness out and cry together, everyone will feel the tension ease. This can be particularly difficult for many men who are unaccustomed to revealing their vulnerability. It's difficult for a father who's always been the provider and protector of the family to be now in need of support and care. It's not a sign of weakness to cry with one's family. It's part of belonging to a family.

Children might experience other feelings which confuse and bewilder not only themselves, but you, too! If these situations arise, remember they'll pass, and give reassurance to your child (and to yourself). Here's a list of possibilities:

- *Some children will be forever disappearing to the homes of neighbors or their friends to avoid being at home.*
- *Some will be afraid they'll get a life-threatening disease too.*
- *Some children will behave badly to cover up their real feelings.*
- *Some will laugh at everything to cover up their real feelings.*
- *Some children will retreat into their own world and won't let you in.*
- *Some will withdraw, unconsciously trying to become more independent in case something happens to you.*
- *Some children will become angry and resentful of you needing their care when previously the opposite was true.*
- *Some will pretend to be sick in order to get the attention they feel they're missing.*
- *Some children will pretend to be sick or play up a minor illness in order to spend more time with you.*

- *Some will become very possessive or clingy and won't let you out of their sight in case something happens to you.*

- *Some children will feel sorry for themselves when a parent is ill and then feel guilty about that. Others will wish their parent wasn't there and then feel guilty.*

- *Some will overcompensate for having had "bad" thoughts about you and will be unnaturally good or set unrealistic standards for themselves.*

- *Some children will form strong attachments to the other parent and avoid being with you.*

All these feelings and behavior patterns are common reactions of children who are endeavoring to come to terms with a situation which is stressful to them. For the parent who's feeling tired, anxious, or debilitated these reactions can be extremely difficult to deal with appropriately, and yet anger toward the child is rarely the appropriate response. It's important to realize this behavior will pass and it's just the child's way of coping with the situation. You'll find by talking *your* feelings through, you're able to maintain a larger perspective through which the behavior of the child can be more easily tolerated.

It's not just young children who can behave in this way. Adults who have cancer or any other serious illness can be very difficult for their parents to live with also. Much of my time being sick was spent with my very loving and supportive parents. However, I'd often retreat into my room and close the door. They felt shut out and tended to "tiptoe" around me for fear of upsetting me further. I refused to talk about all the things I was feeling, mostly because I couldn't have articulated what was going on inside myself even if I'd wanted to. Another difficult area involves the parent with an illness who has adult children. There's more on communication within families in other parts of this book (see pages 285-306, 307-317).

One woman, Barbara, whom I visited at home, was very tired and weak and was suffering with digestive upsets. Though she said her tummy was really her only problem, as we talked it became apparent her seventeen-year-old daughter also caused her considerable discomfort. She and her daughter had had a long and unhappy relationship in which, no matter what Barbara said to Claire, it was misinterpreted or misunderstood. Barbara wept as she acknowledged that this relationship was the greatest tragedy of her life. She would do anything to right it.

Claire was very withdrawn and sullen, which wasn't particularly unusual. Having her living in the next bedroom, going in and out of the house solely according to her whims, never doing anything for her mother, not even saying hello or good-bye, let alone, "How are you, Mom?" was really more than Barbara could bear.

After talking it through, Barbara decided to write Claire a letter, a simple letter straight from the heart. Together we talked about what it was she really wanted to say to Claire, and then she wrote it. At times it was hard for her to get past the resentment and anger she felt and go back to speaking simply from the heart. She talked about the pain of not being included in Claire's world, of always aching to know what was in her mind. She acknowledged how different they were and apologized for the times when she'd tried to make her the same as herself. She affirmed she had done everything, always, with love in her heart and she'd done her best as a mother. She was sorry for the times when her words had not conveyed love. She had always, and would always, love her.

Not surprisingly, by the time she'd finished writing her letter the pain and discomfort in her tummy had left her. She said she felt a huge rock had been removed from inside.

The next time I visited Barbara she was in the hospital. Laughter was coming from her room. She looked completely different. There was color in her cheeks and a softness about her I hadn't seen before. Sitting by her bed was Claire, relaxed and happy, obviously content to be where she was.

At a later time, when I spoke to Barbara, she told me they'd completely healed their relationship and that Claire had become a tremendous support and friend to her. It hadn't happened without tears and strong words. But it had happened.

Once a very wise and wonderful little girl called Kate, aged ten, said to me:

"Sometimes hearts have got to break before they heal."

Quiet Times Together

One of the "positives" of having an illness may be that you spend more time with those you love. Often the bonds within a family strengthen as the members share time, thoughts, and feelings. Often you'll see your children grow in maturity and independence, and you'll know this will help them to face other challenging experiences in life. They might develop more compassion and sensitivity toward people. Don't forget to acknowledge their achievements and express your gratitude and pride in them.

If you've chosen meditation techniques to help you, you might find it enriching to have practice sessions together occasionally. I have made a variety of guided imagery tapes which appeal to young children (as well as adults) and, for teenagers and adults, there are tapes on increasing self-esteem, meditation, and visualization techniques. These are available from Dawn Publications (see Cassette Tapes, page 379). Over the years many children have attended our meditation classes with their parents. Many of the teenagers have continued to use these techniques on a regular basis; they find them particularly useful in preparing for examinations and coping with the stresses of being a teenager. To meditate together is a very special experience. The silence shared by two or more people can touch the very depths of our being.

There are many ways you can involve your children so they feel they're actively supporting you at this time. Even the youngest children can have responsibilities—sending you a rainbow every night before they go to bed, bringing a freshly picked flower or leaf from the garden, giving you so many hugs and kisses a day, bringing a book or a meal. Keep it light and fun so the children don't resent having to do things for you *all* the time, and make sure they've sufficient free time to do whatever pleases them.

Here are some additional suggestions for times when you're

in need of quietness and still want to include your children. You can:

- *Read a book or watch TV or a video together.*
- *Write your family history, including major events, pets, holidays, hobbies, and idiosyncrasies of each member.*
- *Draw pictures of the family. Perhaps suggest the child draw pictures of what it's like to have a parent ill.*
- *Share stories, poems, or songs that are meaningful to you.*
- *Use a guided imagery tape together which takes you on a journey using your imaginations.*
- *Give your children the opportunity to express what they feel through role playing. Use dolls to represent the various members of the family and have the child direct the "play." Listen to what is being said in the play and ask questions about how each doll is feeling—if appropriate. Don't push!*
- *Meet with other families who are affected by a life-threatening disease.*
- *Learn about the body and show where your cancer/illness is by reading a picture book about the body.*
- *Make up a family song or saying which encourages you all.*

It can sometimes be a bit of a challenge to entertain children while you're in the hospital. You might not have much energy to entertain with! However, since playing in the elevators or corridors is to be discouraged, here are some suggestions for hospital activities. You can:

- *Use a tape recorder to record a story.*
- *Ask your children to record a message at home to bring to you; you can have one ready for them when they arrive.*
- *Have a computer game, art supplies, other toys, etc., which stay at the hospital (so that the novelty doesn't wear off).*
- *Make drawings for your children and have them do the same.*
- *Ask the children to make a phone call for you.*
- *Practice a meditation together, perhaps using a tape.*

- *Explain how the hospital "works." Indicate the people in their different uniforms and explain what their functions are. Point out the bed, buzzer, meal service, and how each works. There could be intravenous drips and other equipment which your child would like explained. Don't overload; just give enough information so that your child feels you're being well looked after.*

- *Perhaps have them visit you in the lounge, lobby, or garden if appropriate.*

Never make children do something they don't want to do. Rather, try to understand what's behind their refusal. Usually there's anxiety or a fear of some sort. If they don't want to visit the hospital, it could be because they're frightened of the hospital or the illness or the apparatus surrounding the parent, or they simply don't know what to say. If the parent is receiving oxygen, the well parent could bring home an oxygen mask for young children to play with in order to be familiar with it before they visit. Talk to them to see if you can ascertain what the fear is, and encourage them to tell the parent in the hospital about things at school, friends, pets, and so on. It's usually easy for children to talk about such things. You might want to encourage this fearful child to make little gifts at home for her parent.

It's important, too, for young children to keep visits to the hospital short. Try to organize their visits at a time when the parent feels fairly refreshed and/or pain free, perhaps after medication has been given. If the parent is barely conscious, or unconscious, allow the children to spend a short time visiting and reassure them the parent is no longer in discomfort or pain.

Whoever is looking after the children at home while you're in the hospital might want to encourage them to make a "Welcome Home" banner for you. This can be as simple or as elaborate as the child's imagination is capable of. They could help prepare your bedroom, pick some flowers, make some favorite food or drawings for you. Don't forget to notice and appreciate their gestures of love and support.

Seemingly strange behavior isn't always related to your diagnosis; children have fears we can't even guess at. As has been

mentioned before, children are often very literal in their inter-
pretations. I remember that when I was about nine or ten I became a Christian. I believed the Christian message absolutely
literally. If you were a Christian you went to heaven when you
died; if you weren't you went to a place where there was gnash-
ing of teeth and you burned forever. So, I was O.K., but what
about my grandmother whom I adored and who was the spirit of
love and generosity itself, but who certainly wasn't a Christian?
(She married a minister of the church in her later years only on
condition he never mentioned religion in the house!) I be-
seeched her to mend her ways. I couldn't bear the thought of an
eternity of separation from someone I loved, any more than I
could bear the thought of her eternal suffering. She used to hug
me and say, "Never you mind, darling! I'll be with all my
friends." This was no comfort to me at all and I used to lie
awake at nights praying for some miracle of conversion.

Perhaps some children are more literal in their interpretation
of life than others. I believe all we can do as parents is to establish an open and honest line of communication with our children
and to allow *any* questions about *any* subject to be voiced. Just
as we think after diagnosis that every ache and pain is related to
our illness, let us not assume every fear and anxiety our children
show is related to our illness.

A life-threatening or chronic illness is a challenge for any
family. To respond to such a challenge in a creative way requires
inspiration and all the strength the human spirit can muster. It's
important to acknowledge the creative solutions you've found to
your many dilemmas and take pride in your children's ability to
rise above adversity.

When a Parent Dies

For a child to lose a parent is a sad and devastating event. Most
children will go through several intense emotions, which might
not be clearly defined or well understood by those around them.
Remember, children tend to act out their feelings rather than
articulate them. If you're the surviving parent you'll probably be

immersed in your own grief, which might make it more difficult to hear your child's messages.

Obviously, one of the most common feelings children experience is of being abandoned. "Why did Mommy leave me?" Don't underestimate the amount of guilt a young child might carry. It's clear to any adult that the parent's illness had nothing to do with the child, yet the child may well be looking for reasons why her parent left. "Mom used to say she was sick and tired of cleaning up my room. Maybe if I had kept it tidier, she wouldn't have left me." Remember, it's important to reassure your children often that they had nothing to do with their parent's illness; that she didn't want to leave the family.

Because children act out their feelings, it's important to watch for changes in behavior. These could show themselves in a change in performance at school, reverting to bed-wetting or old habits, an inability to concentrate, an illness, or a change in standards, tidiness, or some other behavior.

The most useful gifts you can give to your child after the loss of a parent is consistency and your presence. Many children experience a deep sense of insecurity when one of the central figures in their world has gone. They might well wonder if you're going to leave them, too. You'll need to do everything possible to reduce uncertainty in your children. Don't "cheat" by going out after they're in bed at night. If they waken to find a baby-sitter or even Grandma, but not you, they'll be distressed. Make small contracts with your children. If you say you'll be back at 3:00 P.M., then make certain you are. If you say bedtime is at 8.30 P.M. then start the bedtime ritual at 8.15 P.M. so they can be in bed at 8.30 P.M. They might request a night light again, even though they haven't needed one for years. They might smuggle themselves into your bed at night; if you can, let them fall asleep there, returning them to their own beds once they're asleep. If sending rainbows has been a feature of the bedtime ritual before the death of the parent, then it might still be a means of communication which they'll want to continue. You can wrap them in the rainbows as always, place your hand over their hearts and send the rainbows out through the air to wherever mom or dad is now. One little child I know believes that mommy is now a star in the heavens and every night he sends a rainbow to her before he falls asleep.

Peter, then age four, had a very special response to the death of his mother, Vivien. She died at home very peacefully after a long and difficult time with cancer. In her last hours, as her body changed, Peter was full of questions. "Why are her hands white?" and "Can she still hear me?" and so on. To each of his questions, we gave him simple yet truthful answers. "Her hands are white because the blood isn't flowing through them so much. She doesn't need to use her hands now because we're taking care of her." "Yes, she can still hear you, Peter; would you like to whisper something special in her ear?"

After Vivien died, Peter peered into her eyes and said, "Yep, she's definitely gone." He looked up then and saw a picture of himself and his mother on the dresser. He ran and fetched it and said, "This is how I remember Mommy. The light is in her eyes, but now it's gone." Peter and I have had discussions since; he's asked simple questions like, "How did the light leave her eyes?" "How did she (her spirit) leave the house?" "Did she go through the doorways, out the window or could she go right through the wall?" His level of acceptance of the fact of his mother's death was absolute and his questions were those of the curious and the intelligent. It's good to have such questions. My answers were speculative. "I don't know how the light left her body. It's a mystery! I imagine that the light being so fine could go any- where it pleases. What do you think?" We talked about how, whenever he thinks of his mother, he can feel her soft warm presence and her smile within his heart.

Another little boy had a similar experience. I'd sat with him by his mother's body. We had "tuned-in" to our hearts and had invited the lovely presence of his mother into them. Afterward I told him that any time he sat down quietly and thought of her, he would feel her presence in his heart. A few days later, after the funeral, Damien was running by, playing with some other children. He came over to me and said, "You're wrong, you know. I don't have to sit still to feel her in my heart. I can feel her when I run too!"

In most households, the death of one parent makes major demands on the surviving parent's time, availability, finances, and physical and emotional energy. It isn't realistic to think you can accomplish everything the two of you did before. Try to list clearly your and your children's needs and endeavor to match that list with the offers of friends, family, and neighbors. You might need special help with cooking, housework, baby-sitting, after-school care, and so on. For your sanity and for the sake of your children, you must overcome any hesitation you have about asking for help.

If you feel your child is taking a longer time to grieve than seems healthy or is stuck in one particular behavior mode for too long, don't hesitate to reach out for professional assistance. The hospital with which your partner was associated, or your nearest children's hospital, will be able to put you in contact with someone who can help.

A woman brought her very shy twelve-year-old daughter to see me. Jenny was only just recovering from chronic fatigue syndrome which she developed after glandular fever when she was nine. She had had three years of fluctuating health and wasn't doing particularly well at school. She took prescribed medication every night to get to sleep and had become quite dependent on it. She'd lie awake for hours and be very restless if she didn't take her sedative. She was fairly picky about what she'd eat and her appetite was small. The story unfolded.

At the time of her glandular fever, Jenny's adored Grandma was receiving treatment for cancer. Because of the chemotherapy the grandmother was taking, her immune system was depressed and she was told not to go close to Jenny because she could pick up the child's infection. When Grandma visited, she always came to Jenny's door to talk and blow kisses. Finally, Grandma entered the hospital for the last time. When she had said goodbye to Jenny from the doorway, she'd told her she was getting better—and Jenny believed her. When the phone call came to say she'd died, Jenny only heard the news was "bad." She surmised that her grandmother had died, though no one told her directly.

The relationship Jenny and her Grandma shared was a powerful one and she was sad that she had never said good-bye and that in those last weeks she couldn't even hug or kiss her. She was bewildered by illness, death, loss, and unacknowledged grief.

With Jenny's hesitant and tearful cooperation we discussed how she felt about illness, cancer, not being told directly about her Grandma's death, and not having the opportunity to say good-bye. Then, with more enthusiasm and joy, she spoke of what she loved and missed about her grandmother.

Together we mapped out a plan. First, I reassured Jenny that lots of people felt the way she did, and that even adults have a really hard time talking about losses because they feel the hurt inside when they do.

I suggested she and her mother create a ritual out of going to bed, which would include a warm bath, being wrapped in a rainbow, and then sending another rainbow from her heart to wherever Grandma was. Because she had formed the habit of taking sleeping medication and was afraid to stop, I prescribed a herbal formula to be taken in *addition* to her usual medication. This formula is very good for calming down restlessness in the body and tends to soothe and relax. It's completely harmless and safe for children and adults alike (see Insomnia, page 216). Once Jenny was confident our plan was working, the idea was that she would take her sedative medication on alternate nights. Then, after a period of weeks, she could stop it when she felt ready. After that time, she could begin reducing the herbal formula in the same way. When she was ready to settle for sleep, she could play my guided imagery tape, *Dolphin Magic* (see page 379), a favorite of many children. I also suggested that Jenny might like to make a special "present" for her Grandma. I could tell this immediately captured her attention and curiosity. Her present could consist of a letter telling her Grandma how much she loved her and what she missed about her now; it could perhaps contain a story of a favorite time they'd spent together, or an occasion of love or laughter; she might like to include some drawings or a special photograph of her Grandma and herself or some trinket they had both enjoyed. All this could be placed inside a covered shoe box and tied with ribbons of her Grandma's favorite colors. By now Jenny looked quite animated at the prospect of her secret present to Grandma.

I then suggested she and her mother drive to a nursery and Jenny choose a tree to plant in the garden, perhaps outside her bedroom window. At the base of the tree she could bury her present for Grandma. Then Jenny could shovel in the earth (with or without assistance) and surround its base with cut flowers. This would then be Grandma's tree, and a place where Jenny could always come and have a chat to Grandma. She could watch it grow over the years, as her love continued to grow and deepen for her Grandma.

Jenny's mother telephoned me three weeks later. Jenny was off all medication, had become a much happier child and was sleeping soundly all night every night.

I've used this ritual of letter writing, drawing, tree planting, and so on with many, many children. It gives them several different ways of processing their thoughts and feelings. They have to use their memories of their loved ones and think about what they shared which was of value; in this process they acknowledge what it is they'll miss in this relative; they can create a gift of their very own which is private and therefore sacred; they use their bodies in planting the tree and in caring for it. It always gives me so much joy and encouragement to see the spirit of a child like Jenny beginning to heal. Children live in a world of symbols. Often they only need the appropriate tools or symbols, and it becomes easy for them to transform their grief into something which brings them comfort and resolution.

It's best to communicate with children of all ages with words which are simple and truthful. Avoid statements like God has taken the parent away to heaven, or the parent has gone on a "long trip," or is "lost." Children may worry that if they "get lost" themselves they too will die. And they may be downright angry with God for wanting the parent in heaven when they wanted mom or dad here on earth. Reassure the child that many people become sick but only those who are very, very ill die. It's best not to make *any* association between "sleep" and death. Don't shy away from reminiscing about the past. Children will gain greatly from going through photographs, telling stories, rereading, for example, letters or postcards, and retelling incidents from the past. Videos of family occasions where happy times were being shared are tremendously valuable also in helping children to be aware of and express their feelings. It's sad to recall the good times when they're gone, but it's far better to do that than to pretend you never had them. It won't be possible to hide from your children your grief, and to cry together is healthy. So are hugs and cuddles. You'll want to protect your children from the full force of your grief, and be mindful of what you express in their presence. To say, for instance, "I wish I was dead, too," or "I don't know how I'll ever cope," might be representative of how you're feeling, but will do nothing to help your child feel more secure. To say, "I feel so terribly sad without Daddy, and I miss him so much, but I know I'll feel better soon," might be more appropriate.

It's not uncommon for the child to have thoughts about, and even talk about, wanting to join the parent who has died. Many a partner has had the same thought. Talking to the child at his or her level, listening for the child's thoughts and the feelings behind them, and asking the right questions might be all that is required. And time. However, do not hesitate to reach out for help if you feel he or she is preoccupied with thoughts of death.

Teenagers might spend more time with their friends, listening to music, drawing, writing, or just "hanging out" in their rooms than in articulating to you their innermost thoughts. Encourage them in whatever their creative outlets might be. Make sure they know you're there at specific times to talk with them if they so choose. You might want to instigate some simple activities you both can share: perhaps doing the shopping together, washing the car, or getting involved in pleasurable activities which are new to both of you.

Some older children will want to take over the role of the parent who has died. This is understandable and can help the child to feel needed and valuable. Caution is necessary, nonetheless, as it's important the child is given permission to be a child and to grieve for the loss of the parent in his or her own way. If too many responsibilities are taken on at an early age, it will interfere with the child's natural development.

All these words represent guidelines only. They don't adequately address the pain present throughout the trauma of a life-threatening disease and, in some cases, the untimely death of a loved one. It takes time. It takes faith and, above all, for the surviving parent, it takes patience. We can either choose to grow or wither in our response to the loss of a person we love. We must assist our children in their search for meaning and understanding so that they, too, may grow and flourish.

Chapter Eleven

LIVING WELL WITH HIV

. . . .

David

I was diagnosed HIV positive late in November 1985 and I didn't have a clue what to do about it. The medical profession, then, was at a loss as to how to cope with the dying, let alone the living, and I wasn't ready to die. I was a man of thirty-seven who had a really warped outlook on society and my role in it. Like a lot of homosexual men at the time, I was caught in a patriarchal belief system which told me that not only was I wrong for being me, but to seek any alternative treatment for a physical ailment was akin to condoning witch-doctory or voodooism. I was fortunate in having a very kind doctor who told me that, for a long time, treatment for, or recovery from, life-threatening illnesses had been very much left by the patient in the hands of recognized medical practitioners; but since the onset of HIV/AIDS, treatment and recovery lay to an extent in the hands of the individual. It was then I decided to investigate alternatives. One of my saving graces was skepticism. Firstly, I attended an information night on meditation and dietary changes, then commenced relaxation and guided visualization classes. Although I found this form of meditation a bit weird and difficult to relax into, the other people kept me coming back. By my old standards they were a bit strange, yet they were really nice gentle souls just interested in gaining a bit more peace in their lives and were serious about positively stimulating their immune system. My next move was to take a weekend away with some of these people and, to my amazement, I was shown that there was a possibility one could keep this virus at bay by stimulating the immune system with a healthy diet, vitamins, and regular exercise. Exercise was all right as vanity got me to the gym, appetite had never been one of my problems and I ate reasonably well; what was lacking was balance and understanding of the toxicity of some of the treatments.

I came to Petrea's practice mid- to halfway through 1986 and experienced the dynamics of her therapy. My journey began in earnest. Vitamins, vegetable juice and a new diet were introduced into my daily routine. An addictive nature was helpful in adaptation to this new lifestyle, then after a while the boredom set in and the real work of consistency had to be learned. Junk food binges laced with mega-guilt trips were the go then for a while, and acquiring balance took quite a time. Yet in the end it came as a matter of preference rather than discipline. Meditation and physical maintenance were not the only things which changed.

It was evident that maybe a change of recreational lifestyle was necessary; late nights at smoky bars, dance halls, and sleaze joints started to change. This adjustment didn't come easily either, because I loved what I then considered to be a "free" lifestyle. What became evident was not only was I caught in my own stereotyped prison and that I was getting (to me) embarrassingly too old to play the games, but my health suffered every time I dabbled as I used to. Very slowly changes took place. My journey has sometimes been lonely. The hardest lesson has been to allow other people to follow their own paths; so many loved ones have died.

It's not my intention to dictate how anyone should live. It is a universal law that eventually we all leave the physical body. However, it's now nearly eight years down the line and there have been no major secondaries from my HIV infection. I've needed a few kick starts in the last few years.

For those who have embarked upon your quest for life, you're already on your path by picking up this book. Have a wonderful journey. Enjoy.

Although much of this book is directed to people who've developed AIDS, cancer, or some other life-threatening illness, it also contains much information which will assist those affected by the *potential* of a life-threatening illness. It's my belief, and my hope that, through the implementation of the techniques and philosophy contained here, people who are symptom free, but HIV+, will maintain and improve their health.

Being HIV+ is very different from having AIDS. Contrary to popular opinion, there's clear evidence that suggests that *not* all people who are HIV+ will go on to develop full AIDS. A follow-up of homosexual and bisexual men who were infected ten years previously showed that almost 20 percent had experienced *no* symptoms of their infection. A further 3 percent had asymptomatic generalized lymphadenopathy (enlargement of lymph glands), 19 percent had AIDS-related complex (ARC), and 59 percent had developed AIDS. Of the 59 percent who'd developed AIDS, 49 percent had died.*

In this chapter I haven't attempted to address all of the perplexing situations which people who live with HIV face. The people affected by the virus come from diverse backgrounds and to address the many issues in a single chapter would be quite impossible. I've worked with families where parents and children are infected, with prisoners inside our jails, with single women of differing lifestyles, intravenous drug users, and men, both straight and gay. For seven years I've facilitated a weekly support group for people with the virus at the Albion Street Center in Sydney, and I've counseled almost three thousand HIV+ people in my private practice. As with all the people with whom I'm privileged to work, many of them have become my friends and companions as well as my clients.

One of my clients who developed AIDS and whose T-cell count was very low was told by his doctors to prepare to die. He changed his attitude to life, sold his home, traveled around the world and his T-cells climbed back up to the normal healthy range. Five years later he came to see me to let me know of his progress. Peter had truly discovered the joy of living and, though he is now only 32, he's at peace with all aspects of his life. He spends his time educating nurses and other HIV+ people about

*Rutherford, GW et al. British Medical Journal 1990, Nov 24; 301:1183

life and living and radiates a special kind of joy and vibrancy.

No disease in the history of humankind has ever proved to be 100 percent fatal. Likewise, there are many people who are living well with HIV, even with full AIDS. There's strong and encouraging evidence to show that the *sooner* you begin to take care of yourself and the *better* you look after yourself, the longer you'll stay well. The guidelines set down here are intended to indicate the various areas which many people have found beneficial to address. The important thing is for *you* to find what works best for you. Areas in your life that you can choose to take responsibility for include:

- *Your mental attitude*
- *Stress management*
- *Exercise*
- *Diet*

You can make a difference.

Reaction to Diagnosis

People react differently to the diagnosis of being HIV+. Some people aren't surprised since they already suspected they were infected, while for others it comes as a complete shock. Occasionally people blame the particular person who infected them. There's often denial, anger (or rage), depression, and fear. To have some, many, or all of these feelings is entirely normal. However, to get stuck with them is detrimental to your peace of mind—and therefore your health. You cannot rush through these feelings and there's no set time for the feelings to be processed. You might well find that you go in and out of all these feelings for years. A calm and positive attitude will be your greatest ally in staying well.

The concept of "guilt" and "innocence" has no place in maintaining a positive attitude. Guilt is exhausting and full of negativity. Life's too short to waste on guilt about the past, or worry about the future. Is there any point in claiming responsibility for having been infected with HIV? We *can* take responsibility for our *response* to the situation we're in. This is a point of empowerment. *Then* we're able to move on to take full responsibility for our health and our view of life.

It's important to be as informed as possible about the illnesses to which you may be prone and the treatment options for them. You must become your body's own best guardian. If possible, always get a second opinion about your treatment options. In this way you can make an informed choice as to the appropriate therapies for you.

The first line of defense against AIDS is self-education. Sometimes we can feel overwhelmed by our options and yet it is only we who can make the decisions for a particular therapy. We need to learn to trust in our own ability to discern what is appropriate for us, to listen to our inner voice or intuition.

The relationship you have with your doctor is of great importance. Find a doctor who'll listen to you, explore options, and offer choices. If at *all* possible, find a doctor who'll actively support *your* efforts to stay well. Many doctors are now encouraging their patients to improve their nutritional intake and other lifestyle factors and to deal with the stress they have in their lives. Many people with the virus are better educated about their disease and its treatments than their doctors. Talk to other people to find out as much information as possible so you remain educated about *yourself*.

Each person must find their own path to healing and wholeness. Health is peace of mind. With peace of mind as our main goal, we also create the perfect environment in which our physical body can achieve and maintain health.

How Can I Improve My Mental Attitude?

Your positive mental attitude will be your greatest asset in living with HIV. Much of what has been written in the first few chapters of this book will help you to achieve this. By taking responsibility for your health and, indeed, for your life, you'll be taking

back a sense of control. Everyone feels better when he or she is
in control of his or her life's choices.

You're bound to have questions almost as soon as you're diagnosed as HIV+. The following ones might be among them:

- *Who should I tell?*
- *What should I say?*
- *How long have I got to live?*
- *When am I going to get sick?*
- *What can I do to help myself?*
- *How can I avoid infecting others?*
- *Should I give up work?*
- *Does being HIV+ mean I have AIDS?*
- *How can I tell my family/partner/friends?*
- *Will the people I tell still love me?*
- *Is that the end of my sex life?*

Finding someone with whom to talk through all these questions
will be invaluable in helping to sort yourself out. Most city clin-
ics/hospitals have set up pre- and post-test counseling for this
very purpose. Even if you don't feel you need this kind of support, it's worth your while to talk through your thoughts and
feelings with someone who's experienced in such counseling. If
you live in an isolated area it can certainly be more difficult to
find people you feel you can trust. I would strongly encourage
you to find a nurse, doctor, counselor, or friend with whom you
can discuss your thoughts, feelings, and options.

Talking with others who are in similar situations can also be
invaluable. You'll then realize that others are experiencing the
same thoughts and feelings as yourself and you won't feel so isolated or alone. There are various groups in which you can meet
with others, and most are open to anyone affected by the virus.
The groups are made up of men and women who are newly diagnosed as HIV+ through to people who are quite sick with AIDS.

It can be very encouraging to meet with people who've been living with the virus for years and who haven't experienced any
symptoms. You'll also meet with others who've experienced various illnesses and who've overcome them.

Most cities have groups for people who are *newly* diagnosed
as HIV+. As the epidemic has grown, so has the variety and
"speciality" of support groups. In most Western countries, for
instance, there are groups for newly diagnosed gay men under
twenty-four years of age; other groups cater to positive women,
blood-transfusion affected men and women, sex workers, gay
men, intravenous drug users, narcotics/alcoholics anonymous
HIV+ people, and so on. You might need to shop around for a
group in which you feel comfortable. To find out what groups
are available ask friends, counselors, AIDS councils, and check
notice boards at clinics, drop-in centers, or doctors' offices.

There are also weekly support groups for people who have
life-threatening illnesses. In these groups are people who have
cancer, HIV, AIDS, multiple sclerosis, lupus, and other diseases.
Often people who have HIV feel more comfortable in a general
support group rather than in one which is specifically for people
with HIV. It can be very encouraging and helpful to hear a
woman with breast cancer, or a man the same age as yourself
with bowel cancer, articulating exactly *your* thoughts and feelings. Many unlikely friendships have sprung up in this way.

On one occasion, a young man, Simon, who'd been a prosti-
tute for several years, was talking to the group about his loneliness and sense of abandonment. He was receiving treatment for
an illness associated with his HIV infection and now had to
spend a lot of time at home resting. His doorbell kept ringing
but the only people who came were men wanting sex. No one
came to see how *he* was. As he related his story, Simon began to
cry. Jackie, the woman sitting next to him, reached for his hand
as she too began to weep. Jackie lived with her loving family in
one of Sydney's "better" suburbs, but she also felt very alone
because her family wouldn't allow her to talk about her fears.
Each time she tried to express her fear, her family would tell her
to be "positive," that she was looking well, that she had put on

weight, and make any inane comment to stop her from talking about her anxiety. Jackie and Simon had a good weep together. Over time the bond between them grew; Simon would visit Jackie when she was in the hospital to have chemotherapy for her cancer and she'd deliver chicken soup to him when he was unwell. Their friendship was very deep and was based on honesty and unconditional loving support.

With emotional support we can get through just about any situation. Often the emotional support we experience in a group is more meaningful and helpful than any other.

Many people find it helpful to become involved in some form of voluntary work which helps other people who have the virus. This help can range from being a "buddy" to someone with AIDS to practical activities like transportation, cooking, shopping, and so on. Most AIDS councils will be able to tell you what kinds of services you could become involved in. Helping someone else is one of the best antidotes to feelings of helplessness.

Many of the activities listed in chapter 2, Techniques for Living, will be of great benefit in attaining and maintaining a positive attitude and you're encouraged to read the chapter carefully and adopt those things which appeal to you.

What Techniques Will Help to Deal with Stress?

Stress, of itself, is not the problem. We need stress in our lives in order to give us a sense of challenge. By overcoming these stresses we experience satisfaction and fulfillment. The problem arises when we feel overwhelmed by stress, or we feel we lack the resources to cope with it. Then our peace of mind disappears and our immune system suffers the consequences. All the suggestions of the early chapters, especially in chapter 1, Creating the Environment for Healing, chapter 2, Techniques for Living, chapter 5, Meditation: A Key to Life and chapter 6, In My Mind's Eye, are relevant for *any* person wanting to improve their way of dealing with stress. Read the chapters carefully and select and implement those suggestions which appeal to you.

Tai Chi, Qi Gong, and yoga are three forms of meditative exercise programs which will assist people to deal with stress in an "active" way. And, of course, as already mentioned, a counseling or group support will help enormously in reducing your stress levels.

Many people find that a regular massage provides them with relaxation and nurturing they don't receive anywhere else. Inquire at your local clinic, doctor's rooms, AIDS council, or ask among your friends for someone who can be recommended. Massage can be particularly helpful for those who experience peripheral neuropathy (see chapter 8, Burps, Burning, and the Dreaded Bloats, for more information about peripheral neuropathy).

Reiki is an ancient form of hands-on healing which many find helpful in dealing with stress. Ask at the places mentioned in the preceding paragraph for a reputable practitioner of Reiki.

What Exercise Is Best?

Exercise is an important component of any health program. It's important that you find exercise which you *enjoy* and which is regular. If you *don't* enjoy the form of exercise you've chosen, it's unlikely you'll incorporate it into your lifestyle in any long-term or committed way. If you're looking at a form of regular exercise, you might like to try something which is new to you; perhaps some sport which involves other people who are also endeavoring to maximize their health. Clients have benefited from playing volleyball, tennis, squash, or joining a swimming team. In this way, you can meet other people who are implementing a positive approach to increasing their health and well-being. Many people find that an aerobics class, gym work, or working out with weights suits them best.

The important thing with exercise is that it be moderate. If you're just starting to take up a regular form of exercise, gradually increase its length and intensity. Don't throw yourself into daily aerobic classes!

If you're having any difficulty with weight loss, exercise must

be very gentle and preferably under supervision. You can run the
risk of burning off all the calories that you need in order to *increase* your weight.

For people who are well and who've no problem with their
weight, exercise which increases your pulse rate to over one-
hundred beats per minute and sustains it at that level for at least
twenty minutes, three times a week, is considered ample for the
average person. This level of exercise will increase your breathing rate and depth.

For further references to exercise, please see the index.

What Should I Eat?

Poor dietary habits contribute to more than half the deaths in
the United States. The average diet in the United States is too
high in fat, sugar, "refined" and overcooked food and, increasingly, foods containing additives and preservatives. Although a
healthy diet will not affect HIV itself, it will certainly give your
immune system the kind of nourishment necessary to combat illness. Many people with the virus have experienced some AIDS-
related damage to their digestive system and are therefore
unable to absorb all the nutrients from their food. Others
haven't ever had a healthy diet. People with the virus have a
special need for improved nutrition because of these two factors.
Taking added vitamins is highly recommended also for these
same reasons. It's important to have a vitamin program tailored
to your individual situation, so consult a naturopath or doctor
who's trained in nutritional medicine.

The sooner you improve your nutrition, the sooner your immune system will feel the benefits. However, that *doesn't* mean
you have to go on to a first-class nourishing diet overnight! It
does mean gently moving in the direction of improved nutrition.
There's much information and guidance given in chapter 7,
Recipe for Life (see pages 152-180), and you're encouraged to
read and implement its suggestions.

It will take time and effort to change your eating patterns, so
don't be hard on yourself when you "slip up" or choose to have

the odd treat. Don't eat an ice cream while chastising yourself over the weakness of your will power! Enjoy the ice cream, and *then* reaffirm your desire and intention to improve your nutrition. If you're already under a lot of stress, be particularly gentle to yourself. Don't set unrealistic standards. Deal with the stresses in your life one at a time. Don't decide to give up meat, alcohol, cigarettes, recreational drugs, and sugar all in one day! Gently, gently, move in your desired direction of improved eating and lifestyle habits.

Friends and family can help keep you motivated if you tell them about the changes you wish to make, and why. Mixing with people who are likewise improving their nutrition can help overcome the old eating habits. Some people find that healthy-eating recipe books make for good bedside reading, or that swapping favorite recipes with friends can keep up the inspiration needed to continue with an improved eating program. Avoid friends who are fast-food or sugar junkies. Sugar has no food value at all and, in large amounts, is positively detrimental to your immune system. To increase your energy supply you're far better off eating a piece of fruit, a sandwich, or a plate of pasta.

For most people, cutting out, or certainly reducing, salt intake is recommended. Use herbs, fresh or dried, and a little sea salt (if desired). However, if you experience night sweats or diarrhea you should get expert advice about salt intake as you'll be losing body salts. See also chapter 8, Burps, Burning, and the Dreaded Bloats, for further information about dealing with night sweats and diarrhea.

It's quite likely you'll have heard (or will hear) about the Candida Diet, which is often recommended for people who are HIV+. This diet is quite involved in its application and *should only be used under the supervision of someone who's an expert in nutritional approaches to disease.*

For the rest, be guided by the information in chapter 7, Recipe for Life. Before long you'll begin to feel the benefits of your improved nutrition and, as you experience more energy, you'll feel encouraged to continue further. You'll also find a lot of information about various dietary complications in chapter 8.

If you have any "weak" areas in your health, do something about it *now!* For instance, if you have recurrent respiratory problems, sinusitis, diarrhea, skin problems, indigestion, and so on, attend to them *before* they become cause for serious future problems.

Living with HIV can become an opportunity for personal growth and an improved quality of life. Sadly, there's still a stigma attached to being infected with the virus. Many people find the stress of keeping their status private is very onerous. For some, to go public is unthinkable. As one well-known man said matter-of-factly on his first visit to me, "I've arranged my public schedule so that I can end my life in November." He continued with deep passion, "But be damned if I'll die before I've learned how to love!" Not surprisingly, when he fully discovered love, suicide was no longer felt to be necessary. Peace, love, and serenity filled the room of this man in his final weeks. He had healed and renewed his relationship with all those whom he loved and the world in which he lived and worked. He had learned to trust life and to trust himself.

When we love ourselves, others opinions of us become inconsequential. With this inner freedom we can look the world in the eye and feel whole, complete and loved.

Chapter Twelve

AT WHAT POINT DO WE STOP LIVING AND START DYING?

. . . .

Lois

It seemed nothing serious to me at the time. However, today I bear the scars of two major operations and continuous treatment—often experimental—in my battle with malignant melanoma.

Five years earlier, when I was eighteen, my sister noticed a curious looking mole on my left shin. Being a nurse, she stubbornly insisted the mole be removed. I didn't understand the fuss, but had it excised anyway. The results of this were never learned and I went on without a care.

In late 1989, several lumps appeared in my groin. My local doctor prescribed a course of antibiotics which proved ineffective. A referral to a surgeon meant a biopsy. The biopsy revealed secondary malignant melanoma. A mole had done this? I had trouble believing this.

I was quickly referred to a specialist surgeon who decided on a radical groin dissection—the removal of all the lymph nodes in the left groin. A big operation leaving a large scar from my tummy to half way down my thigh. Fourteen out of twenty-six nodes were cancerous. The chances of survival beyond two to five years were quite slim, ignoring percentages.

It was quite scary being in the hospital in very real pain. One never thinks of oneself being sick and with something such as cancer, that only happens to somebody else. I wasn't the only one who didn't realize the serious nature of this disease: my family had no idea of what was really happening, with the exception of my father, who'd suffered the loss of his parents through cancer. Our relationship is now strengthened.

After the first surgery I was really determined to do my best to prevent the "non-mes" spreading any more. I had lots of support. I began to make meditation part of my daily routine. Listening to tapes is my choice. I considered my diet as well, since cancer is a multi-factorial disease. I listened and read a lot about formulating my diet, which basically eliminates red meat and dairy food. Fruit, vegetables, and grains—I try to stick to it.

My husband, Mark, has taken a personal toll. We'd only recently been married and we were both so much looking forward to starting a family and settling to a wonderful normal life together. But he has chosen to leave his career and look after me full-time. Before this our relationship was strained. I needed more support from him and now I have my wish. Mark would dearly love to have the magic answer like any doting spouse. He's learned to accept it the hard way.

It took a while for me to become mobile again after the groin operation. The peculiar thing is once you feel better, one starts to become laid back: we started to forget about the situation. If anyone asked, we would say, "That's all over and done with." At that time I was having immunotherapy and three monthly scans after eight weeks of radiotherapy on my groin.

So things seemed to be going well for us: I started back at work part-time, but standing on my feet ended in my left leg swelling and I became very tired. Eight months after the operation I found a lump on my shoulder and, after another biopsy, it proved to be metastic melanoma—the cancer had spread!

I'd been having severe back pains and I was seeing a physiotherapist (I put it down to lifting at work); unfortunately yet another scan revealed a tumor in my spine (second and third lumbar vertebrae), lungs, kidneys and numerous subcutaneous deposits. The tumor in my vertebrae was pressing against my spinal cord. If they didn't do something immediately I'd be a paraplegic.

A number of specialists came together to decide how to treat it:

chemo or ray? Thank the Lord they decided to operate. Except for permanent swelling in my left leg, it was a success.

My family had now realized what was happening. Three of my sisters came down to Sydney from as far as the north coast where I grew up, and took turns to look after me in my convalescences. Not being able to look after yourself is perhaps the worst thing anyone has to bear. This time, I was much more prepared for what was to happen. My attitude was very positive. I've always been so capable and even now I find it frustrating not having the energy to do things that before posed no problem. I've learned to let go of pride and not feel guilty over accepting help, especially love, from others. Just because I'm incapacitated doesn't mean I cannot give. I found I can be a mighty prayer warrior. I really believe in the power of prayer and I know it has carried us through this. I have seen it working in people around me. I've learned a lot from Jesus—he gained his courage through prayer and he knew he had to die as this was God's will. Through prayer, God gave him strength to die for us. It's comforting to know that I'm in God's hands receiving the strength that I need.

Have faith all is well and truly believe. Nothing is too good to happen. Don't be frightened to expect great things—be bold when you pray and ask for them. We are God's children: he wants to look after us, he loves us. Never take for granted his "awesomeness."

Life is to be enjoyed and who are we to say if we're going to be here or there tomorrow? I feel the most important thing for anyone to do is live each day as if it were your last.

Help people find peace, love, and joy through the Lord as there are a lot of lost souls out there whom we can find so much happiness in helping. Tell people how you really feel. Knock down those facades people feel they need to hide behind. Truly love people from the heart and accept love from others—you're worth it, enjoy it.

Love is the answer. If we possess this everything else falls into place. Love really is what life's all about. There's no limit, it's endless. Power we cannot fathom. God is love and nothing is impossible for him. I do believe in miracles. After all, God wants us to, that's why he does them.

Editor's Note: Lois wrote these words just days before she died. Lois passed away on March 11, 1991—peacefully in the hospital where she was born twenty-three years before. She was home. It was genuinely sad for family and friends to lose such a bright, giving person.

My grandmother was loved by everyone who knew her. She was one of those generous spirits who made everyone feel welcome, loved, and valuable as a human being. I have childhood memories of her which are as fresh in my mind as yesterday. I remember her cool and pleasant home with its distinctive "Granny" smell, shady verandahs, her jungly garden full of hidden treasures which she'd pilfered from gardens too numerous to mention.

In the quiet and comfortable rooms of her home her treasures presided. Under each and every item she loved was a label with someone's name on it. China, chairs, tables, ornaments, piano, trinkets, and paintings—all had someone's name neatly written underneath. The name represented the person to whom she wished to pass on each particular treasure.

In this way, I grew up with an understanding that possessions were something to be used, enjoyed, and then passed on to others who you thought might also find pleasure in them. There was no sense of the morbid about her. She was the liveliest, most enthusiastic human being I've ever had the joy to know. Unlike many who are diagnosed with cancer, Granny had never experienced a sick day in her life. She was diagnosed at seventy-six years of age with advanced breast cancer which ended her life within six weeks. Her only acknowledgment of her impending death was to say to my mother, "Isn't it a bugger?" When asked if there was anything she'd like, Granny replied she'd like a party with all her favorite people attending.

One week before she died, a wonderful party was held in my parents' home with all the people she loved. There were mutual farewells, exchanged between her and all those who'd enriched her life.

I consider myself most fortunate in having known someone I

loved deeply who demonstrated so powerfully her peace with both life and death. She had no philosophical belief which promised a rosier future after death. She was *never* interested in things philosophical, much to *my* anguish (as I mentioned in chapter 10). Granny simply lived with her whole being right now, with the belief that the future would take care of itself if she took care of the present moment. It makes me smile when I think of all the torment, frustration, questioning, delving, and seeking *I* have done in coming to the same conclusion as my beloved grandmother!

It might appear that to live for seventy-six years is a happy sufficiency. Yet I've worked with many people who are determined to continue into their nineties and beyond, and who would think of seventy-six as far too young an age to leave. Likewise, I've known ten-year-olds who've accomplished all that the human spirit may, and who are ready to depart. The *number* of years seems almost irrelevant. It's the state of the heart which will determine our readiness and peace in leaving all that is familiar and letting go into the unknown.

As human beings we have a tendency to hold fast to the familiar and are fearful of the unknown. This certainly is so when we are speaking of our deaths. That is why I always encourage people to go all out for peace rather than for a cure. Peace is definitely attainable; peace creates the perfect environment for physical healing. If physical healing doesn't occur then we still have peace. We experience peace when we're affirming life in its fullness. We affirm life through our diet, exercise, treatment, positive and uplifting thoughts and attitudes, meditation and relaxation techniques, forgiveness of past actions, visualization techniques, and relinquishing of anger, guilt, blame, fear, and so on. This is not a laid-back, don't-care attitude. That is not peace.

Peace is a dynamic state achieved through conscious choice.

It is not resignation in the face of defeat, it is not a passive acceptance, but rather an attitude of maximizing the possibilities

of life in any given situation in a harmonious way. When we aim
for this dynamic state of peace, we create the perfect environment for healing to take place. When we go all out for a cure,
what we're really saying is that our healing has to be on our
terms. Yet if we don't succeed in curing our disease, we certainly
won't experience peace either. There's a certain frenetic quality
about people who are determined to cure their illness at all
costs. The cost, inevitably, is peace of mind. This attitude rather
misses the point of healing. Health is inner peace. Certainly,
most of us would rather remain in our bodies, with our loved
ones, doing the things which are familiar and which we've always enjoyed. And yet, so many of us resist life—wanting it to
be on our terms. To lose our "clinging" to life *isn't* giving up. It's
more a *giving over* to life. It embodies a trust in the perfect unfolding of each moment—each moment full of potential, full of
healing, full of peace.

Frequently in the business of diagnosis, treatment, and never-
ending tests, the patient as a person can feel totally lost. One of
the most dearly cherished qualities for any individual is that of
dignity. This quality, more than any other, represents the indi-
viduality of the person. Patients' reactions to all that is said or
done to them will be filtered through their consciousness of
their dignity.

As I've mentioned, I spent many months as a teenager, confined to bed in a hospital while undergoing reconstructive surgery to my legs. The agonies I experienced with bedpans are too
awful to describe! For the first time in my life I became severely
constipated, simply because I couldn't bear the lack of privacy
my situation incurred. To the nurses, the fact there was a twenty
centimeter gap where the curtains didn't meet was unnoticed.
But I felt the entire gaze of the world beaming in, not to mention the ears. So insurmountable a problem did it seem to me
that I even took to throwing my food out of the window in the
hope that if nothing went in, then it would be unnecessary for
anything to come out. The agonies of personal vulnerability!
This is not false modesty: it is a deeply felt vulnerability about
our dignity. The importance of respect for the dignity of the

individual must remain of paramount importance. As a nurse, I well remember the frail hands of an elderly woman reaching down to retrieve the sheet which had left her nakedness exposed after she'd been sponged.

Ultimately it's the patients who must choose their doctors, their treatments, and the way in which they'll conduct their lives, and we must accord complete respect to the individual and his or her choices.

Lisa was an artist of considerable renown when she developed emphysema. She lived for several months connected to a long tube which continuously fed her pure oxygen. With this machine and tubing she was able to walk from room to room, paint, draw, and continue a life which had quality and value. I saw her weekly for a massage and counseling in the weeks leading up to her final hospitalization. When she lay in the hospital, I visited and remained by her side till her death.

Lisa had a most distinctive laugh which could be heard at a hundred meters distance and in the hours leading to her death we found much to giggle about. She had a wild and wonderful sense of humor and on this night, her last, it was in fine form. The nursing staff came in from time to time to inquire if everything was all right as her gales of giggles resounded through their corridors. We assured them all was well and continued with our conversations. From time to time Lisa would say things like, "This can't be dying. I feel so wonderful." Having fully lived, she died peacefully with a look of serenity I envied.

Many people die without ever having discussed their impending death. This *doesn't* mean they're necessarily in "denial." Some people never discuss their inmost feelings with anyone, including close family members. Do not judge whether someone has accepted his or her impending death. My grandmother said much about acceptance, and perhaps anger, when she said, "Isn't it bugger?" No long discussions, no tears, no denial, just a simple statement which was typical of her. To have insisted that she fight to stay alive, drink carrot juice, or meditate would have caused nothing but misery and tension for all concerned. Many a person's desire to keep someone they love alive completely overlooks the feelings of the one affected by the illness.

If you desire it, it's possible to write a living will. This will legally binds those in charge of your medical management *not* to do anything which will prolong your life. This means all medical care is given to ensure comfort without any medical intervention which would prolong your life. Many people reach a point where they wish to concentrate all their energies on quality of life.

Sometimes this point isn't reached by all members of the family at the same time. It might be that you feel you've had enough of treatments, doctors, and hospitals and that you'd prefer to be in your own home surrounded by the people and things you love. Your family might wish for you to continue treatment. This situation needs to be talked out thoroughly so that the feelings *behind* the preferred options can be explored. It's likely that there'll be feelings which include fear of impending loss, anger, frustration, powerlessness, resentment, isolation, guilt, relief, and perhaps a sense of being out of control. *These* are the issues which *need* to be addressed. *These* are the issues which are at the heart of relationships.

Practical Aspects

There are many aspects of dying which you might wish to discuss at some time with your family or loved ones. Some people prefer to do this right near the time of diagnosis. It isn't morbid to talk about your wishes and desires for the future. You'll want to "tidy things up" so that there's little unfinished business for your family to manage.

Part of this procedure would be the formalizing of your will, if you haven't already done so. This isn't a negative action, nor does it mean you are affirming death. Any lawyer will suggest this be done at a young age. You might also wish to state certain preferences for the education of your children or even make tapes for them to play when they reach certain stages in their lives, or leave them something in writing.

When talking with your family, you might wish to give expression to any strongly held ideas you might have on how long life-support systems should be continued; how sedated you'd like to be; whether you'd prefer to be at home or in the hospital, and who you'd like to have with you. These conversations can be difficult to get started and yet, once underway, they can be tremendously rewarding. Obviously there will be many practical considerations which need to be addressed. These can be assessed and discussed with your family, doctor, or visiting nurse.

The majority of people prefer to remain at home to die. This used to be the accepted practice. To die comfortably at home requires good support from your loved ones. They also need to feel supported. One aspect of my work now is training what I call "midwives for the dying." It's my belief that we need just as much assistance to leave this world as to enter it. These "midwives" go beyond just the physical care of the patient. They work with massage, techniques of relaxation and visualization, and counseling children and family members, and generally facilitate in the situation so that everyone comes through the experience in as healthy a way as possible. It's no longer surprising to me to hear the family left behind say they felt a kind of "rightness" and joy, as well as sadness, at the passing of their loved one. The chief role of the midwife is to remain calm and at peace while being really open to the situation. When there's a feeling of calmness and competence, the rest of the family, and indeed the patient, relax more easily into each moment.

Be brave enough to face these practical questions so you know these details have been taken care of. In this way you'll be free to enjoy your family, enjoy your relaxation, and flow into the peace of mind which your meditation brings; allow it to play its full part.

I know many people who've orchestrated their funeral well before the event. They've chosen the music, and in some cases have prepared the readings or other content they wish to be included in the services.

Know that as you prepare for the physical fact of death that you'll also experience yet another wonderful and positive aspect of life. We go through many emotions when we contemplate our own death. Elisabeth Kübler-Ross, author of *On Death and Dying* among other books, has done much to enlighten the community about this process. She classifies five distinct stages through which all people who are dying pass. These stages don't come in any particular order. Often we hop from one stage to another within moments. It can be helpful to be aware of these stages so that when we experience them, we know we're not alone in our experience. Many others have passed this way before. At the time when I was sick, I was unaware of this research and yet, looking back at my experience, I certainly passed through each of those stages. When I was actually in some of them, it was very hard to maintain any objectivity. I sometimes seemed to be completely engulfed by the emotions.

The stages that have been clearly identified are:

Denial

This stage may be quite prolonged or very short. The mind may simply scream an inward *NO!* I denied the diagnosis until real weakness set in. Some people who fall into the high-risk groups for infection with HIV may well go through denial before they ever have a confirming blood test. Many people suspect that something is seriously wrong in their body and yet refuse to see a doctor. They play a wait-and-see game even though they *know* they're in need of medical care.

It's quite common for people who are fairly close to death to move between thoughts which seem at variance with each other, for instance, planning an overseas trip to London one day and reminding the family that the fern on the verandah likes tea leaves occasionally and to be watered twice a week.

Anger

This is the classic, "Why didn't it happen to someone else? Why me?" My uncle's reaction to his diagnosis was, "Well, you don't say 'why me?' when you win the lottery, do you?" As in denial, this stage might be very brief or prolonged, depending on the individual. I didn't go through the "Why me?" so much as the frustration of feeling helpless against an unseen monster. I was angry because I felt out of control, unable to exert any influence over my bloodstream.

Often we experience frustration; frustration about our lack of energy, our weight loss, our inability to get motivated about anything.

Bargaining

This one can be very complex. It can become the driving force behind our actions. "If I drink carrot juice three times a day, eat all the healthy food, take my vitamins, exercise, meditate, and relax then, my reward *should* be that I get well." The people who embrace this philosophy are usually unsuccessful in achieving peace of mind. Many of us slide into this thinking periodically, especially when we have found a new lump, or our test results aren't too good. Our reaction can very easily be: "But I've been doing everything right." There's nothing wrong with doing all the above things in order to increase our level of health and well-being. It's the motivation and attitude behind those actions which becomes so important. The above thinking stems from the attitude, "If I'm good enough, maybe I'll make the grade." Remember, many of us have had a life of "If I'm good enough...," so be wary of allowing it to color your motivation.

This can also extend to a renewed vigor in our church attendance: "If I confess all my sins, if I pray regularly, if I attend church weekly, then maybe the Lord, in His infinite wisdom and mercy, will let me get well." It might well be that attendance at your church or regular meditation will bring you great peace of mind and that healing may take place. That's great! Your motivation was probably to reestablish your connection with God and your own inner peace and to cultivate the trust that all was unfolding just as it should. There's no reason why we can't have the preference of wanting to be healed! It's when we've an "addiction" to being healed that the problems arise: "I can't have peace of mind *unless* I'm healed."

I found I slipped in and out of this kind of bargaining. For me, it was the great issue of trust, of letting go of control. I found it difficult at times to do all I could to affirm life and then sit back and trust all was unfolding appropriately. Our motivation is often very subtle in its influence.

Depression

Depression is perhaps one of the most difficult feelings to live with. This is so for both the patient and the family. The family or loved ones can feel quite excluded from the emotional presence of the patient. They might feel very helpless. We tend to be more prone to depression when everything *isn't* going right. It might well result from some subtle influence of the bargaining attitude. "I've been doing it all right—why aren't I getting better?" Often our feelings seem attached to our test results. If we receive a "bad" report, we plummet again to the depths of despair. By resolving the issues which surface through our depression, we can make great gains in knowing ourselves. In fact, I believe more healing can sometimes take place by working through the issues involved in depression than when we're flying high and feeling fantastic. The depressions I experienced were abysmal, and yet I learned greatly from them. It often only takes one day of feeling an improved level in our energy for our spirits to be lifted.

Acceptance

Acceptance is the trust that all is well. Even dying is all right. One mother, Vivien, had been working with her cancer for two years. She had two small boys and a devoted husband. Over those years, she frequently voiced her sadness and depression about the possibility of leaving her little children. We talked of her spiritual beliefs often and these deepened and expanded during that time. The week before she died, I visited her and we spoke again of her leaving the children. She said she felt completely assured that they'd be all right without her and that her husband would also. She said she felt completely healed and well. Vivien spoke of great inner peace, saying she felt part of her had "gone" already. In her last days she took on a beautiful and translucent look. Her acceptance permeated the household. Her parents, husband, and children were fully involved in her passing, and were open and in touch with their own emotions.

In addressing the fears and uncertainties about our own dying, we also expose the fears and uncertainties present in our living. We don't need a life-threatening disease in order to look at the issues around our own death. When we embrace life fully, we're more ably equipped to relinquish our hold on a body which has served its purpose well. One of the greatest keys to living and to dying is the practice of meditation. Through this practice we begin to understand and experience our real and unlimited nature. With this experience comes a deep, unshakable peace and the certain knowledge that we're indeed far more than just our bodies. When we are firmly rooted in this knowledge, derived from experience, our reality becomes one of complete safety and trust, and we experience our true, indestructible nature.

Several years ago I started a voluntary massage program at a major hospital in Sydney for patients with AIDS, with the intention of offering some comfort and support. This was at a time when people were still wary of touching those with the virus, and they were considered "lepers" by many. The first boy with AIDS that I massaged was only seventeen years old. Throughout this gentle massage, James wept quietly into his pillow. I was beginning to wonder whether massage was such a brilliant idea and, when I finished, I asked him if he wanted to talk about his tears. His reply stunned and saddened me. He said, "Nobody has ever touched me like that before. I've only ever been touched when someone wanted something from me." He continued with his story. He'd been told to leave home at fifteen because he was gay. He harbored enormous resentment and anger toward his family and had absolutely no intention of ever telling them where he was or that he was sick.

Over the next four years, James attended our weekly support

group and within its safe confines explored the many issues which caused him pain. These included his guilt around his homosexuality, his anger toward his family, and his grief and sadness about his deteriorating health. James had incorporated meditation techniques into his daily program and had done much to improve his health, with truly remarkable results. However, his immune system was severely impaired and he was constantly fighting off serious infections. Through the groups James accomplished a miracle, in fact, several. He resolved, and let go of, all his guilt about his homosexuality. He learned to forgive himself and his family and came to accept his life *and* his death with peace and dignity.

James called me as he lay in the hospital, close to death. When I entered he room I felt overwhelmed by emotion. James' mother was gently massaging his feet, his father sat by his side holding his hand and his sister was nearby. The love and peace in the room was palpable. James took my hand and beckoned me to bend close so he could talk to me. He said, "Thank you for teaching me about love. These have been the best four years of my life!"

It's sad that James died aged a mere twenty-one years. Yet perhaps he accomplished more in his twenty-one years than some who reach ninety and who've never healed the bitterness of past painful relationships. Perhaps James' life *was* complete in that he'd let go all that stood in the way of his experiencing peace and wholeness. Perhaps *that* is what life is for?

No matter what attempts we might make to improve our health or reverse the process of our illness, for some death will be the final outcome. However, to look upon death as a failure would be to miss the point in living. It's the *spirit* with which we live which is of importance rather than the length of life.

In my experience most people aren't so afraid of dying as they are of the *process* of dying. People express concerns about whether they'll be in pain, alone, or unable to breathe adequately. All these fears are natural and all of them can be allayed. Many people are afraid that if they begin with analgesics (pain killers) early in their illness, there won't be drugs strong enough to deal with pain later on. This is totally inaccurate. There are stronger drugs or dosages which can be used for more severe pain. Often, it is simply a combination of drugs which will alleviate severe pain. Your doctor or palliative or community nurse will be able to assist you in managing your pain (see chapter 9, Beyond Pain).

Some people are afraid they won't be able to breathe properly. This can be helped enormously by the use of oxygen, either in the home or the hospital (see Oxygen at Home, page 244). If you've been practicing techniques of relaxation or meditation, you'll be familiar with "light" breathing and will find that these techniques can be of tremendous assistance. As the breathing becomes lighter, the brain receives less oxygen and the person might become more sleepy, perhaps drifting into unconsciousness. Many people I've sat with in their last hours drift off very peacefully.

Peter was a member of one of our support groups for several years. He was a very private person and wouldn't readily allow people to befriend him. Over time, we became quite close and, when he became sicker, he asked me to be with him at the time of his death.

Though Peter was beyond words in his last hours, he was intensely conscious and his eyes were very focused and "present." I talked to him quietly about life, trust, and letting go. His eyes twinkled back at me and occasionally he squeezed my hand to register his understanding of my comments. I felt a tremendous sense of peace and unity with Peter and this continued for several hours. As the day wore on (I'd been with him since 4:00 A.M.), I was also aware that I was due to give a lecture (on Healthy Lifestyles!) at 4:30 P.M. at a conference about half an hour's drive from the hospital where Peter lay. An hour before the lecture, I leant forward, took his hand and said to him that I would *have* to leave in half an hour in order to make it to the conference on time. Peter's breathing immediately changed. He began to breathe more and more lightly. His eyes sparkled and seemed full of humor and peace. I continued talking to him as he "practiced" not breathing several times, telling him that it was

O.K. to let go and trust. It was such a privilege to accompany Peter on his journey into death. It was such a "life-filled" experience. At 4:00 P.M. on the dot, the sparkle left his eyes as the only sign of his departure. His presence remains in my heart and I think of him with warmth and joy, certainly not sadness or despair. To join so deeply in the heart of another's life is a privilege beyond words.

In the year before his death, Peter had frequently spoken of suicide as one of his options. He suffered greatly as a result of his illness and often spoke of the difficulty in finding meaning in his life. He wasn't alone with his thoughts about suicide. It's a fairly common topic of discussion, especially among people with AIDS. Many people like to know they *have* the option to end their lives if things become too difficult. Knowing they *have* the option is often as close as they actually come to exercising it. It's commonly believed in the general community that if people talk about suicide they've no intention of committing it. *This is not so.* My brother talked about it and tried on several occasions before he finally succeeded. People need a *safe* and *nonjudgmental* environment in which they can talk through their feelings and thoughts. This safe environment often provides sufficient solace for life to be worth continuing.

It can be an overwhelming challenge to find meaning in each day when there's little to bring joy. Many *have* met the challenge with courage and commitment. Some, having completed their relationships in life, having tidied up their affairs, having fully lived, consciously choose to end their lives. Such a one was George.

George first came into my life when he was already very frail with AIDS. He looked as if the next breeze might bear him away. His spirit, however, was strong and his heart was huge! Such a loving, gentle, and wise person was George. His partner, Robbie, is equally wonderful. Robbie and George lived harmoniously, sharing a remarkably loving relationship. They were an inspiration to each other and to all of us who knew them as a couple.

For many months, George suffered terribly with peripheral neuropathy in his feet, legs, hands, and forearms. This made walking, or even a simple activity like buttoning his shirt, unbearably painful. Over the months, he also experienced digestive complaints with Cryptosporidium causing havoc in his gall bladder. A very deep thinker, George often spoke of the love he felt for his family and Robbie and explored thoroughly his philosophy of life. Somehow he *always* managed to bring humor and lightness to his struggles. Over the three years I knew George, he methodically completed all of his relationships with his family. His relationship with Robbie was in a permanent state of completion, in that there was never any unfinished business between them. Their relationship was a continuous source of joy to them. George was equally methodical in attending to all of his legal and other affairs. He spoke of suicide as his preferred option on many occasions, though while his quality of life was tolerable he was content to remain here.

However, there came a time when all was complete in his life and he planned, very carefully, his death. He'd discussed his thoughts with Robbie, who'd initially disagreed with his intentions. In the last three weeks of George's life, his pain left him and his digestion improved. In that time he and Robbie were able to enjoy the things which were meaningful to both of them. Simple things like conversation over coffee in a cafe; shared walks and talks. Both knew that this was but a short reprieve from the ravages of his disease. George and Robbie together had decided that Robbie shouldn't know of the day of George's intended suicide. They felt that Robbie would be tempted to intervene if he knew. In the days preceding George's death they shared deep and emotional conversations about their relationship. Robbie knew in his heart then that George was preparing to leave. He came home one evening to find George dead. Such were George's preparations that the shock for Robbie was minimized. The house was clean and everything was in order; George had left all his keys neatly together, the lights had been turned on so Robbie wouldn't come into a darkened home, money had been left in Robbie's jacket pocket to cover the next month's rent, a blanket had been placed upon the bed under George in case there was any need to protect the mattress.

Robbie's still grieving, but not for the manner in which George died. He's changed his view of suicide, believing it to be an honorable option for those who so choose.

The following section is devoted particularly to those who've lost a partner or close friend through AIDS. However, *most of what is written is equally applicable for people who've experienced any significant loss, regardless of their illness.*

The Loss of a Loved One Through AIDS

To suffer the loss of a loved one at any time is traumatic and painful. However, there are sometimes added stresses for those whose partner or close friend dies of AIDS. The stresses often involve psychological, physical, financial, spiritual, and social issues. These factors might not all apply to you and each person's reaction to his or her loss will be different, so take from them what seems relevant.

Psychological

Even though AIDS and cancer are nearly always long and protracted diseases, the actual death of a friend comes as a shock. Because the illness *is* so protracted, giving you time to get used to the idea of the loss of your loved one, you might not immediately feel overwhelmed by your reaction. However, it's likely you'll experience a mixture of feelings. These might include relief, sadness, despair, meaninglessness, guilt, loneliness, fear, numbness, yearning, anger, confusion, anxiety, disorganization, helplessness, pining, and restlessness.

Initially you'll have a feeling of shock, perhaps an all-consuming numbness. This might last a few days or weeks, but don't be surprised if a let-down comes a little later. It might feel as if part of you has died. Tears might come, they might not. Don't judge yourself on the reaction you're experiencing.

Grief is a very private matter and everyone will have a different experience. There's no time limit on grieving. It will likely continue for years. You might find, six or more months after the death of your partner, that an incident or memory will catapult you back into the full force of your grief. At such times, you might think you'll never recover from this loss. You might never love another in the *same* way. And, if you *do*, you might face guilt, wondering *how* you can love again. Your partner will always hold a special place in your heart wherein will lie the memories of your love.

You might feel pressured by friends, family or, indeed, yourself to "put on a brave face." It's important that you make your needs known to someone whom you can trust. You might need to reach out for help from a counselor, family member, or friend. Sometimes your friends can be so overloaded with their own grief issues that you might find it difficult to share fully your personal pain. This is becoming increasingly evident as the AIDS epidemic continues its relentless onslaught. Many of us in the front line of this war waged against our loved ones, friends, and acquaintances are wearied by our grief. Seek out someone who *can* respond to your need.

For some, bereavement will present the most powerful emotions you might ever experience in your life. For many, this can be very frightening. You might think you'll die of grief or emotion. If you find you're afraid of the depth and intensity of your emotions, seek out professional help.

There might be times when you feel overwhelmed by pangs of yearning for your partner. You think you hear his key in the lock and your heart is full of anticipation; you expect to see him in his favorite chair as always and you find it gaping at you, empty; you see a beautiful sunset, something which you both used to enjoy, and you go to call him to watch it with you. You find yourself talking to him as you prepare yourself for bed. All these reactions are normal. It's fine to continue talking to your partner. You might even feel his reply within your heart. Perhaps he's not really dead, as in finished; perhaps he's just elsewhere. One of our long-term survivors, Peter, had lost over forty friends to AIDS. He used to say, "They're not really dead to me. It's as if they've moved to Melbourne. When your friends move to Melbourne, you don't see them any more. You don't get to hug them or talk to them, but you know they're alive and well—they're just in Melbourne."

Anniversaries, birthdays, and holidays are often particularly painful times. Often couples have created their own rituals or celebrations at this time and to feel the aloneness of such occasions can be devastating. Joy, happiness, or even a vestige of contentment seems impossible at such times. You might prefer to make a point of not being alone on those days. Conversely, your own company might be just what you need. Only you will know what's right for you.

You'll probably feel a need to talk about the feelings you experienced around the time of the death of your partner. Often death occurs when a partner isn't present, and this can cause feelings of guilt and raise questions in your mind like, "Did he die peacefully? Did he ask for me? Was he in pain?" and so on. It's good to talk to those who were with him or, failing that, to talk about any unresolved feelings you might still have.

Physical

It's common to have a preoccupation with your own health after the recent loss of a loved one. This is so for *all* newly bereaved people but will be particularly so if you're likewise infected with the virus. You might find yourself examining your body for blemishes, rashes, or Kaposi's sarcoma. It's common to experience insomnia, nausea, diarrhea, aching muscles, gastrointestinal problems, fatigue, listlessness, or headaches. It's important that you have a supportive doctor to whom you can talk about your health fears at this time. Have him or her check out any symptoms you might experience so that your mind can be put at rest. Remember, *all* newly bereaved people can experience physical symptoms. If you remember this, it will assist you in containing your anxiety. I can highly recommend a massage within the first week or so after the death of your partner to help deal with the muscular aches, as well as for nurturing.

It's easy to let go taking care of yourself when you're newly bereaved. When you're under great stress you're more susceptible to illness so it's particularly important that you don't neglect your health at this time. Even if you don't enjoy food at present, make an effort to eat regularly. Though sleep might be elusive, it's best to avoid sedatives, (unprescribed) drugs, and alcohol as a means of escape from the pain of loss. It's normal and healthy to experience pain at your loss. It's wise to listen to your friends, family, or counselor and if *they* encourage you to see a doctor, even though it might make no sense to you, do so.

Financial Considerations

If you can avoid any major financial decisions in the early weeks and months, so much the better. However, often the death of our partner also signifies a major drop in income. This might be particularly relevant if you've had joint financial commitments which are dependent on two incomes. Most people find it's best to remain in the home they shared with their loved ones until they feel they can make decisions calmly. If you *do* have to make major financial decisions, talk them over first with a professional financial adviser. Often it's good to have more than one professional opinion before embarking on any substantial change to your financial arrangements.

Depending upon your health, you might find that you're throwing yourself more deeply into work as a way of dealing with the pain and the loss you feel. Relationships with family and friends will continue to be important. Don't let your "busyness" distract you from spending quality time with those who are significant to you.

There might also be the added complication of relatives of your partner who wish to make some financial claim against his estate. You might have to deal with the anger and frustration of interacting with your partner's family who've come to claim his belongings. There's a sad but often true saying, "Where there's a will, there's a relative." If his family have never accepted the fact that your partner was gay, then it's exceedingly unlikely they'll acknowledge, in any substantial way, your relationship with him. Often these relatives have been "out of touch"(!) for a long time and were of no significant support during your partner's illness. Suddenly they can appear on the scene with the intent of "taking over the arrangements." This might include the funeral. There have been many instances where the remaining partner was not only *not* consulted about his and his partner's wishes for the funeral, but that he was either not invited or deliberately asked *not* to attend. Much of this pain can be minimized by thought and preparation. I encourage clients to state very clearly their intentions in their will. These intentions can extend from the funeral arrangements to stating their *exact wishes with regard to their property, possessions, assets, collections, and personal belongings.* One client of mine went so far as to write letters to various members of his family explaining exactly why he'd chosen to will his belongings in the manner he did. This certainly cleared up any doubt anyone might have had about his intentions. It also protected his partner from any unnecessary legal trauma.

For some parents, the fact that their son is gay has led to some painful financial decisions. For instance, Geoff has been in a loving and supportive relationship with Tim for fifteen years. Geoff has AIDS. His parents, who'd never acknowledged his relationship with Tim, on discovering that their son had developed AIDS, immediately blamed Tim for a) "corrupting" their son, and b) for infecting him with the virus. As it is, Tim does *not* have the virus. The parents find that hard to believe. They were going to leave a substantial amount of money to Geoff on their deaths. However, if they do that, it's likely the very person who would benefit from their money would be someone they hold in poor regard. Geoff is outraged that his parents refuse to acknowledge the depth and commitment of his relationship with Tim. In his mind, it is every bit as deep and lasting as any successful heterosexual relationship. He refuses to speak to his parents, forbids them to visit, and requests that they do not attend his funeral.

This kind of situation is not confined only to gay relationships. There are as many strained "in-law" relationships outside the gay community as within it. Helen, who was diagnosed with a very curable lymphoma, has experienced almost the identical situation to Geoff and Tim. She's been married for twelve years, is deeply in love with her husband Jim, and has devoted her life to him. Her parents have never approved of the relationship, believing Helen "wasted" herself on a motor mechanic when she could have married "anyone." Throughout her treatment, Jim was a tremendous support to her. Helen's parents would always choose times to visit her when he wasn't around.

On comprehending the possibility of Helen's death, her parents, who were both quite elderly and wealthy, decided to leave their money to a favorite charity. Helen was deeply hurt and angered by their decision. Firstly, she felt it indicated that her parents didn't believe she would survive the cancer. Secondly, she and Jim would have appreciated their financial support so that Jim could finally have his own workshop. He and Helen had been saving and working toward this dream for many years. As with Geoff and his parents, the rift which this action caused was deep. The anger and hurt hasn't been healed, and the relationship the parents treasured with their only daughter is in tatters. I've included Helen's story because I find that often gay people believe that the negative things that happen to them are because of their sexuality. This is *often* the case but it's not *always* so.

There are, of course, many instances where families have regarded the remaining partner as a valued addition to their extended family. Deeply valued relationships have sprung up between the most unlikely people, whose paths would never have crossed without the joint suffering and loss that has been shared. The hurt surrounding loss signifies that we care. Our shared tears are a tribute to the fact that we cared so deeply.

Social Implications

You might feel more lonely and lost after your partner has died than at any other time in your life. There's often only limited understanding and support for the remaining partner in a gay relationship. There mightn't be any support at all. Sometimes the relationship with this person had no "outward form" at all. A secret love, a private relationship held within the heart but unacknowledged by anyone. For these people, grief is particularly painful because it receives no understanding, compassion, or acknowledgment from anyone "outside."

Even if you *do* receive wonderful emotional support and

understanding, it's generally extended most fully in the first weeks after the death of your partner. Perhaps, as the weeks drag into months, family and friends are less readily available. They get on with their lives, often expecting you to do the same. You might need to consciously reach out and let them know how you *are* feeling. They won't be able to guess what's going on for you.

Young people who've had little or no experience of death might feel completely bewildered and confused as to how they *do* feel. The social contacts/venues of the past might now seem to be hollow and fraught with disillusionment. Going to bars or parties doesn't have the same sense of excitement any more. Friends from the past might have no idea at all of how to support you. You might find yourself wanting to fill the emptiness you feel with another relationship. Don't be afraid to reach out to another, but it's best not to rush into a new relationship. You'll probably not be a wise judge of new relationships until you've worked through a lot of your grief. It doesn't work successfully to cover up the pain you feel by losing yourself in another relationship. Your partner is irreplaceable. What you and he shared stands alone. Enjoy people as they are without seeking to recapture the past. You *will* heal but you'll never be the same person again. You will have matured. You'll have found strengths, compassion, understanding, and a greater sensitivity within yourself. All these qualities you'll then take forward with you as an enriched human being.

Spiritual Aspects

Many people find great comfort and support through their spiritual beliefs when they're experiencing the pain of loss. For others, such a loss can sorely test their faith! Both attitudes are normal and neither of them are "unspiritual." Extend to yourself the compassion and care that you would want to see extended to someone else in your situation. Don't be harsh or judgmental toward yourself. Perhaps listen to what your partner would say to you now.

If going to church or attending any other meeting based on

spiritual principles has been part of your routine, you might like to return once more. Some people prefer solitude, with reading and music to accompany them in their grief. Respect what you know about yourself.

Avoid people who wish to hurry you through the process of your grief. They're probably feeling uncomfortable because of fears about their own inadequacy.

Conclusion

It is for each of us to decide upon his or her philosophical beliefs. I have fewer now than ever before in my life. There was a time when I believed in the Resurrection, and another when the laws of karma made excellent sense. Now? I'm much more content with questions. I've less of a need for answers. I understand a little of the power of love and it's this god, the god of love and compassion, whom I favor as my companion. When I feel the presence of love, all's well in my world. Whether things fare exceedingly well or poorly in health, relationships, finances, or work, if I experience the presence of love, all is well. It's when I rail against the outer circumstances of my life, when I don't get my way, when I'm filled with fear, then the world seems a dark and intimidating place. Then I have blinkered my eyes against the light. To experience love means letting go the blinkers—letting go all that stands in the way of light.

As I reflect upon the passion with which each of these heroes lived, I'm at a loss to say at what point they stopped living and started dying.

Was Elizabeth dying when she reached out to her son to embrace him yet once more in the hours before she left us?

Was Stephen dying in the moments before he departed, when he fondly caressed the cheek of his partner as he whispered, "I'm ready to go home now"?

Was Michelle, aged twenty and paralyzed from the neck down, dying when she said, "Petrea, this can't be dying! I feel so strong and alive within myself"?

Was ten-year-old Kate dying when she reached out to her

parents' hands and said, "I want you to love each other the way you've loved me"?

Or Lisa? Her last words, "I don't feel like I'm dying. I feel like I'm being born into light."

Chapter Thirteen

THE TENDER TRAP

. . . .

Trudi

This is a happy story. Don't be confused by the beginning—wait for the end.

My name is Trudi. Married to Desmond, mother of Jeremy, nine, and Jessica, five, running my own business, busy, busy life, almost no time to catch my breath.

Desmond tells me every morning about his bowel movement problems. I say: "Darling, don't tell me—tell the doctor." He says, "But what if I have bowel cancer?" I say, "Don't be ridiculous, darling. Of course you don't have cancer. Other people, yes. Articles in papers and magazines, yes. In our family—no!"

After the first pathology test, the doctor requests a more complicated test. We're all very busy. Then it's a possibility. The doctor says, "Okay, I'll book you in for a colonoscopy."

After the colonoscopy, I have to collect Desmond from the surgery. I've learned from speaking to other people that when I arrive, Desmond should be waiting in the recovery room, and I'll be able to take him home. This is NOT the case. The nursing sister asks if we'll wait. The doctor wants to talk to us both. Hurry up—two weeks before Christmas. I have to be back at work. It's the busiest time of the year. I have to go. Maybe Desmond can take a taxi. No, no—the doctor will talk to you now. We go in. We sit down. Hurry up, tell me what diet Desmond has to be on. Or tell me what medication he needs to take. I have to go back to work.

*The doctor says "I have some bad news. You have bowel cancer."
The bottom drops out of the world—the things that go through your
mind. Time stands still.*

*Desmond says, "See, I told you so." I go into action. Who is this
doctor anyway? When and how will he fix everything? "An operation," he says. "Urgent, serious." The doctor draws pictures. He seems
to think he can do it.*

*We leave the surgery and Desmond says he wants to keep IT a se-
cret. Impossible. Next week he's having a major operation. What about
work? Family? Desmond decides I'm only to tell those who have to
know. I'm also to tell them he doesn't want to talk about it.*

I do all the phoning

*No one calls Desmond about IT. Desmond feels lonely and ne-
glected. I call everyone again and ask them to call Desmond. I have it
all organized for him in no time.*

*Desmond goes to work to clear his desk frantically. I feel I have to
be very nice to him in case he dies during the operation. It crosses my
mind that maybe it'd be better for all of us if he died instead of pro-
longing the agony.*

*I'm worried that Desmond has no pajamas for the hospital. I buy
some.*

*We go to a Christmas party and afterward Desmond breaks down.
He cries in front of the Opera House. I take him home and put him to
bed. I am a practical person.*

Desmond goes into the hospital. No big deal.

Tests done.

*I visit Desmond in the evening. He tells me that the tests show the
cancer has reached his liver. He's almost smug about it, as if he's been
vindicated. I go home and feel desperate.*

*The day of the operation. I get to the hospital at 6:00 A.M., bring-
ing five good books with me. Desmond is calm as he goes into the operating room. I spend eight and a half hours waiting, not reading. I
could go home but I stay there, in case it makes a difference. The doctor comes in and says all went well, and he does some more drawings.
I ask him how one goes about cutting a liver and we go into a lengthy
discussion about surgical instruments. I see Desmond in intensive care,
all wrapped in foil and shivering. There is a reindeer picture on the*

wall above his bed. It's Christmas and all is under control.

Desmond is a model patient. He has chemotherapy. I report on progress to friends and family. I tell the same story so many times that the emotion drains out of it.

Desmond has recovered rapidly and is home by New Year's Eve.

Desmond goes back to work part-time. He's very concerned about hair regrowth in his crotch. It itches. I apply calamine lotion.

Desmond works full-time. We fall back into the familiar patterns, but somehow they feel different. The doctor never tells us what to do about feelings. Desmond is afraid and asks me if he's all right. I put my hand over where his liver is. I tell him I have healing hands. I tell him I KNOW he is well. I'm afraid, too.

We explain about cancer to the children. Jessica is too young to understand and doesn't take much notice. Jeremy understands that Daddy is like a patch of grass in which some weeds are growing. The weeds have to be cut and sprayed so they don't take over. It's simple, and reassures all of us.

Tests are done every four weeks at first, then at longer intervals. I ring the doctor for the results. All is well.

There's an irregularity in one of the tests. The doctor and I decide not to tell Desmond. It might mean nothing. The next test will tell. What I know eats at me the whole month. I feel that lying to him is a betrayal. The thought of telling him the truth is unbearable.

The next test shows the same irregularity. The doctor tells Desmond. He refers us to a liver specialist. I get very depressed, which causes Desmond to feel stronger. I can't face another operation. We talk about refusing to have one. We talk about euthanasia. Desmond makes me promise not to let him suffer. For now, he feels fantastic physically.

We sit in the liver specialist's waiting room cracking jokes and laughing. The specialist looks nonplused at our good spirits. He tells us the cancer appears to be close to the vena cava. It might not be operable. A liver biopsy is needed to locate the cancer precisely.

I feel that conventional medicine has done all it can for us.

Desmond is feeling so well that it all seems unreal. I go to work, busy myself with the children. I'm tired of feeling depressed. I tell myself that right now Desmond is all right and this is what matters. I feel better.

It's a year since it all started. The liver biopsy is inconclusive.

There's no confirmation of cancer. There's no exclusion of it, either. The specialist decides not to operate. We're sent to an oncologist.

The oncologist says that although Desmond might still have cancer, he has no symptoms. He doesn't see any reason at present for more chemotherapy. We're surprised, and relieved!

Here's the promised happy ending. Desmond continues to be well. It's now two years since it all started. Quite often it seems a dream. [The methods in this book] not only provided emotional support and practical help for Desmond: [they] also helped me look at life differently. I'm still a busy person, but I'm far more focused on the present moment, and I get a much greater enjoyment out of life.

The role of caregiver is a very demanding one. How you cope will depend upon your character, personality, background, and ability to adapt to constantly changing circumstances.

The first emotion after the diagnosis of your loved one will most likely be *shock*. In the same way as for the person *with* the diagnosis, your reaction can vary from numbness through to panic. This might last for days or weeks.

During this time of shock or numbness, it's best to avoid making important decisions. Major decisions should be postponed if at all possible. This isn't a time when you should expect yourself to be rational, courageous, stable, or philosophical. It's unrealistic to expect these attributes to be present in the midst of unexpected crisis, but in time your emotions will stabilize and you *will* be able to make calm decisions. Call and rely on friends and relatives during this period. Give yourself time to absorb the shock. Practice the attitude of trust. This *will* pass and you'll again become your usual capable self, but at this stage, allow yourself to swim with the tide, even though it might feel as if you're sometimes drowning.

Much as we love and care for those near and dear to us who are unwell, we too feel fragile and in need of nurturing. This becomes especially evident when an illness is protracted. It's essential that *as much care go into working out a suitable program for the caregiver as for the patient.*

The unseen, and often unacknowledged, juggling act which must go on is demanding, exhausting, and frequently frustrating. The children still have their squabbles, the shopping has to be done, the carrots juiced, and the telephone answered. People are forever dropping in with bits of advice or sympathy. In addition to all the usual activities there are the sometimes frequent visits to doctors and hospitals. It usually falls to the support person to deal with insurance forms, the bank, the hospital and nursing staff, friends, relatives, and neighbors; all this with an overriding uncertainty about the future. Frequently the future represents an anxiety which "cannot" be discussed and this creates its own form of stress. Illness frequently makes patients irritable and unreasonable, and this is usually shown toward family more than anyone else. We can end up feeling incapable, angry, half-witted, and full of frustration. Often we make the mistake of directing all this negativity at ourselves. We know it doesn't help to feel inferior but when circumstances deprive us of our normal pleasures and freedoms it's an easy trap to fall into. Soon we feel our lives have been taken over by the endless round of tests, hospitalization, recovery, and treatments. You might feel totally taken over by some other force too strong to resist and have panicky moments when you feel everything is out of your control. If you create a way to vent your feelings properly and honestly, you'll find they can be released. They can become another guilt-inducing burden if they're left unexpressed. Everyone else's life seems to glide along smoothly while yours is in turmoil. Be gentle with yourself. You've probably never been in this situation before and you certainly didn't invite it. But here it is, and here you are. Staying alive, sane (relatively), and surviving the experience is what this chapter is about.

It's wise to ascertain your needs as soon after diagnosis as practicable. You might find that making lists will help you to clarify things which you once took for granted. These lists might include the physical, emotional, and financial needs of your family. Physical needs can be everything from getting Jenny to her ballet class on Wednesday afternoon to Fluffy's hormones which must be given on Friday nights, from how to

find time to pick up the dry-cleaning and the groceries, to who's
going to mow the lawn. All these things are essentials which
must continue. Jenny's emotional needs will certainly need addressing if you're constantly at the hospital or preoccupied with
the person who's unwell. Your emotional needs might best be
met by setting time aside every day for you to renew your own
inner resources. Perhaps a time for music, meditation, exercise,
prayer, reading, or simply a time to let your mind drift. Time
out for you. Guard it vigorously. You might need to take over
making all the regular financial payments. If you create lists
whereby you know your commitments—physical, emotional, and
financial—you'll be in a better position to match them with the
resources you have among your own family and relatives, and
the offers of help you might have received from friends and
neighbors.

You'll probably wish to remain as self-reliant as possible, but
don't allow that to stop you from reaching out to those who've
offered their support.

When someone asks, "How are you, Diane?" are you the sort
of person who says, "Oh, I'm fine, thanks," regardless of how
you really feel? This reply is all right when you're talking to a
casual acquaintance, but when people are genuinely interested in
your welfare, this sort of reply ends the conversation very
quickly. What can your friends say if you give such a reply? It's
not whining or being negative to say something like, "Frankly,
today isn't one of my better days. Every day seems worse than
the one before and I feel I'm not coping well at all. I hope tomorrow will be a turning point but I'm not holding my breath!"
What you've said, in essence, to your friends is that your relationship is significant enough for you to be "real" with how
things *actually* are. Then they can give you a hug or say whatever seems appropriate, even though they probably won't have
any particular solution to your problem. Usually what we count
as being really important is that someone actually hears what
we're saying and understands. To say, "I'm fine, thanks" when
that isn't the case brings down a wall of noncommunication.
Your friend will probably feel totally shut out. I've always appre-

ciated the kind of relationship in which I feel comfortable enough with a friend to really unburden myself; when someone has let me hear myself think rather than just giving me *his* or *her* solution for *my* problem. Ultimately we all need to find our own solutions for our problems, and though listening to other people's experiences with similar situations can be extremely helpful, the ultimate solution has to be found by us.

Patients will react in many different ways to the stress imposed by a life-threatening disease. In fact, different days will bring different reactions. For those who've always been fiercely independent, it's very difficult suddenly to express their needs. Being unused to communicating their needs, asking for the smallest thing to be done for them can be very traumatic. Some people simply don't know how to do it. A frequent comment in the support groups is we often feel that if our supporters *really* love and understand us, they'll anticipate our needs, preferably before *we* even know we *have* them! We might realize how childish and unreasonable this is, and yet it can be a difficult habit to break. Often there's an undercurrent of anger and frustration in the patient regarding the state of things, and if there's no appropriate channel for all that pent-up energy it's usually directed at those closest to us. The patient knows those nearest are not going to desert him or her and it can become a pattern of behavior which is difficult to break. It can become even more difficult to see behind a person's irritable behavior when the whole household is feeling the stress of diagnosis, treatments, and the ongoing uncertainty.

Almost always, the diagnosis means people are thrown together more than usual. This can be a strain in itself. Many a wife has had her busy and enjoyable routine turned topsy-turvy by the constant presence and demands of a husband who was formerly working (or vice versa). Perhaps there are financial matters which need to be addressed because of the decreased income of the family. Where both partners are working, major adjustments might need to be made in order to accommodate appointments, treatments, hospitalization, and the emotional turmoil which each might include. Even the best marriage can

find this a strain. If it *wasn't* the best marriage at the time of diagnosis, some considerable effort might need to be put in to
making it better at a time when there are other pressing issues.
But there's no doubt that a crisis can also strengthen the bond
between people, and many people have testified to this.

More than ever, at this time, the health of the support person is paramount. Who's going to look after the diet, recreation,
and exercise of the support people unless they do? There are
often good friends and neighbors who offer practical assistance
and yet people resist allowing such help. *Practice accepting their
offered help.* Let someone pick up the children from school or do
a load of washing or ironing; let your neighbor sit with the patient while you go and have a game of tennis or get your hair
done; let your friend do the shopping or cook the occasional
meal. People like to feel included and of real practical assistance
to you, yet it's up to you to allow them this opportunity. Let go
of the fierce independence and allow yourself to feel part of a
community. I'm not suggesting you surrender your self-reliance,
but that you *do* practice common sense.

Often caregivers feel that they're showing their love and
concern by doing *everything* for the patient. Perhaps they also
think that their love can be measured by how much they actually "do" for the patient. And yes, that's a valid attitude. However, when some of the practical details are taken care of by
someone else, it allows you more time to be with the person in a
more intimate capacity.

Many people fall into the trap of "being strong for each
other," in the belief that if one shows true feeling it might trigger off the tears of the other. There's nothing negative about
tears and frequently the most healing therapy possible is the
shared tears of a family. It's a release of tension. If there are
uncried tears it doesn't mean "I'm strong," it might mean, "I don't
feel safe enough to be vulnerable," "I'm not willing to have the
other person be vulnerable with me," "If I start crying, I might
never stop." The truth is the emotions are there, but are
unacknowledged and unexpressed. Remember the saying, "It's
hard to kiss someone who's keeping a stiff upper lip." Suppressed

emotions cause a heaviness in the heart and can lead to illness in the body. The tears *will* stop. Sometimes, paradoxically, letting go control is the quickest way to feeling back in control once more.

Practicalities

Just as for the patient, there are some areas which are vitally necessary for the support person to address. There's no reason why the support person shouldn't have a healthy diet along with the patient, nor should the support person only make the juices for the ill. A multivitamin, or a formula which concentrates on the vitamins that are in high demand when we're under stress, is also invaluable. Adequate rest and time for personal recreation is essential, so you're in good shape to fulfill the function of the caregiver or support person. Time out for self-reflection is helpful and, if possible, practice the techniques of relaxation and meditation along with the patient or in your own quiet time.

My sympathy is often with those who are there to support us! Having been both a cancer patient and a caregiver, I know how difficult it is to meet the demands of those we love. If you get me soup, I'm likely to think, "I want salad." If you don't get me soup and give me salad, I'm likely to think, "You always give me salad; can't you make me soup?" You often won't get it right, even with all the thought and preparation in the world. Try to maintain your sense of humor and perspective. Keep remembering, "This too will pass." The dilemma of the caregiver certainly extends to the kitchen. Sometimes we want our loved ones to get well so much that we prepare the most exquisite morsels for their consumption, only to be confronted with a look of total disinterest (or worse) upon their faces as we tenderly present to them the symbol of our love. It can be very disconcerting. Remember, disapproval of the food is *not* disapproval of you and your efforts.

Your loved one might continue to lose weight, regardless of your efforts. It's not a reflection on the amount of care you've given him or her.

Endeavor not to get the issues confused. You're not responsible for your loved one's recovery. You're only responsible for the love with which you care for him or her.

When the patient is expressing anger, hostility, sullenness, or irritability, try to remember that what's really being expressed is fear; it's a cry for help. Insofar as your compassion will allow, try to understand and meet this need in the best way you can. Be compassionate toward *yourself* when *you're* fed up and irritable.

In many support groups the caregivers are welcome, and they gain much by sharing their own experiences and listening to those of others. There are also support groups for caregivers, and in this environment much understanding and acceptance is gained. Also, much humor is shared and participants leave feeling less alone with their situation. I believe it's very often more difficult for the support person than for the patient. It's a demanding role to put aside our wants and needs for the sake of another. This is especially so if this necessity arises in a marriage or family where relationships between people are already strained.

A family or marriage counselor can be invaluable at this time to sort out priorities and to open lines of communication between members. In this way, we don't just muddle through the situation but can actually repair relationships which can then deepen and become more meaningful.

If playing sports, going to a club, attending classes in some area of interest, or entertaining friends has been part of your life up until now, look at ways whereby you can maintain those activities even if on a more infrequent or curtailed basis. Ask friends over for morning tea instead of dinner or, if your friends offer to bring something, then let them. You can easily say to friends, "We really miss seeing you and we'd love to spend some time together. Mary's on her special diet, though, so why don't you come around after dinner?"

Simple activities like walking the dog can bring a sense of calm and connectedness with others and the world outside the home. If it's been your custom in the past, keep it up. If the patient is well enough to accompany you, it can be a time of quiet conversation and companionship.

It's very important to keep up your supportive contacts, especially if you're a caregiver, and in this way you maintain as normal a life as possible. Many people find that "friends" on whom they thought they could rely suddenly disappear. This can be very disappointing, bewildering, and hurtful. It's useful to remember these people genuinely don't know how to be of any assistance to you. They feel overwhelmed. Your true friends will be able to say, "I'm sorry to hear about Mary. I just don't know what to say. What can I do to be of assistance?" Or, better still, might turn up on your doorstep with a casserole in hand.

To be positive is to be truly realistic about what is going on.

One supporter had the realization one day that it was O.K. not to cope. She had been a "coper" all her life and found the situation of caring for her sick husband was sometimes overwhelming. She found it very liberating to give herself permission not to cope for the day! Remember, the strange thing is that when we give ourselves permission *not* to cope, it's actually the first step toward *coping!* Personally, I'm not fond of the word "cope." When we talk about someone who's coping quite well with a crisis, we often mean he or she is maintaining composure on the outside regardless of how he or she is feeling on the inside. It's far healthier to express feelings of inadequacy, frustration, fear, or sadness. Once these feelings are expressed we're more able to continue with what's necessary in the situation.

Telephones

The incessant ringing of the telephone with people inquiring about the patient can be exhausting. Consider renting, buying, or borrowing an answering machine. Then you can either leave a message saying when it's convenient for you to take calls or you can redirect phone calls to some other person who's willing to fulfill this function. Perhaps this person can give an update on

the patient (and *you*) which will save you having to repeat yourself over and over again.

Tell your friends and family that you need them to ask about you, too!

Often the support person is overlooked in this regard. It is
like balm to a wound to be remembered for your *own* unique
value. If all else fails, unplug the phone. It *is* your home and you
can choose when you wish to be available to people.

Remember, also, that some patients can become monumen-
tally selfish in their demands. This might be due to their disease
or to fear, in which case one needs to develop and display all
the compassion of which one is capable.

On the other hand, it's also possible they've always been this
way. The diagnosis of a life-threatening illness doesn't necessarily sweeten their attitude. It isn't unreasonable or unusual for the
caregiver to feel resentful or frustrated with this situation. *You're
not alone!* Many have walked this particular tightrope before.
They seem to do it with a combination of inner fortitude, a
sense of humor (if possible!), outside interests, and building an
immunity to other's expectations. One needs to retreat into self-
preservation. You might find it particularly helpful to seek out a
caregiver's support group or find an individual counselor who'll
help you live with the situation.

There's no easy solution to the problems faced by the support person. There'll be days when nothing seems to go right
and disappointments are in the air. Be gentle with yourself.
Avoid having to "cope"! With some thought and effort, create
your *own* support system. The very best thing you can bring to
your loved one is your own peace of mind and calmness. To
achieve the qualities of serenity will certainly take an effort.

To serve others effectively, we must respect and care for ourselves. In this way we retain our own inner calm and strength
and are thus able to give these qualities to others. It's these
qualities which assist us in true healing. A frazzled partner is of
limited assistance to someone who's unwell. A calm and positive
caregiver can bring healing and wholeness to those they're with.

The following list provides possible ways of creating support for yourself. Choose the things which seem to feel 'right' for you. They're not in any preferential order; some will feel right and others won't. Good luck with your efforts!

Remember These Points:

1. *Regular relaxation and recreation are essential. We "recreate" ourselves during practices.*

2. *A good nourishing diet which provides all necessary nutrients for health is a must.*

3. *Appropriate vitamin or mineral supplements provide us with necessary nutrients.*

4. *A regular massage, perhaps with a therapist who'll visit the home and "do" both of you is a great release for stress.*

5. *If it's your partner who's sick, arrange some time for just the two of you to be together or, conversely, you might need to arrange time for the two of you to be apart.*

6. *Enlist the willing aid of neighbors and friends to do many of the mundane physical tasks.*

7. *Continue contact with supportive friends.*

8. *Despite the tiring onslaught of stress, retain your own self-image by having your hair done, exercising, attending your classes, etc.*

9. *Never miss the opportunity to see a funny movie.*

10. *Practice meditation—remember, that can be the glazed state that comes over ardent gardeners when watering their plants at sunset.*

11. *Take time alone for self-reflection.*

12. *It's O.K. not to cope. Be gentle with yourself on those uphill days.*

13. *Let go of maintaining the "perfect image" of being a supporter.*

14. *Feel free to express your emotions. Remember tears are healing.*

15. *Don't hesitate to get professional counseling if there are difficulties in communication. If there were problems in the relationship before the illness, they probably haven't disappeared because of it.*

16. *Look for humor. Even black humor is better than none.*

17. *If finances permit, arrange to have someone come to clean your home regularly, so your time can be better spent.*

18. *Find an affirmation which will help you get through the tough times. An old favorite is, "This too will pass."*

19. *This might sound crazy but—do something for someone else. It somehow lifts the spirits and broadens our perspectives to reach beyond our familiar world of care and extend assistance to another.*

20. *Above all, respect yourself and know you're doing your very best!*

Pointers for Visitors to Sick People

Many people who visit those who have a serious illness are at a loss as to how to relate to or support their friends. They often feel inept in their inability to express their distress, or they're unsure of what might be helpful to their friends. Here are some pointers which might help:

1. *Stop outside the door, take some deep breaths, center yourself, and leave your "busyness" at the door.*

2. *Your tone of voice and your eyes will convey more than the words themselves.*

3. *Be yourself. Be who you've always been with your friend. Those who are unwell are especially sensitive to phoniness.*

4. *Be sensitive to your friend's needs, moods, feelings, and especially to signs of tiredness. Don't overstay your welcome. The patient can feel like a sitting duck and might feel uncomfortable about asking you to leave.*

5. *Listen to your friend—how he or she feels or what he or she needs.*

6. *Equally, sick people might not want to tell you any of the above. They might prefer to hear about you and your activities. You can reminisce, plan, or simply discuss current events in your life. Be flexible. Don't make heavy weather of your visit.*

7. *Don't lie to your friend—hardly the act of a friend!*

8. *Nonverbal communication is as important as anything you might say to your friend. A touch, gesture, smile, or massage might convey more of your love and empathy than all the words in the world. Never underestimate the power of loving touch.*

9. *Give empathy, not sympathy, to your friend. To empathize is to "feel with," whereas sympathizing is to "feel sorry for."*

10. *Don't share your problems or ailments with your friend. Your friend has enough on his or her plate at present without worrying about you.*

11. *Smoking in the presence of sick people might be very distressing for them. Never smoke where oxygen is being used. Strong smells such as perfume, after-shave, incense, can all be upsetting to someone who's feeling sick.*

12. *Don't be afraid of silence. Conversation might be difficult for someone who's seriously ill. You might like to take a book or your knitting and enjoy a companionable silence instead.*

13. *Let your friend dictate the "pace" of your visit. Don't hurry him or her.*

14. *Don't make promises to your friend which you can't keep.*

15. *You don't have to be cheerful all the time with your friend. Allow tears from each of you if that's more appropriate.*

16. *Visiting your friend doesn't have to be a somber occasion either! Laughter and light-heartedness can lift the pall of depression and allow another perspective to be shared.*

17. *If your friend is unconscious, remember he or she can still hear you. Tell him or her whatever is in your heart. You do not need to speak loudly to be heard by an unconscious person. Use your normal voice and rely on touch and tone to convey your feelings.*

18. *Never say to your friend, "I know how you feel." You don't!*

19. *Don't say, "You look wonderful!" (even if he or she does). Your friend might be feeling horrid and everyone keeps telling him or her how wonderful he or she looks. It's better to say, "Do you feel as good as you look?" This gives your friend the option of saying, "No, I feel awful!"*

20. *Don't make assumptions about how your friend feels. Your friend might be very seriously ill and yet deeply at peace with him- or herself and the world. Let your friend tell you how he or she feels.*

Acknowledgments

. . . .

There's no way this book would have been possible without the continuing support I've received from my family and friends.

I am eternally grateful for my parents Geoff and Rae, who've always supported me.

I took four weeks out of my schedule to revise extensively and expand this completely new edition of *Quest for Life*. The only way it could be done was to remove myself from the proximity of the telephone. I'd like to extend my deep gratitude to my mother Rae, my friend and companion. To my brother Ross and his wife Dianne who live in California, my special thanks for opening their home and hearts to Rae and me while this book was being written.

My children Kate and Simon deserve special thanks and appreciation for their patience and willingness to share me with so many others.

I'd like to acknowledge with thanks Gina Misiroglu, who translated the Australian version of this book into a language that Americans would understand.

My deep gratitude to Daryl, who saw me through one of the darkest nights; to Phil, who claims to be only an innocent bystander; and to Dr. David Farrar for his willingness to contribute his medical expertise.

I also want to acknowledge the committee, volunteers and staff at the *Quest for Life Center*, who live the message in this book.

Love and healing to you all in your quest for life.

Petrea King
Quest for Life Center
Sydney NSW
Australia 1994

The Quest for Life Foundation

. . . .

The purpose of the Quest for Life Foundation is to provide emotional support and education for people with life-threatening illnesses, for their families and loved ones, and for the health professionals who care for them. Although the medical facilities within our community provide up-to-date technology and expertise, they're sorely lacking in the ability to give adequate practical and emotional support which will help alleviate the tremendous shock and confusion a diagnosis of a life-threatening illness inevitably brings. Our society is desperately short of people and facilities geared to engender a sense of peace, hope, and encouragement.

The *Quest for Life Center* offers an oasis wherein can be found sensitive and caring people who are trained to assist, and who often have been touched by the experience of a life-threatening illness themselves.

The *Quest for Life Center* has grown out of the work of Petrea King and has been created in order to further her work by offering hope and encouragement to those who seek its services.

At present the following services are offered at the *Quest for Life Center*, which is based in Sydney, Australia.

Emotional Support For:

- *Those diagnosed with a life-threatening illness, their loved ones, family members, and friends*
- *People under stress*
- *Health professionals who care for people with life-threatening illnesses*
- *Parents of HIV+ people*
- *Those dealing with loss and grief*
  (This support is in the form of group work and/or individual counseling.)

- *Families affected by HIV (the virus which causes AIDS)*
  (This is in the form of providing individual counseling, financial assistance, and/or respite care for HIV+ children or parents.)

Educational Programs Include:

- *Several classes each week to teach skills in relaxation, visualization, and meditation techniques*
- *Skills development programs for doctors, nurses, and other health professionals working with people with life-threatening illnesses*
- *The production of educational videos*
- *Training of facilitators for support groups*

Regular Seminars Are Held Throughout Australia on the Following Topics:

- *Structure and function of support groups*
- *The art of living with a life-threatening illness*
- *Palliative care of people with a life-threatening illness*
- *Meditation/visualization and relaxation techniques*
- *Control of symptoms and side effects of disease and its treatments*
- *Stress-management and skills development for health professionals involved in the care of people with cancer/AIDS*

Other Programs Include:

- *Voluntary massage schemes for parents of very sick children and the staff who are under stress within various hospitals in Sydney*
- *Regular residential weekends near Sydney for people with life-threatening illnesses and their caregivers*
- *The CLOWN project. Clown stands for Compassion and Love Offered When Needed. Once a month people who have a life-threatening illness dress up as clowns and visit the Camperdown Children's*

Hospital in Sydney to give gifts to the children there. This project has been very successful and there are plans to expand into other hospitals.

How is Quest for Life Funded?

Quest for Life relies upon financial contributions from people who believe in its work. These contributions take the form of bequests, interest-free loans, and donations. The Quest for Life Foundation is a non-profit company, registered as a charity.

Occasionally, grants from the federal and state government have partially funded specific projects, for example:

- *The First National HIV+ Women's Conference in 1991*
- *Skills development programs for doctors working in HIV medicine*
- *The training of group facilitators*

As greater financial support becomes available, *Quest for Life* will expand its existing services and introduce new ones.

Future Plans for Quest for Life

Quest for Life has outgrown its present home and is raising funds to enable it to move to a larger center which will provide greater support for more people. Once the Center is established in its new premises, *Quest for Life* plans to build a facility in the country which will provide accommodation for seven-day residential programs and retreats. Initially, there will be two programs offered. These are:

Quest for Life Program

This seven-day program is designed for people who have a life-threatening illness and for their support people. It will cover all the aspects mentioned within this book and will be an expansion on the weekend seminar which is run at present.

The Peace in Living Program

A seven-day program designed for health professionals who are working with people with life-threatening illness. This program is designed to improve the self-care skills of health professionals as well as developing their patient skills.

Retreat Accommodation

Small self-contained cabins will be made available for those who wish to spend some quiet time in a beautiful environment.

For further information about *Quest for Life* and its many activities and services please write to:

Quest for Life Foundation
P.O. Box 267
Cammeray NSW 2062
Australia

Telephone: (011 612) 906 3112
Fax: (011 612) 906 1203

For information on Petrea King's programs and workshops in the United States, please call or write to:

Dawn Publications
14618 Tyler Foote Road
Nevada City, CA 95959
1-800-545-7475

Recommended Reading

. . . .

Achterberg, Jeanne, *Imagery in Healing*, Shambala
Benson, Herbert, *The Relaxation Response*, Avon Books
Borysenko, Joan, *Minding the Body, Mending the Mind*, Bantam Books
Brennan, Barbara, *Hands of Light*, Bantam Books
Campbell, Joseph, *The Hero with a Thousand Faces*, Princeton University
Campbell, Joseph, *The Power of Myth*, Doubleday
Chopra, Deepak, *Quantum Healing*, Bantam Books
Cousins, Norman, *Anatomy of an Illness*, Bantam Books
Cousins, Nornam, *The Healing Heart*, Avon Books
Faraday, Ann, *The Dream Game*, Harper & Row
Frankl, Viktor, *Man's Search for Meaning*, Pocket
Furth, Gregg, *The Secret World of Drawings: Healing through Art*, Sigo Press
Gawain, Shakti, *Creative Visualization*, Bantam Books
Hay, Louise, *You Can Heal Your Life*, Hay House
Hay, Louise, *The AIDS Book: Creating a Positive Approach*, Hay House
Jampolsky, Gerald, *Love Is Letting Go of Fear*, Celestial Arts
Jampolsky, Gerald, *Teach Only Love*, Bantam Books
Jampolsky, Gerald, *There Is a Rainbow Behind Every Dark Cloud*, Celestial Arts
Jampolsky, Gerald, *Goodbye to Guilt*, Bantam Books
Jung, Carl, *Man and His Symbols*, Dell
Kübler-Ross, Elizabeth, *On Death and Dying*, Macmillan
Kübler-Ross, Elizabeth, *Death: The Final Stage of Growth*, Prentice-Hall
Kübler-Ross, Elizabeth, *To Live Until We Say Goodbye*, Prentice-Hall
Kushner, Harold, *When Bad Things Happen to Good People*, Avon Books
LeShan, Lawrence, *How to Meditate*, Bantam Books
Levine, Stephen, *Who Dies*, Doubleday
Levine, Stephen, *Meetings at the Edge*, Doubleday
Locke, Steven, *The Healer Within*, E. P. Dutton
Melton, George, *Beyond AIDS*, Brotherhood
Myss, Carolyn, *AIDS: Passageway to Transformation*, Stillpoint
Moody, Raymond, *Life after Life*, Bantam Books
Pelletier, Kenneth, *Mind as Healer, Mind as Slayer*, Delta
Roberts, Jane, *The Nature of Personal Reality*, Prentice-Hall
Rodegast, Pat, *Emmanuel's Book*, Friend's Press
Schuchman, Helen, *A Course in Miracles*, Foundation for Inner Peace
Siegel, Bernie, *Love, Medicine and Miracles*, Harper
Siegel, Bernie, *Peace, Love, and Healing*, Harper
Simonton, Carl, *Getting Well Again*, Bantam Books
Walters, J. Donald, *Affirmations for Self-Healing*, Crystal Clarity
Walters, J. Donald, *Yoga Postures for Higher Awareness*, Crystal Clarity
The Bible

Index

· · · · ·

Contentment 39
Cookies 205
Corn 198
Corticosteroids 226, 244
Coughs 200-201
Counseling 360, 365
Cow's milk–see Milk
Crackers 164, 171, 226, 240, 241
Cramps 201-202
Cream 170, 205
Crispbread 164, 171
Cysteine 214

D
Dairy products 205, 224, 234
    see also milk, cream, sour cream, cheese
Dandelion coffee 206
Decision-making 65-73
Dehydrated 198
Denial 314, 332
Depression 1, 5, 29, 30, 92, 98, 100, 209,
        222, 225, 248, 266, 292, 314, 334
Despair 15, 29, 33, 142, 282
Determination 116
Diagnosis 11, 68, 88, 91, 280
    reaction to 314-315
    diarrhea 71, 174, 188, 198, 202-209,
        221, 236, 321, 342
Diet 25, 70, 153, 155, 160-162, 233, 240-
        242, 311, 312, 314, 320-322, 324,
        327, 361
    foods to avoid 162, 198, 233
Digestive enzymes 189-191, 224, 245
Digestive problems 223
Diuretics 227
Discipline 296
Disease 23, 31, 45, 52
    cause of 8-11
Distress 58, 82
Doctors
    communication with 59-64
    notes for 63-64
Drawing 52-53, 95, 144, 145, 301, 308
Drugs
    addiction 77, 87, 221

therapy 71, 175, 215
Dry mouth 194-197

E
Educational programs 366
Eggs 165, 176, 178, 210
    cooked 165, 187, 224, 234
Emotional
    energy 41
    intimacy 81
    stress 198
    traumatization 100
Emotions 248-249
    expression of 37-41, 112
Empathy 77, 81, 362
Enemas 200
Energy 50, 106, 114, 321
    lack of 183
Enthusiasm 2, 23, 44, 61, 71, 210, 307, 326
Environment, supportive 77
Enzymes 170, 205
Equilibrium 5, 108
Exercise 25, 41, 95, 160, 244, 264-266,
        312, 314, 318-320, 327, 354
Exhaustion 248

F
Facilitator 94
Failure 5, 132
Faith 25, 269, 281, 310
Fast foods 165-166
Fatigue 209-211, 342
Fats 224, 233
Fear 17, 42, 41, 44, 58, 79, 92, 102, 110,
        231, 235-238, 256, 302, 314, 327,
        358
Ferments/molds 166
Fiber 199
Fight or flight response 4-6, 38
Fish 153, 169, 178, 180, 191, 198, 214
    canned 164, 210
Flatulence 212-214, 245
Float tanks 160
Flushes 211-212
Folic acid 186, 210, 214, 216

Petrea King Cassette Tapes

Learning to Meditate

This tape is for both the beginner and experienced meditator. On side one, there are guidelines for meditation, and an explanation of stress and relaxation. The second side has a practical exercise in meditation. There's also an extended version of this tape available. $9.95, 60 and 90 minutes

Learning to Visualize

The perfect complement to the meditation tape. The principles and practice of visualization are set out, and guided imagery is used to bring the listener into a calm healing state. $9.95, 60 minutes

Sleep Easy

No one has ever heard the end of this tape! It's designed for both the chronic insomniac and those who are having temporary difficulty finding deep and restful sleep. $9.95, 60 minutes

Relaxation

For people who are practicing techniques of relaxation, this tape has guided imagery to enhance the function of the immune system. It's used widely in hospitals around Australia, especially for patients with cancer or those who are HIV+. $9.95, 60 minutes

Working with Pain

This tape is for people who suffer with acute or chronic pain. There are two techniques on the tape which are effective in alleviating pain: one is an investigation into pain, the other a rotation of awareness around the body. $9.95, 60 minutes

Increasing Self-Esteem

What IS self-esteem? How does low self-esteem affect health? You can learn to improve your self-esteem, and this tape offers suggestions and guidance for learning to love yourself, so you're more open to receiving love, as well as giving love to others, thus bringing an extra special quality to life. There's a practical exercise on the second side of the tape designed to improve your self-esteem. **$9.95**, 60 minutes

Living Well with Cancer

This tape explains the many positive responses a person can have to the diagnosis of cancer. It includes an explanation of the positive role attitude, diet, relaxation, visualization, and meditation can play, as well as how to prepare for treatments and procedures, and how to live with uncertainty. The second side of the tape has a practical exercise which thousands have found useful in maintaining a positive outlook while living with cancer. **$9.95**, 60 minutes

Living Well with HIV

This tape explains the many positive responses a person can have to the diagnosis of HIV/AIDS. It includes an explanation of the positive role attitude, diet, relaxation, visualization, and meditation can play, as well as how to prepare for treatments and procedures, and how to live with uncertainty. The second side of the tape has a practical exercise which thousands have found useful in maintaining a positive outlook while living with HIV/AIDS. **$9.95**, 60 minutes

Living Well with Breast Cancer

This tape explains the many positive responses a woman can have to the diagnosis of breast cancer. It includes an explanation of the positive role attitude, diet, relaxation, visualization, and meditation can play, as well as how to prepare for treatments and procedures, and how to live with uncertainty. The second side of the tape has a practical exercise which thousands have found useful in maintaining a positive outlook while living with breast cancer. $9.95, 60 minutes

Rainbows to Heal

All of us love the magic and mystery of rainbows. The practise on this tape enables the listener to focus healing energies for the good of themselves and/or others. An invaluable technique which everyone finds useful. This tape is very popular with children as well as adults. **$9.95**, 60 minutes

Forgiveness

All of us need to forgive ourselves or others at various times in our lives. This tape has two techniques which enable you to let go the pain of unforgiving and to allow release from the past. Once set free from the patterns and pain of the past, the listener can more easily embrace the present with enthusiasm. **$9.95**, 60 minutes

Guided Imagery Tapes

Soar Like an Eagle

An opportunity to travel beyond normal boundaries using your imagination. Experience deeper levels of peace and relaxation as you "soar like an eagle!" **$9.95**, 60 minutes

Zen Garden

Meet your own wise inner being in this lovely Japanese garden. Enjoy the cherry blossom and peace in the garden as Petrea guides your imagination on its creative journey to relaxation. **$9.95**, 60 minutes

Dolphin Magic

Explore the depths of your imagination as you journey deep beneath the sea with your special friend, the dolphin, to guide you to a crystal cavern of peace and healing. **$9.95**, 60 minutes

Starlight Voyage

Leave planet earth and visit your own special star, bathed in silver light. Walk through a silvery forest and meet a magical unicorn which can answer your questions and help you with guidance. **$9.95**, 60 minutes

Nurturing Mother

For mothers-to-be and new mothers, to create a better bonding with your baby. Motherhood is a time of joy, and a time of stress, so prepare yourself with this tape during your pregnancy, and after the birth. By nurturing yourself, you're nurturing your child. **$9.95**, 60 minutes

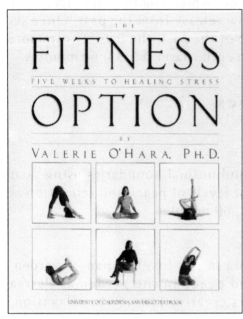

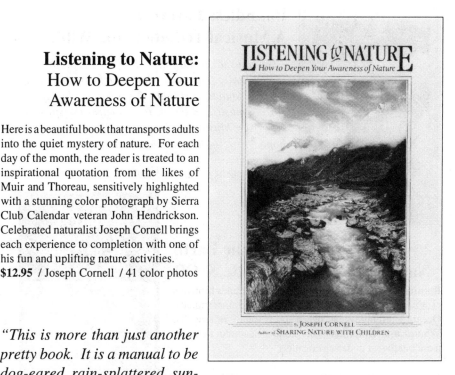

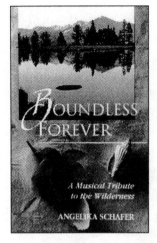
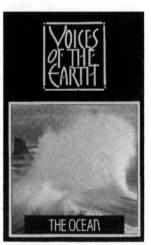

DAWN PUBLICATIONS
Order Form

QTY	TITLE		UNIT COST	TOTAL AMT
	Quest For Life		$12.95	
	Audio Cassettes by Petrea King			
	Sleep Easy	(PK-2)	9.95	
	Learning to Meditate	(PK-3)	9.95	
	Learning to Meditate (Extended)	(PK-3E)	9.95	
	Learning to Visualize	(PK-4)	9.95	
	Relaxation	(PK-5)	9.95	
	Working with Pain	(PK-6)	9.95	
	Increasing Self Esteem	(PK-7)	9.95	
	Living Well With Cancer	(PK-8)	9.95	
	Living Well with HIV-AIDS	(PK-9)	9.95	
	Living Well with Breast Cancer	(PK-10)	9.95	
	Rainbows to Heal	(PK-11)	9.95	
	Forgiveness	(PK-12)	9.95	
	Soar Like an Eagle	(PK-13)	9.95	
	Zen Garden	(PK-14)	9.95	
	Dolphin Magic	(PK-15)	9.95	
	Starlight Voyage	(PK-16)	9.95	
	Nurturing Mother	(PK-17)	9.95	

7.25% tax in California _____

Shipping: $3.75 for 1 or more items; $4.75 for more _____

Please charge to credit card: TOTAL _____

❑ VISA ❑ Master Card # _____ Exp.Date _____

Name_____

Address_____

City_____

State_____Zip_____

Phone_____

> **Please send payment and order to:**
> DAWN Publications
> 14618 Tyler Foote Road,
> Nevada City, Calif. 95959
> 1-800-545-7475
> FAX (916) 292-4258